NHA CCMA Study Guide 2025-2026

Latest CCMA Exam Prep with Review and 750+ Questions along with Detailed Answer Explanations for the Certified Clinical Medical Assistant Exam (5 Full-Length Practice Tests)

Priscilla Lipsey

Matilda Shortle

© 2024-2025

Printed in USA.

Disclaimer:

CONTENTS

The Certified Clinical Medical Assistant (CCMA) exam is a crucial step for anyone aspiring to work in the medical field as a clinical assistant. This credential demonstrates your knowledge, skills, and abilities to perform essential tasks in various healthcare settings.

Understanding the CCMA Credential:

What is CCMA?

The CCMA certification is designed for individuals who perform clinical duties under the supervision of licensed medical professionals. Responsibilities may include taking patient histories, assisting with examinations, working with medical equipment, and ensuring patient comfort. This position is vital in promoting efficient and compassionate healthcare delivery, making the CCMA credential highly valuable in today's job market.

Importance of the CCMA Certification:

Obtaining your CCMA certification signals to employers that you are competent and knowledgeable in clinical procedures. It can enhance your career prospects, increase earning potential, and provide opportunities for advancement. Many employers prefer or require certification for clinical assistants, making it essential for anyone serious about a career in healthcare.

CCMA Exam Overview:

Exam Structure

The CCMA exam consists of 150 multiple-choice questions encompassing various aspects of clinical practice. The questions are designed to evaluate your knowledge in the following key domains:

- **Foundational Knowledge in Basic Science**
- **Anatomy And Physiology**
- **Clinical Patient Care**
- **Enhancing Patient Care Coordination**
- **Administrative Assisting**
- **Communication And Customer Service**
- **Medical Law And Ethics**

Ultimate Guide to Acing the CCMA Exam

Preparing for the Certified Clinical Medical Assistant (CCMA) exam can be both exciting and daunting. However, with the right strategies in place, you can navigate this journey successfully. Here are some effective tips to help you pass the CCMA exam with confidence.

1. Grasp the Exam Format

Understanding the layout of the CCMA exam is the first step towards solid preparation. Dive into the various sections and topics covered in the exam. This knowledge will allow you to tailor your study sessions and allocate your time wisely, ensuring a more focused approach to your preparation.

2. Design a Comprehensive Study Schedule

A structured study plan is your roadmap to success. Craft a realistic timeline that outlines what topics to cover daily or weekly. This structured layout not only helps you manage your time but also ensures that you systematically address each area of the syllabus. Incorporate specific goals for each study session, and don't forget to leave room for review and self-assessment.

3. Develop Effective Time Management Skills

Time management is critical when it comes to the CCMA exam. Practicing with timed quizzes can enhance your ability to think quickly and accurately under pressure. Allocate a specific amount of time for each practice question during your study sessions, helping you to build the stamina and strategy necessary for the real exam day.

4. Engage in Regular Practice Exams

Simulating the exam experience through practice tests can provide a wealth of insight into your preparation. Not only do these assessments reveal your understanding of key concepts, but they also help you identify weaker areas that require additional focus. Regularly taking practice exams allows you to become familiar with the structure and types of questions you'll encounter, reducing anxiety on exam day.

5. Cultivate a Positive Mindset

Maintaining a calm and positive attitude is paramount on the day of the exam. Make sure to rest well the night before, fuel your body with a nutritious breakfast, and arrive early to the testing location. Remind yourself of your preparation and abilities; confidence can significantly impact your performance. Visualization techniques can also be beneficial—picture yourself succeeding!

In summary, passing the CCMA exam hinges on thorough preparation, structured study tactics, and a determined mindset. By employing these strategies, analyzing your progress, and utilizing quality study materials, you can enhance your chances of success. Stay committed, and soon you'll find yourself on the rewarding path to becoming a Certified Clinical Medical Assistant. Wishing you the best on this important endeavor!

Reasons to Choose This Essential Guide for the CCMA Exam:

Current Material:

Discover a thorough study aid specifically designed for the CCMA Exam. This guide is filled with up-to-date information and a wide array of practice questions, ensuring you're thoroughly equipped for success. Frequent updates maintain its relevance to the latest testing requirements.

Professional Expertise:

Crafted by industry experts who have successfully navigated the CCMA Exam, this book offers priceless advice and effective strategies to enhance your exam performance. Leverage the authors' extensive knowledge to approach the exam with assurance.

In-Depth Explanations:

Enhance your grasp of the subject matter through comprehensive explanations accompanying each question. By exploring the reasoning behind the answers, you'll deepen your understanding and be more prepared to tackle tough questions on test day.

True-to-Format Practice:

Experience practice questions that reflect the actual CCMA Exam's format, enabling you to get comfortable with the testing structure and build your confidence. Engaging with material that replicates the real exam will set you up for success on exam day.

Developed Critical Thinking Skills:

Working through the questions, answers, and explanations in this book will hone your critical thinking abilities, allowing you to analyze and respond to exam challenges with finesse. Elevate your problem-solving skills as you get ready for the CCMA Exam.

Straightforward Presentation:

This CCMA Prep is written in a clear, approachable manner that breaks down complex topics, ensuring you grasp crucial concepts without feeling overwhelmed by jargon. Tackle the material with confidence, knowing this guide will support your preparation and help you thrive on the exam.

CCMA

GUIDE

1   Foundational Knowledge in Basic Science:

Foundational Knowledge and Basic Science encompass the essential scientific principles and core knowledge required for clinical practice. This includes an understanding of human anatomy, physiology, and pathology, which form the basis for recognizing normal versus abnormal health conditions. It also covers microbiology, which is crucial for comprehending infection control and disease transmission. Basic pharmacology is included to help understand medication actions, side effects, and interactions. The principles of nutrition and wellness are integral for advising patients on lifestyle modifications. Additionally, knowledge of medical terminology is necessary for effective communication within healthcare settings. Mastery of these areas ensures that medical assistants can support patient care effectively and contribute to a collaborative healthcare environment.

1.1 Knowledge Of:
1.1.1 Health Care Systems Overview:

Health care systems encompass the organized network of institutions, resources, and individuals delivering medical services to populations. These systems vary globally, including public, private, and hybrid models, each with unique structures and funding mechanisms. Health care settings refer to the environments where medical services are provided, such as hospitals, clinics, outpatient facilities, and long-term care institutions. Each setting serves specific patient needs and has distinct operational protocols. Understanding these systems and settings is crucial for medical assistants to navigate patient care efficiently, coordinate with health professionals, and ensure compliance with regulations. Mastery of this knowledge enhances patient outcomes and optimizes health service delivery.

1.1.1.1   MA and Healthcare Team Roles:

Medical Assistants (MAs) perform both administrative and clinical tasks to support healthcare providers. They schedule appointments, maintain patient records, and assist with examinations. MAs must adhere to protocols and ethical standards while ensuring patient comfort. Other healthcare providers, such as physicians and nurses, diagnose, treat, and manage patient care, often relying on MAs for efficient operations. Allied health personnel, including radiologic technologists and physical therapists, specialize in diagnostic, therapeutic, and preventive services. Their roles complement the healthcare team by providing expertise in specific areas of patient care. Effective collaboration among these professionals is crucial for delivering comprehensive and quality healthcare services.

1.1.1.2   Scope Of Practice:

The scope of practice for medical assistants encompasses the range of duties and responsibilities they are legally permitted to perform under state regulations and the supervision of physicians. It includes administrative tasks such as scheduling appointments, maintaining patient records, and billing. Clinically, it involves taking vital signs, preparing patients for examinations, drawing blood, and administering medications as directed by a physician. Understanding the scope of practice is crucial to ensure compliance with legal standards and to provide safe, effective patient care. Medical assistants must stay informed about state-specific laws and any changes in regulations to avoid performing unauthorized tasks, which could lead to legal consequences or compromise patient safety.

1.1.1.3   Titles And Credentials:

In the healthcare field, titles and credentials denote an individual's qualifications, expertise, and scope of practice. Medical assistants can earn the title of Certified Clinical Medical Assistant (CCMA) by passing a recognized certification exam, which demonstrates proficiency in clinical and administrative tasks. Credentials such as the CCMA validate a medical assistant's skills and knowledge, enhancing employability and professional credibility. They also ensure adherence to industry standards and practices. In addition to the CCMA, medical assistants may pursue other certifications, such as the CMA (Certified Medical Assistant) or RMA (Registered Medical Assistant), each with specific requirements. Understanding these titles and credentials helps medical assistants navigate career advancement opportunities within diverse healthcare settings.

1.1.1.4   Licensing And Certification:

Licensing and certification are crucial components of the healthcare profession, ensuring that medical assistants meet specific standards of competence and ethics. Licensing is a mandatory process regulated by state law, granting legal permission to practice as a medical assistant. Certification, while often voluntary, is highly recommended as it validates an individual's expertise and knowledge through standardized exams, such as the CCMA. Certification enhances job prospects and professional credibility and can lead to higher wages. It requires ongoing education to maintain, ensuring that medical assistants remain current with evolving medical practices and technologies. Together, licensing and certification uphold the quality and safety of patient care within healthcare systems.

1.1.1.5   Healthcare Delivery Models:

Healthcare delivery models are systems for organizing and providing care. Health Maintenance Organizations (HMOs) require members to use a network of providers, emphasizing preventive care. Preferred Provider Organizations (PPOs) offer more flexibility in choosing providers but at higher costs. Point of Service (POS) plans combine features of HMOs and PPOs, allowing out-of-network care at higher costs. Patient-Centered Medical Homes (PCMH) focus on coordinated primary care. Accountable Care Organizations (ACOs) incentivize quality over quantity, linking payments to performance. Hospice provides end-of-life care that focuses on comfort. The Collaborative Care Model integrates mental and physical healthcare, enhancing overall patient outcomes through teamwork among healthcare professionals.

1.1.1.6   General vs. Specialty Services:

In healthcare, general services refer to primary care provided by family medicine or internal medicine practitioners who address a broad range of health issues. These practitioners offer preventive care, diagnose common ailments, and manage chronic conditions. In contrast, specialties focus on specific areas of medicine, such as cardiology, dermatology, or orthopedics, where healthcare professionals have advanced training to manage complex conditions within their field. Specialty services often require referrals from general practitioners for targeted treatment. Understanding the distinction between general and specialty services is crucial for medical assistants to effectively coordinate patient care, facilitate referrals, and ensure comprehensive healthcare delivery across various medical settings.

1.1.1.7 Ancillary Services:

Ancillary services encompass a wide range of supportive healthcare services that supplement primary care. These services include diagnostic, therapeutic, and custodial care designed to enhance patient treatment processes. Examples include laboratory tests, radiology, physical therapy, and home health services. Ancillary services are crucial in ensuring comprehensive patient care by providing essential information and support for diagnosis and treatment plans. They help reduce hospital stays and improve patient outcomes by offering specialized care outside the primary physician's office. Medical assistants should understand the role of ancillary services to facilitate coordination between various healthcare providers and ensure efficient patient management within healthcare systems.

1.1.1.8 Alternative Therapies:

Alternative therapies encompass a variety of treatment approaches used in place of conventional medicine. These therapies include practices such as acupuncture, chiropractic care, herbal medicine, and homeopathy. They focus on holistic healing, emphasizing the connection between the mind, body, and spirit. Alternative therapies often aim to enhance the body's natural healing processes and promote overall well-being. While some alternative therapies have gained acceptance within mainstream healthcare for their benefits, others remain controversial due to limited scientific evidence supporting their efficacy. As medical assistants, understanding these therapies is essential for providing informed patient care and respecting diverse patient preferences within the healthcare setting.

1.1.1.9 Insurance Fundamentals:

Insurance fundamentals encompass the basic principles and types of health insurance plans, which are essential for medical assistants to understand. Health insurance is a contract in which an insurer provides financial coverage for medical expenses in exchange for premiums. Key types of health insurance include Health Maintenance Organizations (HMOs), Preferred Provider Organizations (PPOs), and Exclusive Provider Organizations (EPOs). Each plan varies in terms of network restrictions, cost-sharing, and coverage flexibility. Medical assistants must comprehend policy terms such as deductibles, copayments, and coinsurance to effectively assist patients with billing inquiries and insurance claims processing. Understanding these fundamentals ensures accurate management of patient information and facilitates seamless healthcare delivery within diverse healthcare settings.

1.1.2 Medical Terminology:

Medical terminology is the specialized language used by healthcare professionals to ensure precise and effective communication. It consists of root words, prefixes, and suffixes derived primarily from Greek and Latin. Understanding medical terminology is crucial for medical assistants, as it enables them to accurately interpret and document patient information, communicate with colleagues, and understand medical procedures and diagnoses. This terminology often describes the human body's anatomy, conditions, procedures, and treatments. Mastery of this language aids in minimizing errors in patient care and enhances the ability to follow physician instructions. Familiarity with these terms is essential for success on the CCMA exam and in daily clinical practice.

1.1.2.1 Common Abbreviations, Acronyms & Symbols:

In the medical field, abbreviations, acronyms, and symbols are essential for efficient communication. They streamline documentation and ensure clarity among healthcare professionals. Common abbreviations include BP for blood pressure, HR for heart rate, and Rx for prescription. Acronyms like CBC stand for complete blood count, while symbols such as ↑ indicate an increase and ↓ indicate a decrease. Understanding these elements is crucial for medical assistants to accurately interpret medical records and convey information. Mastery of these terms minimizes errors and enhances patient care by ensuring that all team members understand the patient's condition and treatment plan comprehensively and promptly.

1.1.2.2 Conditions, Procedures, And Instruments:

Conditions refer to medical states or disorders affecting the body, such as hypertension or diabetes. Procedures are clinical interventions performed to diagnose, treat, or manage these conditions, including blood tests or surgeries. Instruments are the tools used in these procedures, ranging from stethoscopes for auscultation to scalpels for surgical incisions. Medical assistants must understand these elements to assist effectively in patient care. Recognizing conditions helps prioritize tasks; knowing procedures ensures proper preparation and support during clinical activities; and familiarity with instruments aids in maintaining sterility and functionality. Mastery of these components is essential for providing comprehensive patient care and ensuring successful clinical outcomes.

1.1.2.3 Medical Word Formation Essentials:

Medical word building involves understanding the components of medical terms, primarily prefixes, suffixes, and root words. Prefixes are added to the beginning of a word to modify its meaning, such as hyper-, which indicates excessive or above normal. Suffixes are placed at the end of a word to alter its meaning or indicate a procedure, condition, or disease, such as -itis, which denotes inflammation. Plurals in medical terminology often deviate from standard English rules; for example, bacterium becomes bacteria. Mastery of these elements is crucial for medical assistants to accurately interpret and communicate medical information, ensuring effective patient care and documentation.

1.1.2.4 Positional And Directional Terminology:

Positional and directional terminology is essential for accurately describing the location and orientation of structures in the human body. Terms such as anterior (front) and posterior (back) help specify the position relative to the body's axis. Superior refers to a structure that is closer to the head, while inferior indicates proximity to the feet. Medial describes closeness to the midline, whereas lateral denotes a position further from it. Proximal and distal indicate closeness or distance from the trunk, respectively, particularly in the limbs. Understanding these terms is crucial for medical assistants to communicate effectively in clinical settings, ensuring precision in patient assessment and documentation.

1.1.3 Basic Pharmacology:

Basic pharmacology is the study of drugs, their properties, effects, and interactions within the body. It involves understanding drug classifications, mechanisms of action, therapeutic uses, side effects, and contraindications. Medical assistants must grasp pharmacokinetics (absorption, distribution, metabolism, and excretion) and pharmacodynamics (how drugs affect the body). Knowledge of common medications, including analgesics, antibiotics, antihypertensives, and insulin, is essential. Recognizing drug interactions and adverse reactions ensures patient safety. Basic pharmacology also covers dosage calculations and administration routes, such as oral, intravenous, or topical. Mastery of this topic enables medical assistants to assist in medication management and patient education effectively, ensuring optimal therapeutic outcomes.

1.1.3.1   Common Medications and Abbreviations:
Medical assistants must be familiar with commonly prescribed medications and their abbreviations to ensure accurate communication and patient safety. Common medications include antihypertensives like Lisinopril, antibiotics such as Amoxicillin, and analgesics like Acetaminophen. Each medication has a specific purpose, dosage, and potential side effects that medical assistants should know. Approved abbreviations facilitate efficient documentation and communication; for example, BID means twice a day, PRN indicates as needed, and PO stands for by mouth. Understanding these abbreviations is crucial in preventing medication errors and ensuring proper administration. Mastery of this knowledge is vital for the CCMA exam and effective clinical practice.

1.1.3.2   Drug Classifications & Schedules:
Drug classifications categorize medications based on their therapeutic effects, chemical characteristics, or mechanisms of action. These classifications help medical assistants understand drug interactions and contraindications. Common classifications include analgesics, antibiotics, antihypertensives, and antidiabetics. Drug schedules, determined by the Controlled Substances Act, categorize drugs based on their potential for abuse and medical use. Schedule I drugs have a high potential for abuse and no accepted medical use, while Schedule V drugs have a low potential for abuse with accepted medical uses. Understanding these schedules is crucial for ensuring compliance with legal regulations and safe patient care, as it guides the prescription and dispensing of controlled substances.

1.1.3.3   Understanding Side Effects and Contraindications:
Side effects are unintended, often mild reactions to a medication, such as drowsiness or nausea. Adverse effects are more severe and potentially harmful reactions, such as allergic responses or organ damage. Indications refer to the medical conditions or symptoms for which a drug is prescribed, ensuring that its therapeutic purpose aligns with patient needs. Contraindications are specific situations in which a drug should not be used due to potential harm, such as pre-existing conditions or interactions with other medications. Understanding these aspects is crucial for ensuring patient safety and effective treatment outcomes, guiding medical assistants in monitoring and educating patients about their medications.

1.1.3.4   Measurement and Dosage Calculations:
Medical assistants must accurately measure medication using both metric and household systems. The metric system, which is preferred in healthcare, uses units such as milliliters and grams, while the household system includes teaspoons and tablespoons. Mathematical conversions are essential for translating between these systems to ensure precise dosages. For example, 1 teaspoon equals 5 milliliters. Dosage calculations involve determining the correct amount of medication based on the prescription and patient parameters, such as weight or age. This requires an understanding of formulas like Dose = (Desired Dose / Available Dose) x Quantity Available. Mastery of these skills ensures safe and effective patient care, which is a critical competency for certified clinical medical assistants.

1.1.3.5   Forms Of Medication:
Forms of medication refer to the physical form in which a drug is produced and administered. Pills and capsules are solid forms, with pills being compressed powders and capsules containing medication within a gelatin shell. These forms are convenient for oral administration, allowing for precise dosing. Ointments are semi-solid preparations applied topically, providing localized treatment by delivering active ingredients directly to the skin or mucous membranes. Each form is designed to optimize the drug's absorption, distribution, and action in the body. Understanding these forms helps medical assistants ensure accurate administration and patient compliance, as well as anticipate potential variations in drug onset and duration of action.

1.1.3.6   Look-Alike/Sound-Alike Medications:
Look-alike/sound-alike (LASA) medications are drugs that have similar names or appearances, which can lead to medication errors if not carefully managed. These errors occur when a healthcare professional mistakenly administers the wrong drug due to confusion over the drug's name or packaging. Such mistakes can result in adverse patient outcomes. To mitigate these risks, medical assistants should employ strategies such as using tall man lettering (e.g., hydrOXYzine vs. hydrALAzine), double-checking prescriptions, and confirming patient information with the medication label. Awareness and vigilance are crucial, as is maintaining open communication with pharmacists and other healthcare team members to ensure patient safety and effective medication management.

1.1.3.7   Routes of Administration:
Routes of administration refer to the various pathways through which medications are delivered into the body. These routes are chosen based on factors such as drug properties, desired effects, and patient conditions. Common routes include oral (swallowed), sublingual (under the tongue), and buccal (inside the cheek) for systemic effects. Parenteral routes bypass the gastrointestinal tract and include intravenous (IV), intramuscular (IM), and subcutaneous (SC) injections for rapid absorption. Topical routes involve application to the skin or mucous membranes for localized action, while inhalation delivers drugs directly to the respiratory system. Each route has unique considerations regarding absorption rate, onset of action, and potential side effects, which are crucial for effective patient care.

1.1.3.8   Pharmacokinetics:
Pharmacokinetics involves the study of how drugs move through the body, encompassing four key processes: absorption, distribution, metabolism, and excretion. Absorption refers to the process by which a drug enters the bloodstream from its site of administration. Distribution describes how the drug spreads throughout the body's tissues and fluids. Metabolism is the biochemical modification of the drug, primarily occurring in the liver, to facilitate its elimination. Excretion is the removal of the drug and its metabolites from the body, primarily through urine or feces. Understanding these processes is crucial for medical assistants to ensure optimal therapeutic outcomes and minimize adverse effects in patients.

1.1.3.9   Rights Of Drugs/medication Administration:
The Rights of Medication Administration are fundamental principles that ensure safe and effective drug delivery to patients. These rights include the right patient, right medication, right dose, right route, right time, right documentation, and right reason. Each step is critical in preventing medication errors. The right patient involves verifying the patient's identity using two identifiers. The right medication requires checking the drug label against the prescription. The right dose ensures accuracy in quantity. The right route

confirms the correct method of administration. The right time involves adhering to prescribed schedules. Accurate documentation records all details, while the right reason ensures that the medication's purpose aligns with the patient's condition.

1.1.3.10   Physicians' Desk Reference & Digital Tools:

The Physicians' Desk Reference (PDR) is a comprehensive drug reference guide used by healthcare professionals, including medical assistants, to access detailed information about prescription medications. It includes drug indications, contraindications, side effects, dosages, and manufacturer details. Online resources complement the PDR by providing up-to-date information through platforms like Epocrates and Drugs.com, which offer real-time updates on drug interactions and new approvals. These resources are crucial for medical assistants to ensure safe medication administration and patient education. Familiarity with both the PDR and online tools enables medical assistants to support physicians effectively, ensuring accurate medication management and enhancing patient care outcomes.

1.1.3.11   Storage and Disposal Principles:

The principles of storage and disposal of medications are crucial for ensuring safety and efficacy. Medications must be stored according to manufacturer guidelines, typically in a cool, dry place away from direct sunlight to maintain their stability and effectiveness. Controlled substances require secure storage in locked cabinets to prevent unauthorized access. Proper labeling is essential for easy identification and to avoid medication errors. For disposal, follow federal and state regulations, utilizing take-back programs or DEA-authorized collectors for controlled substances. Never flush medications unless specified; improper disposal can lead to environmental contamination. These practices ensure patient safety and environmental protection, aligning with CCMA standards.

1.1.4 Nutrition:

Nutrition is the science that examines the relationship between diet, health, and disease. It involves the intake and utilization of food substances through which growth, repair, and maintenance of the body are accomplished. Essential nutrients include carbohydrates, proteins, fats, vitamins, minerals, and water. Each of these plays a critical role in bodily functions such as energy production, cellular repair, immune function, and overall development. A balanced diet is vital for maintaining optimal health and preventing chronic diseases like obesity, diabetes, and cardiovascular disorders. Medical assistants must understand nutritional principles to educate patients on healthy eating habits and support dietary management in clinical settings.

1.1.4.1   Dietary Nutrients:

Dietary nutrients are essential substances found in food that the body requires for energy, growth, repair, and overall health maintenance. They are categorized into macronutrients and micronutrients. Macronutrients include carbohydrates, proteins, and fats, which provide energy and support bodily functions. Carbohydrates are the primary energy source; proteins are crucial for tissue repair and enzyme production; fats supply energy and assist in hormone synthesis. Micronutrients, comprising vitamins and minerals, facilitate various biochemical reactions and physiological processes. Vitamins support immune function and cellular health, while minerals contribute to bone strength and fluid balance. A balanced intake of these nutrients is vital for optimal health and disease prevention.

1.1.4.2   Patient Education on Dietary Needs:

Medical Assistants play a crucial role in educating patients about dietary needs, both generally and in relation to specific diseases and conditions. General dietary education involves teaching patients about balanced nutrition, portion control, and the importance of consuming a variety of food groups. When addressing specific conditions such as diabetes or hypertension, education focuses on tailored dietary modifications, such as reducing sugar intake or limiting sodium. Effective patient education involves clear communication, providing practical examples, and ensuring that patients understand how diet impacts their health conditions. This empowers patients to make informed food choices, adhere to dietary recommendations, and ultimately improve their overall health outcomes.

1.1.4.3   Vitamins And Supplements:

Vitamins are organic compounds essential for various metabolic processes, growth, and overall health. They are classified into two categories: water-soluble (e.g., B-complex and C) and fat-soluble (e.g., A, D, E, and K), each serving distinct physiological functions. Supplements are products taken orally that contain one or more ingredients, such as vitamins, minerals, or amino acids, intended to supplement the diet. Medical assistants must understand the role of each vitamin in maintaining health and preventing deficiencies. They should also be aware of potential interactions with medications and the risks of excessive intake. This knowledge aids in advising patients on appropriate dietary choices and supplement use.

1.1.4.4   Eating Disorders:

Eating disorders are serious mental health conditions characterized by abnormal or disturbed eating habits that significantly impact physical health and psychosocial functioning. The most common types include Anorexia Nervosa, Bulimia Nervosa, and Binge Eating Disorder. Anorexia involves severe food restriction leading to extreme weight loss, while Bulimia is marked by cycles of binge eating followed by purging through vomiting or laxatives. Binge Eating Disorder involves uncontrollable overeating without purging behaviors. These disorders often coexist with psychological issues such as anxiety and depression. Treatment typically requires a multidisciplinary approach, including medical, nutritional, and psychological interventions to address both the physical and mental aspects of the disorder.

1.1.4.5   Food Labels:

Food labels are essential tools that provide detailed information about the nutritional content of packaged foods. They include data on serving size, calories, macronutrients (such as fats, carbohydrates, and proteins), and micronutrients (vitamins and minerals). Food labels help consumers make informed dietary choices by indicating the percentage of daily values based on a standard 2,000-calorie diet. They also list ingredients in descending order by weight, alerting consumers to potential allergens. Understanding food labels is crucial for medical assistants to guide patients in managing dietary needs, ensuring balanced nutrition, and preventing chronic diseases. Accurate interpretation aids in promoting healthier lifestyle choices among diverse patient populations.

1.1.5 Psychology:

Psychology is the scientific study of behavior and mental processes, encompassing a wide range of topics, including perception, cognition, emotion, personality, and social interactions. For medical assistants, understanding psychology is crucial for effectively communicating with patients, recognizing emotional and psychological cues, and providing compassionate care. It involves comprehending how mental health affects physical health and vice versa. Psychology also explores developmental stages across the lifespan, which influence patient interaction strategies. Medical assistants can apply psychological principles to enhance patient compliance, manage stress, and support patient education. This foundational knowledge aids in fostering therapeutic relationships, ensuring holistic care that addresses both the physical and psychological needs of patients.

1.1.5.1 Developmental Stages:
Developmental stages refer to the distinct phases of growth and development that individuals experience throughout their lifespan. Each stage is characterized by unique physical, cognitive, and psychosocial changes. Key stages include infancy, childhood, adolescence, adulthood, and old age. During infancy, rapid physical growth and the development of basic motor skills occur. Childhood involves cognitive advancements and the acquisition of social skills. Adolescence is marked by puberty and identity exploration. Adulthood focuses on career establishment and family life. Finally, old age encompasses reflection and coping with physical decline. Understanding these stages aids medical assistants in providing age-appropriate care and anticipating patient needs across different life phases.

1.1.5.2 End-of-Life and Grief Stages:
End-of-life care involves medical and emotional support for individuals nearing death, focusing on comfort and quality of life. Medical assistants play a crucial role by providing compassionate care and effective communication. The stages of grief, as outlined by Elisabeth Kübler-Ross, include denial, anger, bargaining, depression, and acceptance. These stages represent the emotional responses individuals experience when facing loss. Understanding these stages helps medical assistants support patients and families through empathetic listening and appropriate interventions. Recognizing that grief is non-linear and individualized is essential for offering effective support, ensuring that patients' dignity is maintained during their final moments.

1.1.5.3 Psychological Insights on Disability and Disease:
This area of psychology focuses on understanding the mental and emotional challenges faced by individuals with physical disabilities, developmental delays, and chronic diseases. It examines how these conditions impact self-esteem, social interactions, and overall mental health. Patients may experience heightened anxiety, depression, or social isolation due to their conditions. Medical assistants should recognize these psychological aspects to provide empathetic care and effective communication. Supporting patients involves fostering a positive environment, encouraging independence where possible, and connecting them with appropriate resources, such as counseling or support groups. Understanding these psychological dynamics is crucial for holistic patient care and improving quality of life.

1.1.5.4 Environmental And Socio-economic Stressors:
Environmental and socio-economic stressors are external factors that can adversely affect an individual's mental and physical health. Environmental stressors include pollution, noise, and poor living conditions, which can lead to chronic stress responses. Socio-economic stressors encompass financial instability, unemployment, and lack of access to healthcare or education. These stressors can exacerbate mental health issues such as anxiety and depression, impacting overall well-being. Medical assistants must recognize these factors when assessing patients, as they may influence health outcomes and treatment adherence. Understanding these stressors is crucial for providing holistic care and supporting patients in managing their health amidst challenging circumstances.

1.1.5.5 Mental Health Screening:
Mental health screening is a crucial process for identifying individuals who may be experiencing mental health issues. It involves the use of standardized tools and questionnaires to assess symptoms related to conditions such as depression, anxiety, and other psychological disorders. Medical assistants play a vital role in administering these screenings, ensuring confidentiality and accuracy. The screening facilitates early detection, allowing for timely intervention and treatment planning. It is essential for medical assistants to understand the importance of cultural sensitivity and effective patient communication during this process. Proper documentation and referral to appropriate healthcare professionals are key components in managing patients' mental health effectively.

1.1.5.6 Defense Mechanisms:
Defense mechanisms are unconscious psychological strategies employed by individuals to cope with reality and maintain their self-image. They help reduce anxiety arising from unacceptable or potentially harmful stimuli. Common defense mechanisms include denial, where a person refuses to accept reality; repression, which involves pushing distressing thoughts into the unconscious; and projection, where one attributes their own undesirable traits to others. Rationalization involves justifying behaviors or feelings with logical reasons, even if they are not appropriate. Understanding these mechanisms is crucial for medical assistants, as it aids in recognizing patient behaviors and facilitating effective communication and care. Mastery of this concept enhances patient interaction and supports mental health awareness in clinical settings.

2 Anatomy And Physiology:
Anatomy and physiology are fundamental sciences in the medical field that focus on understanding the human body's structure and function. Anatomy is the study of the body's physical structure, including organs, tissues, and cells, detailing their locations and relationships. Physiology examines how these structures operate and interact to sustain life, covering processes such as metabolism, respiration, and reproduction. Together, they provide a comprehensive understanding of how the body maintains homeostasis and adapts to changes. This knowledge is crucial for medical assistants to accurately assess patient conditions, assist in diagnostics, and support effective treatment plans, ensuring optimal patient care and safety in clinical settings.

2.1 Knowledge Of:
2.1.1 Body Structures & Organ Systems Overview:
Body structures and organ systems form the foundation of human anatomy and physiology. The body is organized into cells, tissues, organs, and systems, each serving specific functions essential for maintaining life. Organ systems are groups of organs that work together to perform complex functions. Key systems include the circulatory system, which is responsible for blood transport; the respiratory system, which facilitates gas exchange; the digestive system, which processes nutrients; and the nervous system, which controls body activities through electrical signals. Understanding these systems is crucial for medical assistants to accurately assess patient conditions, assist in diagnostic procedures, and provide effective care within a clinical setting. Mastery of this knowledge is vital for CCMA certification.

2.1.1.1 Anatomical Structures and Positions:
Anatomical structures refer to the distinct parts of the body, such as organs and tissues, each with specific functions. Locations describe where these structures are situated within the body, often categorized by regions (e.g., the thoracic cavity for the heart

and lungs). Positions relate to the body's orientation, using standard terms like anterior (front), posterior (back), superior (above), and inferior (below) to specify relationships between structures. Understanding these concepts is crucial for medical assistants to accurately communicate findings, assist in procedures, and comprehend medical documentation. Mastery of anatomical terminology ensures clarity in identifying and describing the physical layout and function of body systems.

2.1.1.2   Major Body Systems: Structure and Function

The human body comprises several major systems, each with distinct structures and functions. The circulatory system, which includes the heart and blood vessels, transports nutrients and oxygen. The respiratory system, with lungs located in the thoracic cavity, facilitates gas exchange. The digestive system, spanning from the mouth to the intestines, breaks down food for nutrient absorption. The nervous system, consisting of the brain and spinal cord, coordinates body activities. The musculoskeletal system provides support and movement through bones and muscles. The urinary system, which includes the kidneys and bladder, removes waste. Each organ's location is crucial for its function within these interconnected systems, ensuring homeostasis.

2.1.1.3   Organ Systems and Homeostasis Interactions:

Homeostasis is the body's ability to maintain a stable internal environment despite external changes. Organ systems interact intricately to achieve this balance. For instance, the respiratory and circulatory systems work together to regulate oxygen and carbon dioxide levels. The nervous and endocrine systems coordinate to control body temperature, metabolism, and fluid balance. The kidneys in the urinary system filter blood, maintaining electrolyte balance and blood pressure, while the digestive system provides necessary nutrients. Feedback mechanisms, such as negative feedback loops, are crucial in these interactions, detecting deviations from normal states and initiating responses to restore equilibrium. Understanding these interactions is essential for medical assistants to support patient care effectively.

2.1.2 Pathophysiology And Disease Processes:

Pathophysiology refers to the study of how normal physiological processes are altered by disease. It involves understanding the functional changes that occur within the body as a result of a disease or injury. Medical assistants must grasp these concepts to effectively support patient care. Disease processes encompass the progression and stages of diseases, including initiation, development, and resolution. This includes recognizing symptoms, identifying risk factors, and understanding mechanisms such as inflammation, infection, and genetic mutations. A solid understanding of pathophysiology enables medical assistants to assist in diagnosis, treatment planning, and patient education, ensuring comprehensive care and improved health outcomes.

2.1.2.1   Signs, Symptoms, and Etiology of Common Conditions:

Signs are objective evidence of disease observable by others, such as a rash or swelling. Symptoms are subjective experiences reported by the patient, like pain or fatigue. Etiology refers to the cause of a disease or condition. Understanding these aspects is crucial for diagnosis and treatment. For instance, diabetes presents signs such as elevated blood glucose and symptoms like excessive thirst. Its etiology involves insulin resistance or deficiency. Recognizing the signs and symptoms alongside the etiology aids in accurate diagnosis and management. Medical assistants must be adept at identifying these elements to support effective patient care and facilitate communication with healthcare providers.

2.1.2.2   Diagnostic Measures & Treatment Modalities:

Diagnostic measures involve procedures and tests to identify diseases, including imaging (X-rays, MRIs), laboratory tests (blood and urine analysis), and biopsies. These tools provide critical information about the patient's condition, aiding in accurate diagnosis. Treatment modalities refer to the methods used to manage or cure diseases, encompassing pharmacological treatments (medications), surgical interventions, physical therapy, and lifestyle modifications. Medical assistants play a crucial role in preparing patients for diagnostic tests, ensuring compliance with treatment plans, and educating patients about their conditions. Understanding these concepts is essential for medical assistants to support healthcare providers effectively and ensure optimal patient care outcomes.

2.1.2.3   Incidence, Prevalence, and Risk Factors Overview:

Incidence refers to the number of new cases of a disease occurring in a specific population during a defined time period. It helps in understanding the rate at which new illnesses develop. Prevalence indicates the total number of existing cases, both new and pre-existing, in a population at a given time, providing insight into the overall disease burden. Risk factors are attributes or exposures that increase the likelihood of developing a disease, such as genetics, lifestyle, or environmental influences. Understanding these concepts aids medical assistants in identifying trends, planning interventions, and educating patients on prevention strategies to effectively mitigate health risks.

2.1.2.4   High Mortality and Morbidity Risk Factors:

Risk factors leading to high mortality and morbidity include lifestyle choices, genetic predispositions, and environmental exposures that increase susceptibility to diseases. Complications such as hypertension and diabetes can exacerbate existing conditions, elevating mortality risks. Accompanying diseases, such as cardiovascular disorders and chronic respiratory illnesses, further compound health challenges. Socioeconomic factors, including limited access to healthcare and poor nutrition, also contribute significantly. Age and gender may influence disease progression and outcomes. Understanding these risk factors is crucial for medical assistants in identifying at-risk patients and implementing preventive strategies to mitigate complications, ultimately improving patient prognosis and reducing healthcare burdens.

2.1.2.5   Epidemics And Pandemics:

Epidemics refer to the rapid spread of infectious diseases within a specific population or geographic area, causing a significant increase in the number of cases above what is normally expected. They can arise from novel pathogens or from existing ones that become more virulent. Pandemics, however, are epidemics that extend beyond national borders, affecting a large number of people globally. They often result from new infectious agents to which the population has little immunity, such as H1N1 influenza or COVID-19. Understanding these phenomena is crucial for medical assistants to effectively support public health measures, manage patient care during such events, and contribute to prevention efforts through education and vaccination advocacy.

2.1.3 Microbiology:

Microbiology is the scientific study of microorganisms, which are tiny, often microscopic entities, including bacteria, viruses, fungi, and protozoa. This field is crucial for medical assistants, as it underpins the understanding of infection control, disease causation, and laboratory diagnostics. Microorganisms can be pathogenic or beneficial; thus, knowledge in microbiology aids in identifying infectious agents and implementing appropriate sterilization techniques. It also involves understanding microbial growth, reproduction, and the impact of antibiotics and vaccines on these organisms. Proficiency in microbiology enables medical assistants to assist in specimen collection and processing while ensuring adherence to safety protocols to prevent contamination and ensure accurate test results.

2.1.3.1   Cell Structure:
Cells are the basic structural and functional units of life. The nucleus, a membrane-bound organelle, houses genetic material and controls cellular activities. The cell wall, found in plant cells, provides structural support and protection. The cell membrane, a phospholipid bilayer, regulates the passage of substances in and out of the cell. The cytoplasm is the gel-like substance where cellular components reside. Ribosomes are responsible for protein synthesis. Mitochondria, known as the powerhouse of the cell, generate ATP through respiration. Lysosomes contain enzymes for digestion and waste removal. The nucleolus, located within the nucleus, is involved in ribosomal RNA synthesis and ribosome assembly.

2.1.3.2   Common Pathogens And Non-pathogens:
Pathogens are microorganisms that cause disease, including bacteria, viruses, fungi, and parasites. Common bacterial pathogens include *Streptococcus pyogenes*, which causes strep throat, and *Escherichia coli*, which can lead to urinary tract infections. Viral pathogens like the influenza virus and HIV are known for causing the flu and AIDS, respectively. Fungal pathogens such as *Candida albicans* can result in yeast infections. Non-pathogens, on the other hand, are microorganisms that do not cause disease and can be beneficial. For example, *Lactobacillus* species in the gut aid digestion and maintain a healthy microbiome. Understanding these distinctions is crucial for medical assistants to effectively prevent the spread of infections and promote patient health.

2.1.3.3   Organisms And Microorganisms:
Organisms are living entities that can function independently, encompassing a wide range of life forms from simple bacteria to complex humans. Microorganisms, or microbes, are microscopic organisms that are invisible to the naked eye, including bacteria, viruses, fungi, and protozoa. These tiny life forms play crucial roles in various ecosystems and human health. Bacteria can be beneficial, aiding in digestion and nutrient cycling, or pathogenic, causing diseases. Viruses require host cells to replicate and are responsible for illnesses such as the flu. Fungi can decompose organic matter or cause infections. Protozoa are single-celled organisms that can lead to diseases such as malaria. Understanding these entities is essential for diagnosing and treating infections effectively.

2.1.3.4   Infectious Agents:
Infectious agents, also known as pathogens, are microorganisms capable of causing disease in humans. These include bacteria, viruses, fungi, protozoa, and helminths. Bacteria are single-celled organisms that can multiply rapidly in suitable environments. Viruses are smaller than bacteria and require a host cell to replicate. Fungi can be unicellular or multicellular and often cause superficial infections. Protozoa are single-celled eukaryotes that can lead to diseases such as malaria. Helminths are parasitic worms that affect various body systems. Understanding these agents is crucial for medical assistants to implement infection control measures effectively and to assist in diagnosing and treating infectious diseases, thereby ensuring patient safety and the quality of health care.

2.1.3.5   Chain Of Infection:
The Chain of Infection refers to the sequence of events that enables the spread of infections. It consists of six links: infectious agent, reservoir, portal of exit, mode of transmission, portal of entry, and susceptible host. The infectious agent is the pathogen causing the disease. The reservoir is where the pathogen resides, such as in humans or on surfaces. The portal of exit is the path through which the pathogen leaves the reservoir. The mode of transmission is how the pathogen spreads, either directly or indirectly. The portal of entry is how it enters a new host. A susceptible host is an individual who is vulnerable to infection. Breaking any link in the chain can prevent the spread of infection, which is crucial for infection control in healthcare settings.

2.1.3.6   Conditions For Growth:
Microorganisms require specific conditions to thrive, which include optimal temperature, pH, moisture, and nutrient availability. Temperature influences enzymatic activities; most pathogens prefer body temperature (37°C). The pH level affects microbial enzyme function, with many bacteria favoring a neutral pH of around 7. Moisture is crucial as it facilitates nutrient absorption and metabolic processes. Nutrients such as carbon, nitrogen, and minerals are essential for energy production and cellular functions. Oxygen requirements vary: obligate aerobes need oxygen, while obligate anaerobes grow without it. Facultative anaerobes can survive in both conditions. Understanding these growth conditions helps medical assistants in infection control and sterilization practices in clinical settings.

3   Clinical Patient Care:
Clinical patient care involves the direct interaction between medical assistants and patients to ensure optimal health outcomes. It encompasses a range of duties, including taking vital signs, recording medical histories, assisting physicians during examinations, and administering medications as directed. Medical assistants must demonstrate proficiency in clinical skills, maintain patient confidentiality, and adhere to ethical standards. They play a crucial role in patient education, ensuring that patients understand their treatment plans and medication instructions. Effective communication and empathy are essential components, as they enhance patient trust and compliance. Mastery of these skills is vital for medical assistants aiming to excel in the Certified Clinical Medical Assistant (CCMA) certification exam.

3.1 General Patient Care:
General patient care encompasses a wide range of responsibilities aimed at ensuring the well-being and comfort of patients. It involves conducting initial patient assessments, taking vital signs, and documenting medical histories. Medical assistants must proficiently perform basic clinical tasks such as administering medications, assisting with minor procedures, and providing wound care. Effective communication is crucial for educating patients about their conditions and treatment plans. Additionally, maintaining a clean and safe environment, adhering to infection control protocols, and ensuring patient confidentiality are fundamental aspects of general patient care. This role requires empathy, attention to detail, and a comprehensive understanding of medical protocols to support patient health and facilitate efficient healthcare delivery.

3.1.1 Tasks:
3.1.1.1   Identify Patient:
Identifying a patient accurately is a critical task in clinical patient care to ensure safety and proper treatment. It involves verifying the patient's identity using at least two identifiers, such as their full name and date of birth, before any medical procedure or medication administration. This process helps prevent errors such as misdiagnosis or incorrect treatments. Medical assistants must

cross-check these identifiers with the patient's medical records and confirm them verbally with the patient whenever possible. Additionally, checking identification bands or documents is essential. Proper patient identification fosters trust, reduces risks, and enhances the overall quality of care, aligning with best practices and regulatory standards in healthcare settings.

3.1.1.2   Prepare Examination/procedure Room:

Preparing an examination or procedure room involves ensuring it is clean, organized, and equipped with the necessary supplies for patient care. Start by disinfecting surfaces and equipment to prevent infection. Arrange instruments, gloves, and other materials in an accessible manner. Verify that all medical tools are functioning and sterile. Stock the room with essential items such as gowns, drapes, and specimen containers. Adjust the lighting and temperature for patient comfort. Confirm that patient records and consent forms are ready for review. This preparation ensures a smooth workflow, enhances patient safety, and supports efficient clinical operations, reflecting the professionalism expected of Certified Clinical Medical Assistants (CCMA).

3.1.1.3   Enhancing Patient Safety in Clinical Settings:

Ensuring patient safety within the clinical setting involves implementing protocols and practices to prevent harm and promote well-being during healthcare delivery. Medical assistants must adhere to infection control measures, such as proper hand hygiene and the use of personal protective equipment (PPE), to minimize the risk of infections. They should verify patient identity before procedures and medications to ensure accurate treatment. Maintaining a clutter-free environment reduces fall risks, while clear communication with patients and staff prevents misunderstandings. Regularly checking equipment functionality and promptly reporting hazards are crucial. By fostering a culture of safety, medical assistants contribute significantly to the overall quality of patient care.

3.1.1.4   Comprehensive Clinical Intake Process Overview:

A comprehensive clinical intake process involves systematically gathering essential patient information prior to consultation. This includes verifying personal details, medical history, current medications, and allergies. The purpose of the visit is crucial, as it guides the healthcare provider in understanding the patient's primary concerns and expectations. Medical assistants play a vital role by accurately documenting these details and ensuring all necessary forms are completed. This process facilitates effective communication between the patient and the healthcare team, enhancing diagnostic accuracy and treatment planning. Thorough intake procedures ensure that the visit is efficient and focused, ultimately improving patient care outcomes and satisfaction.

3.1.1.5   Measure Vital Signs:

Vital signs are crucial indicators of a patient's health status and include temperature, pulse, respiration, and blood pressure. Medical assistants must accurately measure these vital signs to assess and monitor patients effectively. Temperature can be taken orally, rectally, axillary, or tympanically. Pulse is measured at various sites, most commonly at the radial artery, where beats are counted per minute. Respiration involves observing the rise and fall of the chest to count breaths per minute. Blood pressure is measured using a sphygmomanometer and stethoscope to determine systolic and diastolic pressures. Accurate measurement ensures effective diagnosis and treatment planning, emphasizing the importance of precision and consistency in clinical practice for patient safety.

3.1.1.6   Obtain Anthropometric Measurements:

Anthropometric measurements are critical in assessing a patient's nutritional status and growth patterns. These measurements include height, weight, body mass index (BMI), and, in some cases, skinfold thickness. Medical assistants must ensure accuracy by using calibrated equipment and standardized procedures. Height is measured with a stadiometer, while weight is taken using a digital or beam balance scale. BMI is calculated by dividing weight in kilograms by height in meters squared. Accurate anthropometric data are essential for diagnosing obesity, malnutrition, and other health conditions. It is crucial to record these measurements precisely in the patient's medical record for ongoing monitoring and evaluation of health interventions.

3.1.1.7   Abnormal Signs and Symptoms Reporting:

Medical assistants play a crucial role in recognizing and managing patient health concerns. Identifying abnormal signs and symptoms involves observing deviations from normal physiological parameters, such as unusual vital signs, skin discoloration, or altered mental status. Documentation requires accurately recording these findings in the patient's medical record, ensuring that details such as onset, duration, and severity are included. Reporting involves promptly communicating these abnormalities to the supervising healthcare provider for further evaluation and intervention. This process ensures a timely medical response, enhances patient safety, and supports effective treatment planning. Mastery of this skill is essential for CCMA certification and contributes significantly to quality patient care.

3.1.1.8   Assist Provider in Physical Exam:

Assisting a provider with a general physical examination involves preparing the examination room, ensuring that all necessary equipment and supplies are available, and maintaining a sterile environment. Medical Assistants must verify the patient's identity, obtain vital signs, and document the medical history accurately. They should provide patient comfort by explaining procedures and addressing any concerns. During the exam, assistants hand instruments to the provider, manage patient positioning, and record findings as directed. Post-examination duties include cleaning the examination area, disposing of used materials safely, and updating patient records. Effective communication and organizational skills are essential to facilitate a smooth examination process and ensure optimal patient care.

3.1.1.9   Supporting Specialty Exam Providers:

Assisting providers with specialty examinations involves preparing both the patient and the examination room, ensuring that all necessary equipment and supplies are available and functioning. Medical assistants must be knowledgeable about specific procedures related to various specialties, such as cardiology, dermatology, or orthopedics. They play a critical role in obtaining patient history and vital signs, providing patient education on the procedure, and ensuring patient comfort throughout the exam. Additionally, they may assist in specimen collection, documentation, and follow-up care instructions. Understanding the nuances of each specialty ensures seamless support for the provider, enhances patient care, and facilitates efficient clinical workflow during these specialized assessments.

3.1.1.10   Prepare Patient For Procedures:

Preparing a patient for procedures involves several critical steps to ensure safety and comfort. Medical Assistants must first verify the patient's identity and confirm the procedure to be performed. They should review the patient's medical history, allergies, and current medications to identify any potential risks. Providing clear instructions and answering any questions helps alleviate patient anxiety. The assistant must ensure that all necessary equipment and supplies are ready and that the procedure area is clean and organized. Proper positioning of the patient is crucial for both comfort and optimal access for the healthcare provider. Documentation of all preparatory actions is essential for maintaining accurate medical records.

3.1.1.11   Medication Administration Techniques:

Medical assistants are tasked with the precise preparation and administration of medications via various routes. Non-parenteral routes include oral (swallowing), buccal (between the gums and cheek), and sublingual (under the tongue), ensuring accurate dosage and patient compliance. Parenteral routes, excluding intravenous, involve intramuscular (deep muscle tissue), intradermal (between skin layers), and subcutaneous (under the skin) injections, which require sterile techniques to prevent infection. Topical application involves the direct placement of medication on the skin, while transdermal patches deliver medication through skin absorption. Inhalation methods administer drugs via the respiratory tract, demanding correct device usage for efficacy. Understanding these routes ensures safe and effective patient care.

3.1.1.12   Staple and Suture Removal Techniques:

Staple and suture removal is a critical task for medical assistants, involving the careful extraction of staples or sutures from a patient's wound to facilitate healing. This procedure requires an understanding of wound healing stages and the ability to recognize signs of infection. Before removal, verify the physician's order and ensure that the wound is ready for staple or suture removal, typically after 5 to 14 days, depending on the location and type of wound. Use sterile techniques to prevent infection: cleanse the area with antiseptic, and then use appropriate tools such as a staple remover or suture scissors. Gently lift each staple or cut each suture knot, pulling carefully to avoid tissue damage while ensuring patient comfort throughout the procedure.

3.1.1.13   Administering Eye, Ear, and Topical Medications:

Administering eye, ear, and topical medications involves applying medication directly to the affected area to treat local conditions. For eye medications, ensure the patient is seated or lying down. Gently pull down the lower eyelid to create a pocket, and apply drops or ointment without touching the eye. For ear medications, have the patient tilt their head or lie on their side. Pull the ear upward and outward for adults (downward for children), and instill the drops. Topical medications are applied to skin surfaces; clean the area first, then apply as directed. Always follow proper hygiene practices and verify medication orders to ensure patient safety and efficacy.

3.1.1.14   Ear and Eye Irrigation Techniques:

Ear and eye irrigation are essential procedures for removing debris, discharge, or foreign bodies from these sensitive areas. Ear irrigation involves gently flushing the ear canal with a warm saline solution to clear cerumen (earwax) or other obstructions. This procedure helps prevent infections and improve hearing. Eye irrigation, on the other hand, is performed to cleanse the eye of irritants or chemical splashes using a sterile saline solution. It is crucial for preventing damage to the cornea and maintaining ocular health. Medical assistants must ensure proper technique, maintain sterility, and monitor patient comfort throughout the procedure to achieve effective and safe outcomes.

3.1.1.15   First Aid & Basic Wound Care:

Administering first aid and basic wound care involves initial treatment to prevent infection, control bleeding, and stabilize the patient until further medical help is available. Medical assistants should first assess the situation for safety and then evaluate the wound's severity. Cleanse the wound with saline or clean water, gently removing any debris. Apply antiseptic if available, and cover the wound with a sterile dressing to protect it from contaminants. For bleeding, apply direct pressure with a clean cloth and elevate the injured area, if possible, to reduce blood flow. Ensure you follow universal precautions to prevent cross-contamination. Document the care provided and monitor for signs of infection or complications.

3.1.1.16   Emergency Response Identification:

In clinical settings, medical assistants must promptly identify and respond to emergencies or priority situations to ensure patient safety. This involves recognizing signs of distress, such as difficulty breathing, chest pain, or severe bleeding. Medical assistants should follow established protocols, including alerting the healthcare team immediately and providing basic life support if necessary. They must remain calm, communicate effectively, and document the incident accurately. Understanding triage principles helps prioritize care based on severity. Continuous training in emergency procedures enhances preparedness. Quick and decisive action can stabilize patients until further medical intervention is available, underscoring the critical role of medical assistants in emergency response.

3.1.1.17   Perform CPR:

Cardiopulmonary resuscitation (CPR) is an emergency procedure performed to manually preserve brain function in a person experiencing cardiac arrest until further medical help arrives. Medical assistants should ensure scene safety, check for responsiveness, and call for emergency assistance. Begin CPR with chest compressions at a rate of 100-120 compressions per minute, pressing down at least two inches deep in the center of the chest. Allow complete chest recoil between compressions. For rescue breaths, open the airway using the head-tilt-chin-lift method and deliver two breaths after every 30 compressions, if trained to do so. Continue CPR cycles until professional help takes over or the patient shows signs of life.

3.1.1.18   Assisting Providers in Minor & Traumatic Injuries:

Medical assistants play a crucial role in supporting providers when patients present with minor and traumatic injuries. This involves preparing the examination room, ensuring that all necessary supplies and equipment are available, and maintaining a sterile environment to prevent infection. They assist by obtaining the patient's history, documenting vital signs, and describing the mechanism of the injury. During the examination, medical assistants may help with wound cleansing, dressing application, or immobilization of injured areas. Effective communication is vital for accurately relaying patient concerns to the provider. Additionally, they provide post-care instructions to patients, ensuring that they understand follow-up care and medication adherence for optimal recovery.

3.1.1.19   Assist With Surgical Interventions:

Medical assistants play a crucial role in assisting with minor surgical interventions such as sebaceous cyst removal, toenail removal, colposcopy, and cryosurgery. Their responsibilities include preparing the surgical area by ensuring sterility, setting up necessary instruments, and assisting the physician during the procedure. They must maintain patient comfort and safety by explaining procedures, monitoring vital signs, and providing post-operative care instructions. For sebaceous cyst or toenail removal, they prepare local anesthetics and dressings. In colposcopy, they assist with biopsy tools. During cryosurgery, they manage cryogenic equipment. Proficiency in these tasks ensures an efficient workflow and enhances patient outcomes in clinical settings.

3.1.1.20   Patient Discharge Instructions Review:

Medical assistants play a crucial role in ensuring that patients understand their discharge instructions and plan of care. This involves reviewing the provider's instructions with the patient, which may include medication management, follow-up appointments, dietary restrictions, activity limitations, and signs of potential complications. It is essential to communicate clearly and confirm patient comprehension by asking them to repeat the information back. Additionally, medical assistants should provide written materials when necessary and encourage questions to clarify any uncertainties. Ensuring that patients understand their care plan helps promote adherence, reduces the risk of readmission, and supports positive health outcomes. Effective discharge instruction review is integral to comprehensive patient care.

3.1.1.21   Prescription Order Submission Guidelines:

Medical assistants must adhere to strict protocols when sending prescription orders and refills through telephone, fax, or email to ensure patient safety and compliance with legal regulations. This involves verifying the patient's identity and medication details, ensuring that the prescriber's authorization is documented, and confirming the pharmacy's contact information. Communication must be clear and precise to prevent errors. When using email or fax, secure channels should be employed to protect patient confidentiality in accordance with HIPAA guidelines. Telephone communications should be documented in the patient's medical record, including the date, time, and details of the conversation. Adhering to these guidelines minimizes risks and ensures efficient medication management.

3.1.1.22   Patient Care Documentation in Records:

Accurate documentation in patient records is essential for effective clinical patient care. It involves recording comprehensive details of a patient's health status, treatments, and care plans. Medical Assistants must ensure that entries are clear, concise, and reflect the latest interactions with the patient. This includes vital signs, symptoms, medications administered, and any procedural interventions. Proper documentation supports continuity of care, facilitates communication among healthcare providers, and serves as legal evidence of care provided. It is crucial to adhere to confidentiality protocols and use standardized medical terminology to avoid misinterpretation. Consistent and precise documentation enhances patient safety and improves healthcare outcomes.

3.1.1.23   Basic EHR/EMR Operations:

Electronic Health Records (EHR) and Electronic Medical Records (EMR) are digital versions of patients' paper charts. Operating these systems involves accessing, updating, and managing patient information efficiently. Medical assistants must be proficient in navigating the software to input data such as patient demographics, medical history, and treatment plans. They should also know how to schedule appointments, manage billing codes, and generate reports. Understanding privacy regulations like HIPAA is crucial for safeguarding patient information. Familiarity with EHR/EMR systems enhances workflow efficiency, improves patient care coordination, and facilitates communication among healthcare providers. Mastery of these functions is essential for effective clinical support and administrative duties.

3.1.1.24   Enter Orders Into CPOE:

Computerized Provider Order Entry (CPOE) is a system that allows healthcare providers to enter and manage orders for patient services electronically. Medical Assistants play a crucial role in this process by accurately inputting orders such as medications, laboratory tests, and imaging studies into the CPOE system. This ensures clear communication among healthcare team members and minimizes errors associated with handwritten orders. Familiarity with the CPOE interface and an understanding of order protocols are essential for efficiency and accuracy. Medical Assistants must verify patient information, confirm order details with the provider, and follow institutional guidelines to ensure compliance with regulatory standards, ultimately enhancing patient safety and the quality of care.

3.1.2 Knowledge Of:
3.1.2.1   Patient Identifiers:

Patient identifiers are critical pieces of information used to accurately identify and match a patient with their health records, ensuring safe and effective care. Common identifiers include the patient's full name, date of birth, medical record number, and sometimes additional details such as address or phone number. These identifiers help prevent errors, such as administering incorrect treatments or tests. In clinical settings, verifying at least two patient identifiers before any procedure or medication administration is standard practice. This process is vital for maintaining patient safety and confidentiality. Medical assistants must be diligent in confirming these identifiers to avoid potential harm and uphold the integrity of the healthcare system.

3.1.2.2   Components of Patient History:

A comprehensive patient history is crucial for effective clinical assessment and care planning. Medical history includes past and current illnesses, allergies, medications, and immunizations. Surgical history covers previous surgeries, complications, and recovery outcomes. Family history identifies hereditary conditions by noting relatives' health issues. Social history examines lifestyle factors such as occupation, smoking, alcohol use, and living situation that impact health. Each element provides insight into risk factors and guides diagnostic and therapeutic decisions. Understanding these components enables medical assistants to gather accurate information, aiding in comprehensive patient evaluation and fostering informed healthcare delivery.

3.1.2.3   Vital Signs Measurement Methods:

Obtaining blood pressure is crucial for assessing cardiovascular health. Manually, it involves using a sphygmomanometer and a stethoscope. The cuff is placed on the patient's upper arm, inflated to occlude arterial blood flow, and then slowly deflated while listening for Korotkoff sounds. The first sound indicates systolic pressure, while the disappearance of sound marks diastolic pressure. Electronically, automated devices use oscillometric methods to detect blood flow vibrations through the cuff. These devices provide digital readings of systolic and diastolic pressures, offering convenience and reducing human error. Both methods require the proper cuff size and placement to ensure accuracy. Understanding these techniques is essential for effective patient assessment.

3.1.2.4   Vital Signs Assessment:

Respiration refers to the process of inhaling oxygen and exhaling carbon dioxide. Medical assistants must accurately count breaths per minute to assess respiratory health. Temperature measurement is crucial for detecting fever or hypothermia, using oral, tympanic, or temporal methods. Pulse is the rhythmic expansion of arteries as blood is pumped by the heart; it should be measured at various sites, such as the radial artery, to determine heart rate and rhythm. Pulse oximetry measures oxygen saturation in the blood, providing vital information about a patient's respiratory efficiency. Mastery of these assessments is essential for identifying potential health issues and ensuring effective patient care.

3.1.2.5   Vital Signs: Normal vs. Abnormal

Vital signs are critical indicators of a patient's health status, including temperature, pulse, respiration, and blood pressure. Normal ranges vary by age but typically include a temperature of 97°F to 99°F, a pulse rate of 60 to 100 beats per minute, respiratory rates of 12 to 20 breaths per minute, and blood pressure around 120/80 mmHg for adults. Abnormal vital signs may indicate underlying health issues; for instance, fever (above 100.4°F), tachycardia (pulse over 100 bpm), bradypnea (respirations under 12), or hypertension (blood pressure above 140/90 mmHg). Recognizing deviations from normal ranges is crucial for timely intervention and effective patient care management.

3.1.2.6   Height, Weight, and BMI Measurement Methods:

Height is measured using a stadiometer, ensuring that the patient stands straight with their heels together and their back aligned to the wall. Weight is measured with a calibrated scale, ensuring that the patient removes heavy clothing and shoes for accuracy. Body Mass Index (BMI) is calculated using the formula: weight in kilograms divided by height in meters squared (kg/m²). It assesses body fat based on height and weight, categorizing individuals as underweight, normal weight, overweight, or obese. Accurate measurement of these parameters is crucial for assessing overall health, monitoring growth in children, and managing conditions such as obesity or malnutrition. Proper technique ensures reliable data for clinical decisions.

3.1.2.7   Age, Health, Status, and Disability Considerations:

Medical assistants must tailor care to accommodate patients' diverse needs based on age, health status, and disabilities. Age-specific considerations involve understanding developmental stages and age-related physiological changes. For instance, pediatric patients require different communication techniques and dosages than adults. Health status necessitates assessing chronic conditions or acute illnesses and adjusting interventions accordingly. Disabilities require modifications in communication methods and physical accessibility to ensure effective care delivery. Socioeconomic status impacts access to resources and adherence to treatment plans. Sensitivity to these factors enhances patient-centered care, promoting safety and efficacy. Understanding these considerations is crucial for medical assistants to provide equitable and compassionate healthcare services.

3.1.2.8   Growth Chart:

A growth chart is a tool used in pediatric healthcare to monitor a child's physical development over time. It consists of percentile curves that illustrate the distribution of body measurements, such as weight, height, and head circumference, in children. Medical assistants utilize growth charts to assess whether a child's growth pattern aligns with standard benchmarks for their age and sex. By plotting these measurements on a growth chart, healthcare providers can identify potential health issues, such as malnutrition or developmental disorders. Regular monitoring allows for early intervention if deviations from typical growth patterns are observed, ensuring timely management and support for the child's health and development.

3.1.2.9   Positioning & Draping for Exams & Treatments:

Positioning and draping are critical components in medical examinations, procedures, and treatments, ensuring patient comfort, privacy, and access for healthcare providers. Proper positioning involves placing the patient in a specific posture to facilitate examination or treatment; for instance, the supine position for abdominal exams or the lithotomy position for gynecological procedures. Draping involves covering the patient with a cloth or paper sheet to maintain modesty while exposing only the necessary areas. Each specialty may have unique requirements; thus, understanding these nuances is essential for medical assistants to enhance procedural efficiency and uphold professional standards of care during patient interactions.

3.1.2.10   Essential Equipment for Examination Room Setup:

The preparation of an examination or procedure room requires specific equipment, instruments, and supplies to ensure efficiency and patient safety. Essential equipment includes an examination table, adequate lighting, and a sink with soap and hand sanitizer for hygiene. Instruments such as stethoscopes, otoscopes, and blood pressure cuffs must be readily available. Supplies like gloves, gowns, drapes, tongue depressors, and sterile swabs are necessary for various procedures. Proper organization of these items in designated areas ensures quick access during examinations. Regular inventory checks and maintenance of equipment are crucial to avoid disruptions in patient care and to maintain a sterile environment conducive to medical assessments.

3.1.2.11   Essential Equipment for Physical Examinations:

In a general physical examination, medical assistants must ensure the availability of essential equipment and supplies to facilitate a thorough assessment. This includes a stethoscope for auscultation, a sphygmomanometer for blood pressure measurement, and a thermometer for temperature checks. An otoscope and ophthalmoscope are vital for ear and eye examinations, respectively. A reflex hammer assesses neurological function, while a tuning fork evaluates auditory acuity. Examination gloves, gowns, and drapes maintain hygiene and patient modesty. Additionally, tongue depressors assist in oral examinations, and alcohol wipes ensure the sterilization of equipment. Accurate preparation of these instruments enhances diagnostic efficiency and patient care during physical exams.

3.1.2.12   Specialty Exam Equipment & Supplies:

Specialty examinations necessitate specific equipment, supplies, and instruments to ensure accurate diagnosis and treatment. For instance, an ophthalmic examination requires a tonometer, ophthalmoscope, and slit lamp for assessing eye health. Dermatological exams may require dermatoscopes and biopsy punches. Gynecological assessments utilize speculums and colposcopes, while cardiovascular evaluations often require EKG machines and sphygmomanometers. Each instrument serves a distinct purpose, aiding in precise examination and diagnosis. Medical assistants must be proficient in identifying, preparing, and maintaining these tools to support physicians effectively. Understanding the function and handling of each piece of equipment is essential for patient safety and optimal care delivery during specialty examinations.

3.1.2.13   Patient Instructions for Procedures:

Patient instruction specific to procedures involves educating patients about what to expect before, during, and after medical procedures. Pre-procedural instructions may include fasting guidelines, medication adjustments, or activity restrictions to ensure patient safety and optimal outcomes. Post-procedural instructions focus on recovery, including wound care, signs of complications, medication adherence, and follow-up appointments. Clear communication is crucial for empowering patients, reducing anxiety, and promoting compliance with care plans. Medical assistants must ensure that patients understand these instructions by using layman's terms when necessary and confirming comprehension through teach-back methods. Proper patient education enhances procedural success and supports patient-centered care.

3.1.2.14 Patient-Centric Care Modifications:

Modifications to patient care involve adapting healthcare practices to meet individual patient needs, ensuring safety and comfort. For frail and disabled patients, this includes assisting with ambulation and transfers. Medical assistants must assess the patient's mobility level and use appropriate techniques, such as gait belts or transfer boards, to prevent injury. Clear communication with the patient is essential to understand their limitations and preferences. Providing support during ambulation may involve guiding or physically supporting the patient while walking. For transfers, proper body mechanics are crucial for safely moving patients between beds, chairs, or wheelchairs. Tailoring care to each patient's capabilities enhances their independence and quality of life.

3.1.2.15 Child-Friendly Terminology for Pediatric Care:

When communicating with pediatric patients, it is crucial to use simple, age-appropriate language that they can easily comprehend. This involves breaking down complex medical terminology into words and concepts familiar to a child's everyday experiences. For instance, instead of saying injection, you might say a quick pinch or medicine shot. The goal is to alleviate fear and anxiety by making the conversation relatable and less intimidating. Additionally, using visual aids or storytelling can enhance understanding. By ensuring clarity and comfort in communication, medical assistants can foster trust and cooperation from young patients, which is essential for effective healthcare delivery and positive patient experiences.

3.1.2.16 Consent Requirements: Written and Verbal

Consent is a fundamental patient right and a legal requirement in healthcare. Written consent involves obtaining the patient's signature on a document after explaining the procedure, risks, benefits, and alternatives. It is crucial for invasive procedures or those with significant risks. Verbal consent, while less formal, involves the patient agreeing to a procedure after receiving adequate information. It is typically used for minor, low-risk procedures. Both forms of consent ensure patient autonomy and comprehension. Medical assistants must ensure that patients understand the information provided and voluntarily agree to the procedure, documenting the consent process accurately in the patient's medical record.

3.1.2.17 Immunization Schedules And Requirements:

Immunization schedules and requirements are structured timelines and criteria established by health authorities, such as the CDC, to ensure that individuals receive vaccinations at appropriate ages. These schedules are designed to provide immunity before individuals are exposed to potentially life-threatening diseases. Medical assistants must understand these schedules to effectively educate patients and ensure compliance with state and federal regulations. They include vaccines for diseases such as measles, mumps, rubella, and influenza. Requirements may vary based on age, health status, and geographic location. Medical assistants play a critical role in accurately documenting immunizations, managing vaccine inventory, and recognizing contraindications or adverse reactions to maintain patient safety.

3.1.2.18 Overview of Allergies: Drug and Non-Drug Types

Allergies are hypersensitive immune responses to substances that are typically harmless. Common allergens include drugs (e.g., penicillin) and non-drug substances like latex and bee stings. Upon exposure, the immune system overreacts, releasing chemicals such as histamine, which can lead to symptoms ranging from mild (hives, itching) to severe (anaphylaxis). Medical assistants must recognize the signs of allergic reactions and understand emergency protocols, such as administering epinephrine for anaphylaxis. Knowledge of a patient's allergy history is critical for preventing exposure. Documentation and communication with the healthcare team are essential to ensure patient safety and effective management of allergic reactions.

3.1.2.19 Allergic Reactions: Response Levels

Allergic reactions vary in severity: mild, moderate, and severe. Mild reactions may include skin rashes or itching, and their management typically involves antihistamines and monitoring. Moderate reactions can involve respiratory distress or swelling, which may require bronchodilators or corticosteroids. Severe reactions, such as anaphylaxis, are life-threatening and are characterized by airway obstruction, hypotension, and shock. The immediate response includes administering epinephrine, ensuring airway patency, and calling emergency services. Medical assistants must recognize symptoms quickly and act promptly to prevent escalation. Continuous monitoring and supportive care are crucial until professional medical help arrives. Understanding these responses ensures patient safety and effective management of allergic emergencies.

3.1.2.20 Signs Of Infection:

Signs of infection are clinical indicators that suggest the presence of pathogenic microorganisms in the body. Common signs include redness, swelling, warmth, and pain at the infection site, often accompanied by fever. These manifestations result from the body's inflammatory response to fight off pathogens. Additional systemic signs may include fatigue, malaise, and lymphadenopathy. In some cases, pus formation or discharge may occur if the infection is localized. Medical assistants must recognize these signs promptly to ensure timely intervention and treatment. Accurate identification aids in preventing complications and promoting effective patient care, aligning with the role of a Certified Clinical Medical Assistant in a healthcare setting.

3.1.2.21 Sterile Techniques in Medical Procedures:

Sterile techniques are critical for preventing infection during medical examinations, procedures, injections, and medication administration. These techniques involve creating an environment free of microorganisms. Key practices include hand hygiene, the use of sterile gloves and instruments, and the maintenance of a sterile field. Sterile drapes and barriers are employed to protect areas from contamination. Medical assistants must ensure that all equipment is properly sterilized and that aseptic techniques are strictly followed. During injections and medication administration, it is essential to use alcohol swabs to clean the skin and to ensure that needles and syringes are sterile. Adhering to these protocols minimizes the risk of infection and ensures patient safety.

3.1.2.22 Oral and Injectable Dosage Calculations:

Dosage calculations are critical in ensuring patient safety and therapeutic efficacy. For oral medications, calculations involve determining the correct tablet or liquid dose based on the prescribed amount and the available medication concentration. This requires an understanding of units of measurement, conversion factors, and the application of formulas. For injectables, calculations must account for the volume of liquid needed to deliver the prescribed dose, considering the concentration of the drug in vials or ampoules. Mastery of these calculations is essential to prevent underdosing or overdosing. Medical assistants must be proficient in interpreting prescriptions, using calculation formulas accurately, and double-checking their work to ensure precise medication administration.

3.1.2.23 Oral and Parenteral Medications Overview:

Oral medications are typically administered in forms such as tablets, capsules, or liquids and are packaged in bottles or blister packs. They are ingested through the mouth and absorbed via the gastrointestinal tract. Parenteral medications bypass the digestive system and are administered through injections, including intravenous (IV), intramuscular (IM), and subcutaneous (SC) routes. These medications are often packaged in vials, ampoules, or pre-filled syringes. The choice of route depends on the medication's properties, the desired speed of action, and patient-specific factors. Understanding these routes and forms is crucial for ensuring proper medication administration and achieving therapeutic effects safely and effectively.

3.1.2.24   Rights Of Medication Administration:
The Rights of Medication Administration is a crucial framework that ensures patient safety and effective medication management. It encompasses verifying the right patient, medication, dose, route, time, and documentation. Medical Assistants must confirm patient identity using at least two identifiers. They check the medication label against the prescription to ensure accuracy in both the drug and dosage. The correct route (oral, intravenous, etc.) and timing are verified to optimize therapeutic effects. Documentation involves recording every administered dose in the patient's medical record. Adhering to these rights minimizes errors, enhances patient safety, and ensures compliance with legal and ethical standards in healthcare practice.

3.1.2.25   Storage:
Storage in a medical setting refers to the systematic organization and safekeeping of medical supplies, equipment, and patient records. Proper storage ensures accessibility, prevents contamination, and complies with regulatory standards. Medical assistants must understand the protocols for storing medications, which often require specific temperature controls to maintain efficacy. Equipment should be stored in designated areas to avoid damage and facilitate easy retrieval. Patient records must be securely stored to protect confidentiality, adhering to HIPAA regulations. Effective storage practices minimize waste, optimize space, and enhance workflow efficiency. Mastery of storage techniques is crucial for maintaining a safe and efficient healthcare environment.

3.1.2.26   Labeling:
Labeling in the clinical setting involves accurately identifying and marking specimens, medications, and patient information to ensure safety and proper handling. It is a critical task for medical assistants to prevent errors in patient care. Proper labeling includes the patient's full name, date of birth, unique identification number, date and time of collection, and the type of specimen or medication. This practice ensures that all healthcare providers have access to accurate information, reducing the risk of misdiagnosis or incorrect treatment. Medical assistants must adhere to strict protocols and double-check labels against patient records to maintain accuracy and compliance with healthcare regulations, ultimately safeguarding patient safety and the quality of care.

3.1.2.27   And Medication Logs:
Medication logs are detailed records that track the administration of medications to patients. They serve as a critical tool for ensuring patient safety, maintaining accurate medication histories, and facilitating communication among healthcare providers. These logs typically include information such as the patient's name, medication name, dosage, route of administration, time and date of administration, and the initials or signature of the administering medical assistant. Accurate documentation in medication logs helps prevent medication errors, supports compliance with legal and regulatory requirements, and provides a reliable reference for future medical care. Medical assistants must ensure that these logs are meticulously maintained and updated to support optimal patient outcomes.

3.1.2.28   Techniques And Injection Sites:
Understanding techniques and injection sites is crucial for safe and effective medication administration. Techniques vary based on the type of injection: intramuscular (IM), subcutaneous (SC), or intradermal (ID). IM injections are administered at a 90-degree angle into muscle tissue, typically in the deltoid, vastus lateralis, or ventrogluteal sites. SC injections are given at a 45 to 90-degree angle into the fatty tissue, commonly in the upper arm, thigh, or abdomen. ID injections are administered at a 10 to 15-degree angle into the dermis, often on the forearm. Proper site selection minimizes complications and maximizes absorption efficiency, ensuring patient safety and therapeutic efficacy.

3.1.2.29   Injection Supplies and Equipment:
Medical assistants must be proficient with various supplies and equipment used for injections to ensure safe and effective administration. This includes syringes, needles, alcohol swabs, bandages, and sharps containers. Syringes vary in size and type, such as insulin or tuberculin syringes, each suited for specific medications. Needles differ in gauge and length; the selection depends on the type of injection (intramuscular, subcutaneous, or intradermal). Alcohol swabs are used to disinfect the skin before injection to prevent infection. Bandages cover the injection site post-administration. Sharps containers are essential for the safe disposal of used needles to minimize needlestick injuries and maintain a sterile environment.

3.1.2.30   Storage Of Injectables:
Proper storage of injectables is crucial for maintaining their efficacy and safety. Injectables must be stored according to manufacturer guidelines, which are typically found on the packaging or accompanying documentation. Most injectables require refrigeration at temperatures between 2°C and 8°C (36°F and 46°F) to preserve their stability. It is essential to avoid freezing, as this can damage the medication. Some injectables may be stored at room temperature if specified. Always ensure that vials are kept in their original packaging to protect them from light exposure. Regularly monitor storage conditions with calibrated thermometers and document any deviations. Adhering to these guidelines ensures patient safety and medication effectiveness.

3.1.2.31   Suture and Staple Removal Techniques:
Suture and staple removal is a critical skill for medical assistants, involving precise techniques to prevent infection and promote healing. Sutures are removed using sterile suture scissors or forceps, carefully cutting and pulling each stitch without disturbing the wound. Staples require a specialized staple remover, which gently lifts and disengages each staple from the skin. Both procedures demand strict adherence to aseptic techniques to minimize the risk of infection. The medical assistant must assess the wound for proper healing before removal and document the procedure accurately. Understanding skin integrity and the stages of healing is crucial for determining the appropriate timing for suture or staple removal.

3.1.2.32   Suture Types and Sizes:
Sutures are critical for wound closure and healing, and they are available in various types and sizes tailored to specific medical needs. Types include absorbable sutures, which dissolve naturally over time, and non-absorbable sutures, which require removal after healing. Common materials include silk, nylon, and polypropylene. Sizes range from 11-0 (the finest) to 7 (the thickest), denoting diameter; finer sutures are used for delicate tissues such as blood vessels, while thicker ones are used for robust tissues like skin. Understanding the appropriate type and size of sutures is crucial for minimizing the risk of infection and ensuring optimal healing. Medical assistants must recognize these distinctions to assist effectively during surgical procedures.

3.1.2.33   Administration Techniques for Eye, Ear, and Topical Medications:

Administering eye, ear, and topical medications requires precision and adherence to specific techniques to ensure efficacy and patient safety. For eye medications, use sterile droppers or applicators, instructing patients to avoid touching the eye surface. Ear medications necessitate proper positioning of the patient, typically lying on their side, with gentle pulling of the earlobe to straighten the ear canal. Topical medications involve applying creams or ointments directly onto the skin using gloves or applicators to prevent contamination. Supplies include sterile droppers, cotton balls, gloves, and applicators. Mastery of these methods is crucial for effective treatment and the prevention of infections or complications.

3.1.2.34   Eye and Ear Irrigation Tools and Techniques:

Eye and ear irrigation involves the use of specific instruments and supplies to cleanse and remove debris or foreign substances. For eye irrigation, a sterile eye cup or syringe is used with a saline solution to gently flush the eye. Proper technique involves tilting the patient's head to prevent contamination and ensuring that the solution flows from the inner to the outer corner of the eye. Ear irrigation requires an otoscope for examination, a bulb syringe or electronic irrigator, and warm saline or water. The procedure involves tilting the head and gently flushing the ear canal to dislodge cerumen or debris, ensuring patient comfort and safety throughout.

3.1.2.35   Common Injury Types:

Lacerations are deep cuts or tears in the skin or flesh, often requiring stitches for proper healing. Abrasions, commonly known as scrapes, occur when the skin is rubbed away by friction. Fractures are breaks in bones, ranging from hairline cracks to complete breaks, necessitating immobilization and sometimes surgery. Sprains involve the stretching or tearing of ligaments, typically affecting joints such as the ankle or wrist. Each type of injury demands specific first aid and medical interventions to prevent complications and promote recovery. Understanding these injuries enables medical assistants to provide appropriate care and guidance to patients, ensuring effective treatment and rehabilitation processes.

3.1.2.36   Injury Treatment Overview:

Injury treatment involves immediate and appropriate actions to minimize damage and promote healing. Bandaging provides support, reduces swelling, and protects wounds from infection. Proper application ensures that circulation is not compromised. Ice application, typically performed in 15-20 minute intervals, reduces swelling and numbs pain by constricting blood vessels. Elevation above heart level decreases blood flow to the injured area, further reducing swelling and pain. These techniques are crucial for effectively managing sprains, strains, and minor wounds. Medical assistants must assess the type and severity of the injury to apply these treatments correctly, ensuring patient safety and comfort while preventing complications or delays in recovery.

3.1.2.37   Types of Surgical Interventions:

Surgical interventions are procedures performed to treat or diagnose medical conditions. Common types include appendectomy, cholecystectomy, and hernia repair. An appendectomy involves removing an inflamed appendix, often due to appendicitis, to prevent rupture. A cholecystectomy is the removal of the gallbladder, typically due to gallstones causing pain or infection. Hernia repair addresses the protrusion of an organ through a weakened abdominal wall, which can cause discomfort and complications. These surgeries can be performed using open or minimally invasive techniques, such as laparoscopy. Understanding these procedures enables medical assistants to provide effective pre- and post-operative care, ensuring patient safety and recovery.

3.1.2.38   Urgent and Emergency Signs and Symptoms:

Recognizing urgent and emergency situations is crucial for medical assistants. Diabetic shock presents with confusion, sweating, and a rapid heartbeat. Heat stroke is characterized by a high body temperature, hot skin, and an altered mental state. Allergic reactions may involve hives, swelling, and difficulty breathing. Choking is identified by an inability to speak or breathe, along with cyanosis. Syncope involves sudden fainting due to decreased blood flow to the brain. Seizures manifest as convulsions, loss of consciousness, or abnormal movements. Prompt identification and intervention can prevent complications. Understanding these signs ensures a timely response and enhances patient safety in critical scenarios.

3.1.2.39   Emergency Action Plans: Crash Carts & Injectables

Emergency Action Plans (EAPs) are structured protocols designed to manage medical emergencies efficiently and effectively. A crash cart is a mobile unit stocked with essential equipment and medications required during emergencies, such as cardiac arrest. It includes defibrillators, airway management tools, and emergency injectables like epinephrine and atropine. Emergency injectables are critical for immediate intervention in life-threatening situations, providing a rapid pharmacological response to stabilize patients. Medical Assistants must be familiar with the location and contents of crash carts and understand the proper administration of emergency injectables. This knowledge ensures prompt action, potentially saving lives during critical incidents within healthcare settings.

3.1.2.40   CPR, BLS, and AED Procedures:

Cardiopulmonary Resuscitation (CPR) is a life-saving technique used in emergencies when someone's breathing or heartbeat has stopped. Basic Life Support (BLS) encompasses CPR and involves maintaining airway patency, supporting breathing, and ensuring circulation without the use of advanced equipment. To perform CPR, initiate chest compressions at a rate of 100 to 120 compressions per minute and provide rescue breaths in a 30:2 ratio. An Automated External Defibrillator (AED) analyzes the heart's rhythm and delivers an electric shock to restore a normal rhythm. Medical Assistants must ensure scene safety, call for help, start CPR immediately, and use the AED as soon as it arrives to maximize the chances of survival.

3.1.2.41   CPOE Overview:

Computerized Physician Order Entry (CPOE) is a digital system that allows healthcare providers to enter and manage medical orders electronically. This technology replaces traditional paper-based methods, enhancing accuracy and efficiency in patient care. CPOE systems are integrated with electronic health records (EHRs), enabling seamless communication across healthcare teams. They reduce medication errors by providing decision support tools, such as drug interaction alerts and dosage recommendations. For medical assistants, understanding CPOE is crucial, as it streamlines workflow, ensures timely order processing, and improves patient safety. Familiarity with CPOE systems is essential for assisting physicians in managing patient orders effectively and maintaining accurate medical documentation.

3.1.2.42   Referral Authorizations:

Referral authorizations are formal approvals required for patients to see specialists or receive specific medical services beyond primary care. These authorizations ensure that the recommended services are necessary and covered by the patient's insurance plan. As a medical assistant, understanding the process involves verifying insurance requirements, completing necessary paperwork, and communicating with both the referring and receiving providers. Efficient handling of referral authorizations prevents delays in patient care and avoids unexpected costs for patients. It is crucial to maintain accurate records, follow up on pending authorizations, and inform patients about their responsibilities and any potential out-of-pocket expenses associated with the referral.

3.1.2.43   Insurance Authorizations:
Insurance authorizations are formal approvals from a health insurance provider that confirm coverage for specific medical services, procedures, or medications. This process ensures that the proposed healthcare services are deemed medically necessary and covered under the patient's insurance plan. Medical assistants play a crucial role in obtaining these authorizations by submitting required documentation, such as physician orders and patient medical records, to the insurance company. They must be familiar with various insurance policies and guidelines to expedite the process efficiently. Timely authorization prevents delays in patient care and avoids unexpected financial burdens on patients due to denied claims. Understanding insurance authorizations is essential for seamless healthcare delivery and reimbursement.

3.1.2.44   Legal Prescription Content & Transmission Requirements:
Prescriptions must include specific elements to be legally valid: the patient's name, the date of issue, the medication name, the dosage, the route of administration, the frequency, and the quantity. The prescriber's signature and license number are essential. Electronic prescriptions must comply with federal and state regulations, ensuring secure transmission to prevent unauthorized access. The Health Insurance Portability and Accountability Act (HIPAA) mandates confidentiality during transmission. Medical assistants must verify the completeness and accuracy of prescriptions before processing. Understanding the regulations surrounding controlled substances is crucial, as they have stricter requirements. Compliance ensures patient safety and legal adherence, minimizing medication errors and potential legal repercussions for healthcare providers.

3.1.2.45   Prior Authorizations For Medication:
Prior authorizations for medication are a cost-control process used by insurance companies to determine whether they will cover a prescribed medication. This process requires healthcare providers to obtain approval from the insurance company before the patient can receive the medication. It involves submitting detailed information about the patient's condition and the necessity of the prescribed drug. Medical assistants play a crucial role in facilitating this process by gathering the necessary documentation, completing required forms, and communicating with both the insurance company and the prescribing physician. Understanding prior authorizations is essential for ensuring that patients receive timely access to their medications while effectively managing healthcare costs.

3.1.2.46   Electronic Prescribing Software:
Electronic Prescribing Software is a digital tool utilized by healthcare providers to create, modify, review, and transmit prescription information electronically to pharmacies. This software enhances medication safety by reducing errors associated with handwritten prescriptions and facilitates quicker communication between providers and pharmacists. It integrates with electronic health records (EHRs) to provide comprehensive patient medication histories, check for drug interactions, and ensure adherence to formulary guidelines. Additionally, it supports compliance with regulatory requirements and improves efficiency by streamlining the prescribing process. For Certified Clinical Medical Assistants, understanding this software is crucial for assisting in accurate prescription management and ensuring optimal patient care within clinical settings.

3.1.2.47   Essential Elements of Medical Records:
Medical records are essential for documenting patient care and must include specific components to ensure comprehensive and effective communication among healthcare providers. Key components include the patient's personal information, medical history, and current health status. Documentation of clinical findings, diagnoses, treatment plans, and progress notes is crucial for continuity of care. Additionally, records should contain laboratory and imaging results, medication lists, and informed consent forms. Each entry must be dated and signed by the healthcare provider responsible for the care. Proper documentation supports legal compliance, billing accuracy, and quality assurance. Maintaining the confidentiality and security of medical records is paramount to protect patient privacy and comply with regulations.

3.1.2.48   Medical Necessity Guidelines:
Medical Necessity Guidelines are criteria used to determine the appropriateness of healthcare services based on clinical standards. These guidelines ensure that medical interventions, procedures, or tests are essential for diagnosing or treating a patient's condition. They help evaluate whether the provided care is reasonable, necessary, and in alignment with evidence-based practices. Medical Necessity Guidelines are crucial for insurance coverage decisions, ensuring that patients receive appropriate care without incurring unnecessary costs. As a Certified Clinical Medical Assistant (CCMA), understanding these guidelines aids in accurate documentation and communication with healthcare providers to support the delivery of justified and effective patient care.

3.2 Infection Control:
Infection control refers to the systematic approach used to prevent and manage the spread of infections within healthcare settings. It involves implementing practices and procedures that aim to protect patients, healthcare workers, and visitors from infectious diseases. Key components include hand hygiene, the use of personal protective equipment (PPE), proper sterilization and disinfection of medical instruments, and isolation protocols for contagious patients. Medical assistants play a crucial role by adhering to these guidelines, ensuring a clean environment, and educating patients on infection prevention strategies. Effective infection control minimizes the risk of healthcare-associated infections (HAIs), promotes safer healthcare delivery, and improves patient outcomes.

3.2.1 Tasks:
3.2.1.1   Infection Control Compliance:
Medical assistants must strictly follow established infection control regulations and guidelines to prevent the spread of infectious diseases. These protocols are set by organizations such as the CDC and OSHA and include practices like hand hygiene, the use of personal protective equipment (PPE), proper sterilization techniques, and safe disposal of sharps and biohazardous waste. Adhering to these guidelines is crucial for maintaining a safe healthcare environment for both patients and staff. Medical assistants should be well-versed in these standards, regularly update their knowledge, and ensure compliance in all clinical procedures to minimize infection risks, thereby effectively safeguarding public health.

3.2.1.2 Hand Hygiene Guidelines Compliance:
Hand hygiene is a critical component of infection control, aimed at preventing the transmission of pathogens in healthcare settings. Medical assistants must adhere to established guidelines, such as those from the CDC and WHO, which emphasize washing hands with soap and water when they are visibly soiled or using an alcohol-based hand sanitizer for routine decontamination. Proper technique involves covering all surfaces of the hands and fingers and rubbing them for at least 20 seconds. Hand hygiene should be performed before and after patient contact, after contact with potentially infectious materials, and after removing gloves. Compliance with these guidelines reduces healthcare-associated infections, thereby protecting both patients and healthcare workers.

3.2.1.3 Perform Disinfection/Sanitization:
Disinfection and sanitization are critical tasks in infection control, aimed at reducing or eliminating pathogenic microorganisms on surfaces and instruments. Disinfection involves using chemical agents to destroy bacteria, viruses, and fungi, ensuring that surfaces are free from harmful pathogens. Sanitization, on the other hand, refers to cleaning surfaces to lower the number of germs to safe levels as determined by public health standards. Medical assistants must follow protocols for selecting appropriate disinfectants and sanitizing agents, ensuring that the contact time is sufficient for effectiveness. Proper disinfection and sanitization prevent healthcare-associated infections (HAIs), safeguarding patient health and maintaining a sterile environment in clinical settings.

3.2.1.4 Sterilization of Medical Equipment:
Sterilization of medical equipment is a critical task that involves eliminating all forms of microbial life, including bacteria, viruses, and spores, to prevent infection and ensure patient safety. This process is achieved through methods such as autoclaving, which uses steam under pressure, or chemical sterilants like ethylene oxide. Medical assistants must meticulously clean instruments before sterilization to remove organic material and debris. They must also adhere to manufacturer guidelines and facility protocols to maintain the integrity and functionality of the equipment. Proper documentation and handling are essential to ensure that all items are accounted for and remain sterile until use, safeguarding both patients and healthcare providers from potential infections.

3.2.1.5 Aseptic Techniques in Clinical Settings:
Aseptic techniques are critical practices used to prevent contamination and infection during clinical procedures. These techniques include hand hygiene, the use of personal protective equipment (PPE), sterilization of instruments, and maintaining a sterile field. In various clinical situations, such as wound dressing or catheter insertion, medical assistants must ensure that all tools are sterilized and that hands are washed thoroughly. Gloves, masks, and gowns should be worn as necessary to protect both the patient and the healthcare provider. The sterile field must be maintained by avoiding contact with non-sterile surfaces. Proper disposal of used materials is essential to minimize infection risk and ensure patient safety.

3.2.1.6 OSHA Biohazard Waste Disposal:
Disposing of biohazardous materials is crucial for maintaining a safe healthcare environment. The Occupational Safety and Health Administration (OSHA) mandates strict guidelines to prevent exposure to infectious agents. Biohazardous waste, such as used needles and contaminated materials, must be placed in puncture-resistant sharps containers and sealed in red bags. These containers are designed to prevent leakage and injury. Medical assistants must ensure that these items are disposed of promptly in designated areas for proper handling and treatment. Compliance with OSHA regulations not only protects healthcare workers and patients but also ensures legal adherence, minimizing the risk of fines or sanctions for the healthcare facility.

3.2.2 Knowledge Of:
3.2.2.1 Universal Precautions:
Universal Precautions are a set of guidelines aimed at preventing the transmission of bloodborne pathogens and other infectious materials in healthcare settings. These precautions require healthcare workers, including medical assistants, to treat all human blood and certain body fluids as potentially infectious, regardless of the perceived risk. Key practices include the use of personal protective equipment (PPE) such as gloves, masks, and gowns; proper hand hygiene; safe handling and disposal of sharps; and surface decontamination. By adhering to these protocols, medical assistants minimize the risk of exposure to infectious agents, thereby ensuring their safety and that of their patients. Understanding and implementing Universal Precautions is essential for maintaining a safe clinical environment.

3.2.2.2 Hand-washing Techniques:
Effective handwashing is a critical practice for infection control in clinical settings. It involves using soap and water to remove dirt, bacteria, and viruses from the skin. Begin by wetting your hands with clean, running water, then apply soap. Rub your hands together vigorously for at least 20 seconds, ensuring that you scrub all surfaces, including the backs of your hands, between your fingers, and under your nails. Rinse thoroughly under running water and dry with a clean towel or air dry. Handwashing is essential before and after patient contact, after touching potentially contaminated surfaces, and after removing gloves. Proper technique significantly reduces the risk of healthcare-associated infections.

3.2.2.3 Alcohol-based Rubs/sanitizer:
Alcohol-based rubs or sanitizers are hand hygiene products containing ethanol, isopropanol, or n-propanol as the active ingredients, used to reduce microbial flora on the skin. They are essential in healthcare settings for preventing the spread of infections, especially when soap and water are unavailable. These sanitizers work by denaturing proteins and disrupting the cell membranes of microorganisms, effectively killing bacteria, viruses, and fungi. For optimal efficacy, a concentration of 60-95% alcohol is recommended. Medical assistants must ensure proper application by covering all hand surfaces and rubbing until dry, which typically takes around 20 seconds. Regular use helps maintain hand hygiene compliance and patient safety.

3.2.2.4 Blood-borne Pathogens: Transmission & Precautions
Infectious agents are microorganisms, such as bacteria, viruses, fungi, and parasites, that cause disease. Transmission occurs through direct contact, droplets, airborne particles, or vectors. Blood-borne pathogens, including HIV, HBV, and HCV, spread via blood and bodily fluids. Medical assistants must adhere to standard precautions, which include using personal protective equipment (PPE) like gloves and masks to minimize exposure risk. Proper hand hygiene and safe needle practices are crucial. Disinfecting surfaces and disposing of sharps in designated containers further prevent transmission. Understanding these principles ensures the safety of both patients and healthcare workers by mitigating the spread of infectious diseases in clinical settings.

3.2.2.5   Personal Protective Equipment (PPE):

Personal Protective Equipment (PPE) refers to specialized clothing or equipment worn by healthcare workers to protect against infectious materials and minimize exposure to hazards. PPE includes gloves, masks, gowns, face shields, and goggles. Each type of PPE serves a specific protective function; for example, gloves prevent contamination of the hands, while masks and respirators protect the respiratory system from airborne pathogens. Proper usage of PPE is crucial in preventing the spread of infections within healthcare settings. Medical assistants must be adept at selecting appropriate PPE based on the situation, ensuring a correct fit, and following protocols for donning and doffing to maintain safety and compliance with health regulations.

3.2.2.6   Sterilization Techniques:

Sterilization is crucial in preventing infections in clinical settings. The autoclave uses pressurized steam to eliminate all microorganisms, ensuring instrument sterility. Instrument cleaners remove organic material before sterilization, enhancing the effectiveness of subsequent processes. Germicidal disinfectants are chemical agents that reduce the microbial load on surfaces and instruments but do not achieve full sterilization. Disposable items are designed for single use to prevent cross-contamination, eliminating the need for sterilization. Each technique serves a specific purpose in infection control, with the autoclave being the most reliable method for complete sterilization. Proper application of these methods ensures a safe environment for both patients and healthcare providers.

3.2.2.7   Aseptic Techniques in Medicine and Surgery:

Medical asepsis, or clean technique, involves procedures to reduce and prevent the spread of microorganisms. This includes hand hygiene, the use of personal protective equipment (PPE), and the cleaning of surfaces. Surgical asepsis, or sterile technique, aims to eliminate all microorganisms from an area. It involves sterilizing instruments, maintaining a sterile field, and using sterile gloves and gowns. Both techniques are crucial in preventing infections in healthcare settings. Medical assistants must understand these principles to ensure patient safety during procedures. Proper aseptic techniques reduce the risk of healthcare-associated infections, thereby improving patient outcomes and maintaining a safe environment for both patients and healthcare providers.

3.2.2.8   Cleaning Order and Product Types:

The order of cleaning in a clinical setting is crucial for maintaining hygiene and preventing cross-contamination. Begin with the least soiled areas, progressing to more soiled zones to avoid spreading contaminants. Start with high-touch surfaces, such as doorknobs and light switches, and then move to larger surfaces, such as countertops and floors. Types of cleaning products include detergents for general cleaning, disinfectants for killing pathogens on surfaces, and sanitizers that reduce bacteria to safe levels. Use EPA-registered disinfectants for effective pathogen control. Always follow the manufacturer's instructions for use and dilution. Proper cleaning order and product selection are essential for maintaining a safe clinical environment.

3.2.2.9   Safety Data Sheets (SDS):

Safety Data Sheets (SDS) are essential documents that provide detailed information about the properties, hazards, handling, storage, and emergency measures related to chemicals used in healthcare settings. As a medical assistant, understanding SDS is crucial for ensuring workplace safety and compliance with Occupational Safety and Health Administration (OSHA) regulations. Each SDS includes sections on chemical identification, hazard identification, composition, first-aid measures, firefighting measures, accidental release measures, handling and storage guidelines, exposure controls/personal protection, physical and chemical properties, stability and reactivity, toxicological information, and disposal considerations. Familiarity with SDS enables medical assistants to effectively manage chemical risks and protect both themselves and patients from potential hazards.

3.2.2.10   Cautions Related To Chemicals:

In the medical setting, chemical safety is paramount to protect patients and healthcare workers. Medical Assistants must be vigilant when handling chemicals, including disinfectants, cleaning agents, and laboratory reagents. Proper labeling and storage are crucial to prevent accidental exposure or misuse. Always use personal protective equipment (PPE), such as gloves and goggles, when handling chemicals. Be familiar with the Material Safety Data Sheets (MSDS) for each chemical, which provide detailed information on hazards and first aid measures. Ensure proper ventilation in areas where chemicals are used. In the event of spills, follow established protocols for containment and cleanup to minimize the risks of exposure and contamination.

3.2.2.11   Disposal Methods:

Disposal methods refer to the systematic procedures for safely discarding medical waste to prevent contamination and ensure environmental safety. Medical assistants must understand the classification of waste, including sharps, biohazardous materials, pharmaceuticals, and general waste. Proper disposal involves using designated containers, such as puncture-resistant sharps containers for needles and red biohazard bags for contaminated materials. Compliance with Occupational Safety and Health Administration (OSHA) regulations and local guidelines is essential. Medical assistants should be trained in handling spills, labeling waste correctly, and coordinating with licensed disposal companies for collection and treatment. Effective disposal methods minimize infection risks and uphold public health standards.

3.2.2.12   Exposure Control Plan:

An Exposure Control Plan (ECP) is a critical component in healthcare settings designed to protect medical staff from occupational exposure to bloodborne pathogens and other infectious materials. It outlines specific procedures and responsibilities to minimize risk, including the identification of job roles with potential exposure, the implementation of safety devices, and mandatory training programs. The ECP mandates the use of personal protective equipment (PPE), proper disposal methods for sharps and biohazardous waste, and post-exposure evaluation protocols. Regular updates and reviews ensure compliance with OSHA standards. Medical Assistants must familiarize themselves with their facility's ECP to ensure personal safety and contribute to a safe working environment.

3.2.2.13   Calibration Of Equipment:

Calibration of equipment is the process of adjusting and verifying the accuracy of medical instruments to ensure they provide precise measurements. This is crucial in a clinical setting to maintain the reliability and validity of diagnostic results. Calibration involves comparing the instrument's measurements with a known standard and making necessary adjustments to align with these benchmarks. Regular calibration ensures that equipment functions correctly, preventing diagnostic errors and enhancing patient safety. Medical assistants must understand calibration procedures, recognize signs indicating the need for recalibration, and document calibration activities accurately. Adhering to manufacturer guidelines and institutional policies is essential for maintaining equipment integrity and compliance with regulatory standards.

3.2.2.14   Essential Logs for Maintenance and Quality Control:
Logs are systematic records essential for maintaining clinical standards and ensuring operational efficiency within a healthcare setting. Maintenance logs track routine checks and repairs of medical equipment, preventing malfunctions and ensuring patient safety. Equipment servicing logs document the servicing history, facilitating timely interventions and compliance with manufacturer guidelines. Temperature logs for refrigerators ensure that vaccines and medications are stored at the correct temperatures, safeguarding their efficacy. Quality control logs monitor and document the performance of laboratory tests, ensuring the accuracy and reliability of results. These logs serve as legal documents, supporting audits and inspections while fostering a culture of accountability and continuous improvement in clinical practice.

3.3 Testing And Laboratory Procedures:
Testing and laboratory procedures encompass a range of diagnostic activities performed by clinical medical assistants to support patient care. These procedures include collecting, handling, and processing specimens such as blood, urine, and other bodily fluids for analysis. Medical assistants must adhere to strict protocols to ensure the accuracy and reliability of test results. This involves understanding the correct techniques for specimen collection, labeling, storage, and transportation. They also operate and maintain laboratory equipment, perform basic tests under supervision, and ensure compliance with safety standards and regulations. Proficiency in these procedures is crucial for accurate diagnosis, effective treatment planning, and monitoring patient health outcomes, thus playing a vital role in healthcare delivery.

3.3.1 Tasks:
3.3.1.1   Non-Blood Specimen Collection:
Collecting non-blood specimens is a critical task for medical assistants, requiring precision and adherence to protocols to ensure accurate diagnostic results. Urine collection involves instructing patients on proper midstream clean-catch techniques or using catheters when necessary. Stool samples are collected in sterile containers, emphasizing hygiene to prevent contamination. Cultures require swabbing specific body sites, such as the throat or wound areas, to identify pathogens. Sputum collection involves obtaining deep cough samples in sterile containers for respiratory analysis. Each procedure demands clear patient communication, proper labeling, and timely transportation to the laboratory to maintain specimen integrity and the reliability of test outcomes.

3.3.1.2   Perform CLIA-waived Testing (labs):
CLIA-waived testing refers to laboratory tests that are simple, carry a low risk of an incorrect result, and are exempt from stringent federal regulatory oversight under the Clinical Laboratory Improvement Amendments (CLIA). Medical assistants performing these tests must ensure proper patient identification, specimen collection, and adherence to the manufacturer's instructions. These tests include glucose monitoring, urine pregnancy tests, and rapid strep tests. Accurate documentation of results and quality control measures is crucial. Medical assistants should understand the limitations of each test and communicate results effectively to the healthcare provider for further evaluation. Mastery of these procedures is essential for ensuring patient safety and maintaining compliance with healthcare standards.

3.3.1.3   Vision and Hearing Test Procedures:
Performing vision and hearing tests involves assessing a patient's ability to see and hear accurately, which are crucial components of routine physical examinations. For vision tests, medical assistants may conduct visual acuity tests using a Snellen chart to evaluate the sharpness of vision and identify any impairments such as myopia or hyperopia. For hearing tests, they might use audiometers to measure hearing sensitivity across different frequencies, identifying potential hearing loss. Medical assistants must ensure that the equipment is calibrated correctly and follow standardized procedures to obtain accurate results. Documenting findings meticulously and reporting any abnormalities to the supervising healthcare provider are essential responsibilities in these assessments.

3.3.1.4   Perform Allergy Testing:
Allergy testing involves identifying specific allergens that trigger allergic reactions in patients. Medical assistants play a crucial role in this process by preparing the patient and assisting with the procedure. Common methods include skin prick tests, where small amounts of potential allergens are introduced to the skin's surface, and intradermal tests, which involve injecting allergens into the dermis layer. Observing and documenting any reactions, such as redness or swelling, is essential for accurate diagnosis. Medical assistants must ensure that all equipment is sterile, follow safety protocols, and educate patients on post-test care. Understanding these procedures aids in effective allergy management and treatment planning.

3.3.1.5   Spirometry/Pulmonary Function Testing:
Spirometry is a critical diagnostic test used to assess lung function by measuring the volume and speed of air that a patient can inhale and exhale. Medical Assistants performing this test must ensure that the patient is seated comfortably, provide clear instructions, and demonstrate the proper technique for breathing into the spirometer. Electronic spirometers provide digital readings, while manual spirometers require the manual recording of results. Accurate calibration of the equipment is essential to ensure reliable data. The results help diagnose conditions such as asthma, chronic obstructive pulmonary disease (COPD), and other respiratory disorders. Proper infection control measures, such as using disposable mouthpieces, are crucial during the procedure.

3.3.1.6   Laboratory Value Recognition and Reporting:
Recognizing, documenting, and reporting laboratory and test values are critical tasks for medical assistants. This involves understanding standard reference ranges for various tests to identify normal and abnormal results. Abnormal values must be promptly documented in the patient's medical record with accuracy and clarity. It is essential to report these findings to the supervising healthcare provider immediately to ensure timely intervention. Medical assistants must maintain confidentiality while handling sensitive information. Proficiency in using electronic health record (EHR) systems is necessary for efficient documentation. This process ensures continuity of care, aids in diagnosis, and contributes to effective patient management.

3.3.1.7   Specimen-Patient Match and Requisition Labeling:
Accurate specimen labeling is critical to patient safety and diagnostic accuracy. Medical Assistants must ensure that each specimen is matched to the correct patient and requisition form. This involves verifying patient identifiers, such as name and date of birth, on both the specimen container and the requisition form. The label should include the patient's full name, identification number, date and time of collection, and the type of specimen. Cross-checking this information prevents errors in diagnosis and treatment. Proper labeling ensures that laboratory results are correctly attributed to the right patient, maintaining the integrity of the testing process and ensuring high standards of care.

3.3.1.8   Specimen Processing and Transport:
Medical assistants must efficiently manage specimens to ensure accurate diagnostic results. Processing involves labeling specimens with patient information, including the date and time of collection, to prevent identification errors. Handling requires adherence to safety protocols, such as wearing gloves and using biohazard containers to minimize contamination and exposure risks. Specimens must be stored at appropriate temperatures to preserve their integrity until analysis. Transporting specimens involves using secure packaging and documentation according to regulatory standards, ensuring timely delivery to laboratories. Following these procedures prevents sample degradation and maintains the chain of custody, which is crucial for reliable test outcomes. Mastery of these practices is essential for medical assistants to support clinical accuracy and patient safety.

3.3.2 Knowledge Of:
3.3.2.1   Point Of Care Testing:
Point of Care Testing (POCT) refers to medical diagnostic testing performed at or near the site of patient care, rather than in a centralized laboratory. This approach allows for rapid results, facilitating immediate clinical decisions and improving patient outcomes. POCT encompasses various tests, including blood glucose monitoring, urinalysis, and rapid strep tests. These tests utilize portable devices or kits that are user-friendly and require minimal training. For medical assistants, proficiency in POCT involves understanding test procedures, quality control measures, and accurate documentation of results. Ensuring compliance with regulatory standards and maintaining equipment are crucial responsibilities to guarantee reliability and accuracy in patient care.

3.3.2.2   Provider Request Form Information Requirements:
A provider request or requisition form is essential for accurately processing laboratory tests, diagnostic procedures, or referrals. Key information includes the patient's full name, date of birth, and identification number to ensure precise patient identification. The form must specify the requested tests or procedures, including any special instructions. The provider's name, contact details, and signature are crucial for authorization and follow-up communication. Additionally, insurance information is required for billing purposes. Accurate documentation of the date and time of the request ensures timely processing. This comprehensive data ensures efficient coordination between healthcare providers and laboratories, minimizing errors and enhancing patient care.

3.3.2.3   Specimen Collection Techniques Overview:
Specimen collection involves obtaining samples such as blood, urine, or tissue for diagnostic testing. Proper techniques ensure accuracy and prevent contamination. For blood draws, use aseptic methods, select appropriate veins, and adhere to the order of draw to avoid cross-contamination. Urine collection may require midstream or 24-hour samples, necessitating patient instruction for accuracy. Tissue samples must be handled with sterile instruments and preserved in suitable media. Label specimens accurately with patient details and test information. Follow institutional protocols and OSHA guidelines to maintain safety and quality. Understanding these techniques is crucial for clinical medical assistants to support accurate diagnosis and patient care.

3.3.2.4   CLIA-waived Testing Regulations:
CLIA-waived testing regulations, established under the Clinical Laboratory Improvement Amendments (CLIA) of 1988, govern simple laboratory tests that carry a minimal risk of erroneous results. These tests are exempt from stringent regulatory oversight due to their low complexity. Medical assistants must ensure compliance by performing tests according to manufacturer instructions and maintaining proper documentation. CLIA-waived tests include glucose monitoring and pregnancy tests, which require periodic quality control checks. Understanding these regulations is crucial for medical assistants to ensure accurate patient results and maintain the integrity of laboratory operations. Compliance with these guidelines ensures patient safety and supports the delivery of high-quality healthcare services.

3.3.2.5   COLA Accreditation Standards:
COLA Accreditation Standards are guidelines established by the Commission on Office Laboratory Accreditation to ensure quality and reliability in laboratory testing. These standards focus on essential aspects such as personnel qualifications, proficiency testing, quality control, and documentation. For medical assistants, understanding these standards is crucial, as they play a key role in maintaining compliance by accurately performing tests and recording results. COLA emphasizes continuous improvement through regular inspections and education, ensuring that laboratories operate safely and effectively. Adherence to these standards not only enhances patient care but also minimizes errors, thereby upholding the integrity of laboratory services within clinical settings.

3.3.2.6   Controls/calibration/quality Control:
Controls, calibration, and quality control are critical components in clinical laboratory settings that ensure accurate and reliable test results. Controls are known samples used to verify the accuracy of test results by comparing them against expected outcomes. Calibration involves adjusting measurement instruments to align with standard values, ensuring precision in readings. Quality control encompasses procedures that monitor and maintain the integrity of laboratory processes, identifying errors and preventing inaccuracies. Medical assistants must understand these concepts to assist in maintaining compliance with regulatory standards and ensuring patient safety through dependable diagnostic testing. Mastery of these practices is essential for effective clinical support and operational excellence.

3.3.2.7   Lab Values: Normal vs. Abnormal
Lab values are numerical results from medical tests that help assess a patient's health status. Normal lab values are reference ranges established by analyzing the results of healthy individuals, indicating typical functioning. Abnormal lab values fall outside these ranges and may signal underlying health issues or the need for further investigation. Understanding these values is crucial for clinical decision-making, as they guide diagnosis, treatment plans, and the monitoring of disease progression or response to therapy. Medical assistants must familiarize themselves with common lab tests such as CBC, BMP, and lipid panels, recognizing deviations that require physician attention to ensure optimal patient care and safety.

3.3.2.8   Vision and Hearing Test Elements:
Vision and hearing tests are crucial for assessing sensory function. Color vision tests determine the ability to distinguish colors, often using Ishihara plates. Acuity tests measure the clarity of vision at various distances, typically employing a Snellen chart for distance acuity. Visual field tests evaluate peripheral vision to detect potential blind spots or field loss, using methods such as confrontation testing or automated perimetry. Hearing tests, such as audiometry, assess auditory function across different frequencies and intensities. These evaluations help identify sensory impairments, guiding further diagnostic or therapeutic interventions to enhance patient care and quality of life.

3.3.2.9 Tone, Speech, and Tympanometry:

Tone, speech, and word recognition are essential components of audiological assessments that evaluate a patient's auditory processing capabilities. Tone recognition tests assess the ability to perceive pure tones at various frequencies, indicating hearing sensitivity. Speech recognition involves understanding spoken language, which is crucial for effective communication. Word recognition tests measure how well individuals can identify and repeat words presented at different volumes. Tympanometry is a diagnostic test that evaluates middle ear function by measuring eardrum mobility in response to changes in air pressure. It helps identify issues such as fluid accumulation or eustachian tube dysfunction. These assessments collectively aid in diagnosing hearing impairments and guiding appropriate interventions for improved auditory health.

3.3.2.10 Peak Flow Rates:

Peak flow rates measure the maximum speed of expiration, reflecting lung function and airway constriction. This is a critical parameter in managing respiratory conditions like asthma. Using a peak flow meter, patients can monitor their lung function by blowing into the device as forcefully as possible after a full inhalation. The measurement helps identify asthma exacerbations early and adjust medication accordingly. Peak flow rates vary based on age, sex, and height; thus, personalized charts are used for comparison. Regular monitoring aids in recognizing patterns or triggers of respiratory distress, ensuring timely intervention. Medical assistants must understand these principles to educate patients effectively on self-monitoring techniques.

3.3.2.11 Common Allergens:

Common allergens are substances that can trigger allergic reactions in sensitive individuals. These include pollen, dust mites, mold spores, pet dander, insect stings, and certain foods such as peanuts, tree nuts, milk, eggs, soy, wheat, fish, and shellfish. Allergic reactions occur when the immune system mistakenly identifies these harmless substances as threats and releases chemicals like histamine. Symptoms can range from mild, such as sneezing and itching, to severe, including anaphylaxis. Understanding common allergens is crucial for medical assistants to effectively assist in patient education and the management of allergic conditions. Identifying allergens helps in creating avoidance strategies and preparing for potential emergency interventions.

3.3.2.12 Scratch vs. Intradermal Allergy Testing:

The scratch test involves placing a drop of allergen onto the skin, which is then lightly pricked or scratched to introduce the substance. This test is used to identify immediate allergic reactions to substances such as pollen, pet dander, or food. A positive reaction typically appears as a raised, red bump. The intradermal allergy test involves injecting a small amount of allergen into the dermis layer of the skin. It is more sensitive than the scratch test and is used when stronger reactions are needed for diagnosis. Both tests require observation for 15 to 20 minutes for reactions and are crucial for effectively diagnosing allergies.

3.3.2.13 Specimen Transportation and Handling Requirements:

Specimen management is critical for accurate diagnosis. Proper labeling with patient identifiers (name, date of birth, medical record number) ensures traceability. Transportation must maintain specimen integrity; temperature-controlled containers should be used if necessary. Diagnostic procedures require adherence to test-specific protocols to prevent contamination or degradation. Storage conditions, such as refrigeration or freezing, are dictated by specimen type and test requirements to preserve viability. Disposal must follow biohazard regulations to prevent exposure risks. Documentation of the site or test specifics is essential for clarity and continuity of care. Compliance with these requirements ensures reliable results and patient safety, fulfilling legal and ethical obligations.

3.3.2.14 Requisition Content: Date, Time, and ICD-10

A requisition form is a formal document used in medical settings to request specific tests or procedures for a patient. It must include the date and time to ensure accurate tracking and scheduling of services. The date and time provide a chronological reference that aids in the timely processing of requests. Additionally, the ICD-10 code, which stands for the International Classification of Diseases, 10th Revision, is crucial as it specifies the diagnosis or reason for the test. Accurate ICD-10 coding ensures appropriate billing and compliance with insurance requirements, facilitating smooth communication between healthcare providers and insurance companies.

3.4 Phlebotomy:

Phlebotomy is the practice of drawing blood from patients for diagnostic, therapeutic, or donation purposes. It is a critical skill for Certified Clinical Medical Assistants (CCMAs) as it involves not only technical proficiency but also patient interaction and care. Phlebotomists must understand venipuncture techniques, properly handle blood samples, and adhere to safety protocols to prevent contamination and ensure accurate results. Additionally, they must maintain patient comfort and confidentiality throughout the procedure. Mastery of phlebotomy requires knowledge of anatomy, particularly the circulatory system, and familiarity with different types of collection equipment such as needles, tourniquets, and vacutainers. Effective communication skills are essential for explaining procedures and alleviating patient anxiety.

3.4.1 Phlebotomy Tasks:

Phlebotomy tasks involve the collection of blood samples for laboratory analysis, which is crucial for diagnosing and monitoring patient health. Certified Clinical Medical Assistants (CCMAs) must proficiently perform venipuncture and capillary punctures while adhering to strict protocols to ensure patient safety and sample integrity. This includes verifying patient identity, selecting appropriate collection tubes, and labeling specimens accurately. CCMAs must also manage equipment, such as needles and tourniquets, ensuring that they are sterile and disposed of correctly to prevent contamination or infection. Additionally, maintaining patient comfort and addressing any concerns during the procedure is vital, along with documenting all procedures accurately in medical records for continuity of care.

3.4.1.1 Verify Order Details:

Verifying order details is a critical task in phlebotomy, ensuring patient safety and accurate test results. Medical assistants must meticulously check the requisition form for completeness, confirming that the patient's full name, date of birth, and identification number match those on the specimen labels. They should verify that the specific tests ordered align with the patient's clinical needs and the physician's instructions. It is also important to cross-check the date and time of collection to adhere to any time-sensitive testing requirements. Additionally, confirm that any special handling or fasting requirements are noted and communicated. This verification process minimizes errors, prevents misidentification, and ensures that specimens are processed correctly, ultimately contributing to reliable patient care outcomes.

3.4.1.2   Choosing Supplies for Ordered Tests:

Selecting appropriate supplies for ordered tests is a critical task in phlebotomy, ensuring accurate and efficient specimen collection. Medical assistants must understand the specific requirements of each test, such as the type of collection tube (e.g., EDTA, heparin, or serum separator tubes), needle gauge, and additional materials like tourniquets or alcohol swabs. Proper selection prevents sample contamination and ensures test integrity. Familiarity with color-coded tube systems is essential, as each color indicates different additives or preservatives necessary for specific tests. Additionally, verifying patient information and test requisitions before gathering supplies minimizes errors, enhances patient safety, and maintains laboratory standards.

3.4.1.3   Venipuncture Site Accessibility by Age and Condition:

Determining venipuncture site accessibility involves assessing the most suitable vein for a blood draw, considering the patient's age and health condition. In adults, the median cubital vein in the antecubital fossa is typically preferred due to its size and accessibility. For infants, scalp or heel punctures are common, given their smaller veins. Elderly patients may present challenges due to fragile veins, necessitating careful selection to avoid complications. Additionally, patients with conditions such as obesity or dehydration may require alternative sites or techniques. Medical assistants must evaluate these factors to ensure a successful venipuncture while minimizing discomfort and the risk of injury to the patient.

3.4.1.4   Prepare Site For Venipuncture:

Preparing the site for venipuncture is a critical step in phlebotomy to ensure patient safety and sample integrity. Begin by confirming the patient's identity and explaining the procedure to alleviate anxiety. Select an appropriate vein, usually in the antecubital fossa, using visual and tactile assessment. Clean the site with a 70% isopropyl alcohol swab in a circular motion from the center outward, allowing it to air dry completely to prevent contamination and ensure the antiseptic's effectiveness. Avoid touching the site after cleansing. Proper preparation minimizes the risk of infection and ensures accurate test results, reflecting adherence to best practices essential for clinical proficiency in venipuncture.

3.4.1.5   Perform Venipuncture:

Venipuncture is the process of obtaining intravenous access for blood sampling or intravenous therapy. Medical Assistants must skillfully identify suitable veins, typically in the antecubital fossa, and use aseptic techniques to prevent infection. The procedure involves applying a tourniquet to engorge the veins, cleansing the site with an antiseptic, and inserting a sterile needle at an appropriate angle into the vein. Proper tube selection and the order of draw are essential to avoid cross-contamination. After the procedure, apply pressure to prevent hematoma formation. Mastery of venipuncture minimizes patient discomfort and ensures accurate specimen collection, which is crucial for diagnostic purposes. Proficiency requires practice, adherence to protocols, and effective patient communication skills.

3.4.1.6   Perform Capillary Puncture:

Capillary puncture, also known as a fingerstick, is a minimally invasive procedure used to obtain small blood samples. This technique involves puncturing the skin, typically on the fingertip or heel, using a lancet to access capillary blood vessels. Medical assistants must ensure proper site selection and preparation, including cleansing with an antiseptic wipe to prevent contamination. The procedure requires gentle pressure to encourage blood flow without excessive squeezing, which can cause hemolysis. Collected samples are used for point-of-care testing, such as glucose monitoring or hematocrit levels. Mastery of this skill ensures accurate results and patient comfort, which are crucial for effective clinical practice and patient care.

3.4.1.7   Perform Post-procedural Care:

Post-procedural care in phlebotomy involves essential steps to ensure patient safety and comfort after blood collection. It includes applying pressure to the venipuncture site to prevent bleeding and hematoma formation. Once hemostasis is achieved, a bandage or adhesive strip is applied. The medical assistant must instruct the patient to keep the bandage on for at least 15 minutes and to avoid heavy lifting with the affected arm for several hours. Monitoring the patient for adverse reactions, such as dizziness or fainting, is crucial. Proper documentation of the procedure, including any complications, is necessary for accurate medical records and continuity of care.

3.4.1.8   Blood Sample Handling for Diagnostics:

Handling blood samples for diagnostic purposes involves several critical steps to ensure the accuracy and reliability of test results. Medical assistants must adhere to proper protocols for collection, labeling, and transportation. This includes using the correct type of collection tube for specific tests, ensuring that patient identification is accurate, and maintaining aseptic techniques to prevent contamination. Once collected, samples must be stored at appropriate temperatures and transported swiftly to the laboratory to preserve their integrity. Additionally, understanding the importance of following guidelines for sample handling helps prevent hemolysis or clotting, which can compromise test outcomes. Proper documentation throughout the process is crucial for traceability and quality assurance.

3.4.1.9   Laboratory Blood Specimen Processing:

Processing blood specimens for laboratory analysis involves several critical steps to ensure the accuracy and reliability of test results. After collection, blood specimens must be properly labeled with patient information, as well as the date and time of collection. They are then transported to the laboratory while maintaining appropriate temperature conditions to preserve sample integrity. In the lab, specimens are logged into a tracking system and may undergo centrifugation to separate components if required. Proper handling techniques, including avoiding hemolysis and contamination, are crucial. Finally, specimens are stored or prepared for specific tests according to laboratory protocols. This process ensures that test results are precise and reflective of the patient's health status.

3.4.1.10   Specimen-Patient Match and Requisition Labeling:

Ensuring accurate matching and labeling of specimens to the patient and the completed requisition is crucial in phlebotomy. This process involves verifying the patient's identity using two identifiers, such as name and date of birth, before collecting the specimen. Once collected, the specimen must be labeled immediately at the bedside or in the collection area with details that match the requisition form, including the patient's name, identification number, date, time of collection, and collector's initials. This practice prevents misidentification errors, ensuring that diagnostic tests are performed on the correct patient. Proper documentation on the requisition form must align with the label to maintain consistency and accuracy throughout the testing process.

3.4.1.11 Managing Abnormal Test Results:
Recognizing and responding to abnormal test results is a critical task for Certified Clinical Medical Assistants. It involves identifying deviations from normal laboratory values that may indicate underlying health issues. Medical assistants must be proficient in interpreting lab results, understanding reference ranges, and discerning significant variances. Upon detecting abnormal results, they must promptly notify the healthcare provider to ensure timely intervention. This process requires attention to detail, effective communication skills, and adherence to protocols for documentation and follow-up actions. Proper responses to abnormal results are essential for patient safety and optimal care outcomes, as they facilitate early diagnosis and treatment of potential health problems.

3.4.1.12 Sample Preparation for External Lab Transport:
Medical assistants must ensure that samples are correctly prepared for transportation to an outside laboratory, following strict protocols to maintain sample integrity. This involves accurately labeling specimens with patient information and test details to prevent misidentification. Samples must be placed in appropriate containers with secure lids to prevent leaks. Use biohazard bags for safety and include requisition forms with the necessary information. Ensure that samples are stored at the required temperature, using ice packs or insulated containers if needed. Follow specific guidelines for time-sensitive specimens to ensure timely delivery. Adhering to these procedures ensures accurate test results and compliance with regulatory standards, thereby safeguarding the quality of patient care.

3.4.1.13 Guidelines for Distributing Lab Results:
This task involves ensuring that laboratory results are accurately and securely delivered to the correct ordering provider. Begin by verifying the patient's identity using two identifiers, such as their name and date of birth, to match them with the correct provider. Adhere to HIPAA guidelines to maintain patient confidentiality during this process. Use secure communication methods, such as encrypted emails or electronic health record systems, to distribute results. Confirm receipt by the provider and document the transaction in the patient's medical record. This ensures that results are reviewed promptly, facilitating timely clinical decisions and maintaining continuity of care while upholding legal and ethical standards.

3.4.2 Knowledge Of:
3.4.2.1 Patient Identifiers in Healthcare:
Patient identifiers are crucial elements used to accurately match a patient to their intended healthcare service, thereby minimizing the risk of errors. These identifiers include personal information such as the patient's full name, date of birth, and medical record number. When specific tests or procedures are involved, additional identifiers, such as the test type or procedure site, must be confirmed to ensure accuracy. For instance, verifying the correct limb for surgery or the proper anatomical site for imaging is essential. This practice is vital for maintaining patient safety and ensuring that the right care is administered to the right patient, thereby upholding high standards of clinical practice.

3.4.2.2 And Content Of Requisition:
A requisition is a formal request for laboratory tests or medical procedures, essential for ensuring accurate patient diagnosis and treatment. It typically includes patient identification details, such as name and date of birth, along with the ordering physician's information. The requisition specifies the required tests or procedures, providing clear instructions to the laboratory or relevant department. Accurate completion of requisitions prevents errors and ensures timely processing. Medical Assistants play a crucial role in verifying the accuracy and completeness of requisitions before submission. Understanding requisition content is vital for maintaining an efficient workflow and effective communication between healthcare providers and laboratory personnel.

3.4.2.3 Patient Preparation for Phlebotomy: Fasting Guidelines
Patient preparation for phlebotomy is critical to ensuring accurate test results. Fasting requirements depend on the type of test ordered. For fasting tests, such as lipid panels or glucose levels, patients must abstain from eating or drinking anything other than water for 8 to 12 hours before the procedure. Non-fasting tests do not require dietary restrictions. Medical Assistants must verify the specific requirements with the laboratory and communicate them clearly to patients. Proper documentation of fasting status is essential. Additionally, assessing the patient's understanding and compliance with these instructions is crucial to avoid rescheduling and to ensure the validity of test results.

3.4.2.4 Patient Comfort and Anxiety Assessment:
Evaluating a patient's comfort and anxiety levels before, during, and after a medical procedure is essential for effective patient care. This assessment involves observing verbal and non-verbal cues, such as facial expressions, body language, and vocal tone. Medical Assistants should engage in active listening, ask open-ended questions about the patient's feelings, and provide reassurance to alleviate fears. Understanding the patient's emotional state aids in tailoring communication and procedural approaches to enhance comfort. This assessment helps identify the need for additional support, such as relaxation techniques or pain management strategies, ensuring a positive patient experience and promoting trust in the healthcare setting.

3.4.2.5 Blood Vacuum Tubes for Testing:
Blood vacuum tubes are essential for collecting and preserving blood samples for laboratory analysis. For chemistry testing, serum separator tubes (SST) with a gel barrier and clot activator are used to separate serum from cells. In hematology, lavender-top tubes containing EDTA prevent clotting and preserve cell morphology for complete blood counts (CBC). For microbiology testing, yellow-top tubes with sodium polyanethol sulfonate (SPS) are used to maintain microbial viability during culture and sensitivity tests. The additives and color coding of each tube ensure proper sample processing, accurate test results, and patient safety. Understanding these tubes is crucial for Certified Clinical Medical Assistants in performing efficient phlebotomy procedures.

3.4.2.6 Blood-borne Pathogens:
Blood-borne pathogens are infectious microorganisms present in blood and other bodily fluids that can cause diseases in humans. These include viruses such as Hepatitis B (HBV), Hepatitis C (HCV), and Human Immunodeficiency Virus (HIV). Medical assistants must understand the modes of transmission, which primarily occur through needlestick injuries, cuts from contaminated sharps, or contact with infected blood on mucous membranes. Adhering to standard precautions, such as using personal protective equipment (PPE) and the proper disposal of sharps, is crucial to preventing occupational exposure. Understanding these pathogens is essential for ensuring safety in healthcare settings and for complying with Occupational Safety and Health Administration (OSHA) regulations.

3.4.2.7   Impact of Medical History on Blood Draw Order:
Certain medical conditions, patient history, and medications can significantly impact the order of draw during venipuncture. Conditions such as coagulation disorders or recent surgeries may necessitate specific tube sequences to prevent contamination or clotting issues. Anticoagulant medications like warfarin or heparin require careful handling to avoid hemolysis or inaccurate results. Additionally, patients with a history of fainting or anxiety may need a modified approach to ensure safety and comfort. Understanding these factors is crucial for medical assistants to ensure accurate laboratory results and patient safety, adhering strictly to the established order of draw guidelines to prevent cross-contamination between tubes.

3.4.2.8   Anatomy:
Anatomy is the study of the structure of the human body, focusing on the spatial relationships between various bodily systems and organs. Understanding anatomy is crucial for medical assistants, as it aids in identifying normal versus abnormal physiological conditions. It encompasses macroscopic structures like organs and tissues, as well as microscopic components such as cells and molecules. Mastery of anatomy ensures accurate patient assessments, effective communication with healthcare providers, and precise execution of clinical tasks.

Skin Integrity:

Skin integrity refers to the health and intactness of the skin, which serves as a protective barrier against environmental threats. Maintaining skin integrity involves ensuring that the skin remains free from wounds, infections, or pressure sores. Medical assistants must assess the skin for signs of damage or disease, provide appropriate wound care, and educate patients on skincare practices to prevent complications. Monitoring skin integrity is vital for preventing infections and promoting overall patient health.

Venous Sufficiency:

Venous sufficiency pertains to the proper functioning of veins in returning blood from the extremities to the heart. It ensures adequate blood circulation and prevents conditions like varicose veins or venous ulcers. Medical assistants should recognize signs of venous insufficiency, such as swelling or discoloration, and understand interventions like compression therapy. Knowledge of venous sufficiency is essential for assisting with vascular assessments and educating patients on lifestyle modifications to enhance circulation.

Contraindications:

Contraindications are specific conditions or factors that render certain medical treatments or procedures inadvisable due to potential harm. Recognizing contraindications is critical for patient safety, as it prevents adverse reactions or complications. Medical assistants must be aware of common contraindications related to medications, procedures, or therapies, ensuring they gather comprehensive patient histories and communicate effectively with healthcare teams to avoid contraindicated interventions.

3.4.2.9   Phlebotomy Site Prep & Order of Draw:
Phlebotomy site preparation is crucial for accurate blood collection and involves cleansing the puncture area with an antiseptic, such as 70% isopropyl alcohol, to prevent contamination. Allow the site to air dry before proceeding. After venipuncture, apply gentle pressure and wrap the site with a sterile bandage to prevent bleeding. The order of draw for microtubes is essential to avoid cross-contamination: begin with blood cultures, followed by coagulation tubes (light blue), then serum tubes (red or gold), heparin tubes (green), EDTA tubes (lavender), and finally, glycolytic inhibitor tubes (gray). This sequence ensures specimen integrity and accurate test results.

3.4.2.10   Insertion And Removal Techniques:
Insertion and removal techniques refer to the standardized procedures utilized by medical assistants for safely inserting and removing medical devices such as catheters, IV lines, and nasogastric tubes. These techniques require a thorough understanding of anatomy, aseptic principles, and considerations for patient comfort. Proper insertion involves choosing the correct device size, maintaining sterility, and ensuring accurate placement to avoid complications. Removal requires careful monitoring of the patient's response, gentle extraction to prevent tissue damage, and appropriate disposal of used equipment. Mastery of these techniques is crucial for minimizing infection risks, ensuring patient safety, and enhancing procedural efficiency in clinical settings. Proficiency in these skills is essential for passing the CCMA exam.

3.4.2.11   Evacuated Tube, Syringe, and Butterfly Techniques:
The evacuated tube method uses a vacuum-sealed tube to draw blood directly from the vein, minimizing contamination and preserving sample integrity. The syringe method involves manually drawing blood into a syringe, offering control over suction pressure, which is beneficial for fragile veins. The butterfly method employs a winged infusion set with flexible tubing, making it ideal for small or difficult veins, such as those in pediatric or geriatric patients. Each technique requires proficiency in handling equipment and an understanding of vein anatomy to ensure patient comfort and accurate results. Mastery of these methods is essential for medical assistants to perform phlebotomy efficiently and safely in clinical settings.

3.4.2.12   Tube Types and Positions: Inversions and Fill Ratios
In phlebotomy, various tubes are used for blood collection, each with specific additives and colors indicating their purpose. Common types include EDTA (lavender top), sodium citrate (light blue top), and serum separator (gold or red top) tubes. Proper tube positioning ensures accurate sample collection and prevents hemolysis. Tube inversions mix the blood with additives; typically, 8 to 10 inversions are needed for anticoagulant tubes, while clot activator tubes require fewer. Fill levels must match the tube's vacuum capacity to maintain the correct blood-to-additive ratio, which is crucial for test accuracy. Understanding these factors is essential for reliable laboratory results and patient safety.

3.4.2.13   Additives And Preservatives:
Additives and preservatives are substances incorporated into blood collection tubes to maintain specimen integrity. Additives, such as anticoagulants (e.g., EDTA, heparin), prevent clotting, ensuring accurate hematological analysis. Preservatives, like sodium fluoride, inhibit glycolysis in glucose testing, thereby maintaining analyte stability. Each tube color indicates specific additives; for instance, lavender tops contain EDTA for complete blood counts (CBCs), while green tops contain heparin for plasma chemistry tests. Understanding the function and appropriate use of these substances is crucial for medical assistants to ensure accurate test results and patient safety. Proper handling and knowledge of these components are essential for effective clinical practice and laboratory procedures.

3.4.2.14   Bandaging Techniques: Allergies & Skin Types
Bandaging procedures involve applying a protective covering to a wound or injury, ensuring proper pressure and support. Medical assistants must assess the patient's skin type and potential allergies to bandage materials, such as latex or adhesives. Sensitive skin may require hypoallergenic options to prevent irritation. Understanding different skin types aids in selecting appropriate bandages that provide adequate protection without causing adverse reactions. Awareness of allergies is crucial to avoid complications, such as contact dermatitis. Proper bandaging technique involves cleaning the area, choosing the right type of bandage, and securing it effectively while monitoring for signs of discomfort or allergic reactions, thereby ensuring optimal healing conditions.

3.4.2.15   Specimen Quality and Consistency Considerations:
Pre-analytical considerations are critical to ensuring specimen quality and consistency, which directly impact diagnostic accuracy. Key factors include proper patient identification, correct labeling, and appropriate collection techniques. Medical Assistants must ensure the use of suitable containers and preservatives while adhering to specific handling and storage conditions to prevent degradation or contamination. Time-sensitive specimens require prompt processing to maintain their integrity. Additionally, understanding patient preparation protocols, such as fasting or medication restrictions, is essential to avoid skewed results. Attention to these details minimizes pre-analytical errors, enhances the reliability of laboratory outcomes, and supports accurate clinical decision-making.

3.4.2.16   Special Collections:
Special collections in phlebotomy refer to the precise collection of specimens that require specific timing or conditions to ensure accurate results. Timed specimens are collected at set intervals to monitor fluctuations, such as in glucose tolerance tests. Drug level assessments evaluate therapeutic medication concentrations, requiring samples to be taken at specific times post-dose. Blood cultures are used to detect bloodstream infections and must be collected using strict aseptic techniques to prevent contamination. Fasting specimens necessitate patient abstinence from food and drink (except water) for a defined period before collection, ensuring baseline metabolic levels. Each type of special collection demands adherence to protocols to maintain sample integrity and provide reliable diagnostic information.

3.4.2.17   Centrifuge And Aliquot:
A centrifuge is a laboratory device used to separate components of a fluid by spinning it at high speed, causing denser substances to move outward. In clinical settings, it is primarily used to separate blood components, such as plasma or serum, from cells. Aliquoting involves dividing a sample into smaller portions after centrifugation. This process ensures that tests can be conducted on precise volumes without contaminating the original sample. Medical assistants must understand the proper operation and maintenance of the centrifuge, as well as accurate aliquoting techniques, to ensure reliable test results and maintain sample integrity. Mastery of these skills is crucial for efficient laboratory workflow and patient care.

3.4.2.18   Test Values: Normal vs. Abnormal
Normal test values are standardized ranges established through population studies that indicate typical physiological functioning. These values serve as a baseline for comparison to detect abnormalities. Abnormal test values fall outside these established ranges and may suggest underlying health issues or the need for further investigation. Control values are used in laboratory settings to ensure the accuracy and reliability of test results. They represent known measurements that validate the testing process, allowing for adjustments and calibration of equipment. Understanding these values is crucial for medical assistants to accurately interpret laboratory results, assist in diagnosis, and provide effective patient care within clinical settings.

3.4.2.19   Equipment Calibration:
Equipment calibration is the process of verifying and adjusting the accuracy of medical instruments to ensure precise and reliable measurements. For medical assistants, understanding equipment calibration is crucial, as it impacts patient diagnosis and treatment. Calibration involves comparing the instrument's output with a known standard and making necessary adjustments to align with established benchmarks. Regular calibration minimizes errors, maintains compliance with healthcare regulations, and enhances patient safety. Medical assistants must be familiar with the specific procedures for calibrating various devices, such as blood pressure monitors, thermometers, and glucometers. Proper documentation of calibration activities is essential to maintain equipment integrity and support quality assurance in clinical settings.

3.4.2.20   Light and Temperature Sensitivity in Storage:
Certain medications and medical supplies require specific storage conditions to maintain their efficacy and safety. Sensitivity to light can cause degradation in some medications, leading to reduced potency or altered chemical composition. These items should be stored in opaque containers or dark environments. Temperature sensitivity is also critical; some medications need refrigeration, while others must be kept at room temperature. Exposure to inappropriate temperatures can result in the loss of therapeutic effectiveness or even toxicity. Medical assistants must understand these requirements to ensure proper storage, handling, and patient safety. Always refer to manufacturer guidelines for specific storage instructions to prevent compromising product integrity.

3.4.2.21   Transportation, Diagnosis, Storage, Disposal Requirements:
The transportation of medical specimens requires leak-proof containers and proper labeling to prevent contamination and ensure accurate diagnosis. During the diagnostic process, medical assistants must adhere to protocols for handling specimens to maintain their integrity and avoid diagnostic errors. Storage involves maintaining specimens at specified temperatures and conditions to preserve their viability until analysis. The disposal of medical waste mandates compliance with OSHA and EPA regulations to prevent environmental contamination and ensure public safety. This includes using designated biohazard containers for sharps and infectious materials. Understanding these requirements ensures the safety of patients and healthcare personnel while maintaining the accuracy and reliability of diagnostic results.

3.4.2.22   Processing And Labeling Requirements:
Processing and labeling requirements are critical protocols in clinical settings to ensure the accuracy and integrity of patient specimens. Medical assistants must adhere to standardized procedures for handling, labeling, and processing samples to prevent errors. Proper labeling includes patient identification details such as name, date of birth, and sample type, ensuring traceability and reducing the risk of misdiagnosis. Processing involves the timely handling of specimens, maintaining appropriate conditions (e.g., temperature), and ensuring that samples reach the laboratory without contamination. Adherence to these protocols is essential for compliance with legal standards and ensures that diagnostic results are reliable, thereby supporting effective patient care and treatment decisions.

3.4.2.23   Utilizing External Databases:
External databases refer to digital repositories and systems outside of a healthcare facility that store and provide access to critical medical information. These include databases from external laboratories, which offer test results and diagnostic data, as well as reference sources such as medical journals and drug databases. Medical assistants utilize these resources to verify patient test results, cross-reference clinical information, and support healthcare providers in decision-making. Understanding how to navigate these databases efficiently ensures accurate data retrieval, enhances the quality of patient care, and maintains compliance with medical standards. Proficiency in using external databases is vital for ensuring timely access to comprehensive and up-to-date medical information.

3.5 EKG And Cardiovascular Testing:
Electrocardiograms (EKGs) and cardiovascular testing are essential diagnostic tools used to assess heart health. An EKG records the electrical activity of the heart, identifying abnormalities such as arrhythmias, myocardial infarctions, and other cardiac conditions. Medical assistants must understand lead placement, patient preparation, and equipment operation to ensure accurate results. Cardiovascular testing may also include stress tests, echocardiograms, and Holter monitoring, each providing critical insights into cardiac function under various conditions. Proficiency in these tests enables medical assistants to assist physicians in diagnosing and managing cardiovascular diseases effectively. Mastery of EKG interpretation and cardiovascular testing protocols is crucial for the CCMA exam.

3.5.1 Tasks:
3.5.1.1   Prepare Patients For Procedure:
Preparing patients for EKG and cardiovascular testing involves several critical steps to ensure accurate results and patient comfort. Begin by verifying the patient's identity and explaining the procedure to alleviate anxiety. Confirm that the patient has followed any pre-test instructions, such as fasting or medication adjustments. Position the patient comfortably, ensuring they are relaxed and free from restrictive clothing. Clean the skin where electrodes will be placed to ensure proper adhesion and signal transmission. Attach the electrodes correctly, following anatomical landmarks, and check the equipment's functionality. Communicate with the patient throughout the process, addressing concerns and confirming their understanding, which enhances cooperation and test efficacy.

3.5.1.2   Cardiac Monitoring: EKG/ECG Tests
Electrocardiography (EKG or ECG) is a critical diagnostic tool used to assess the electrical activity of the heart. Medical Assistants are responsible for preparing patients, explaining procedures, and ensuring the accuracy of electrode placement to capture precise cardiac data. The test involves attaching electrodes to the patient's skin to record the electrical impulses that trigger heartbeats. These impulses are displayed as waveforms on an EKG machine, allowing healthcare providers to evaluate heart rhythm, detect abnormalities, and diagnose conditions such as arrhythmias or myocardial infarctions. Mastery of EKG procedures ensures accurate data collection and enhances patient care by enabling timely diagnosis and intervention in cardiovascular health issues.

3.5.1.3   EKG Equipment Functionality Assurance:
Ensuring the proper functioning of EKG equipment is critical for accurate cardiovascular testing. Medical assistants must routinely inspect the equipment for any signs of wear or damage, such as frayed cables or loose connections. Calibration checks should be performed regularly to maintain accuracy, in alignment with manufacturer guidelines. Before each use, verify that the electrodes and leads are clean and intact, ensuring optimal skin contact to prevent signal interference. Additionally, confirm that the machine's settings match the required test parameters. It is essential to keep the software updated and maintain a log for routine maintenance and troubleshooting. This vigilance ensures reliable results and patient safety during cardiovascular assessments.

3.5.1.4   Identifying Abnormal EKG Results:
Medical assistants must accurately identify abnormal or emergent EKG results to ensure timely intervention. Dysrhythmias and arrhythmias refer to irregular heart rhythms that can range from benign to life-threatening conditions, such as atrial fibrillation or ventricular tachycardia. Recognizing these conditions involves analyzing P waves, QRS complexes, and T waves for abnormalities in rate, rhythm, and morphology. Artifacts, on the other hand, are extraneous signals caused by patient movement or electrical interference that can mimic arrhythmias but do not originate from cardiac activity. Differentiating between true dysrhythmias and artifacts is crucial for accurate diagnosis and management, requiring a keen eye and a thorough understanding of EKG patterns.

3.5.1.5   Non-invasive Cardiovascular Profiling Assistance:
Non-invasive cardiovascular profiling involves procedures that assess heart function without penetrating the body. Medical assistants play a crucial role in facilitating these tests. During a stress test, they prepare the patient by attaching electrodes and monitoring vital signs while the patient exercises. For Holter monitoring, assistants attach a portable device to record heart activity over 24 to 48 hours, instructing patients on proper usage and activity logging. Event monitoring involves a similar setup but is used for intermittent recording over extended periods. Medical assistants ensure equipment functionality, patient comfort, and accurate data collection, supporting providers in diagnosing arrhythmias, ischemia, or other cardiac conditions.

3.5.1.6   Results Transmission to EMR or Paper Chart:
Medical assistants play a crucial role in ensuring the accurate transmission of EKG and cardiovascular test results. This involves entering data into the patient's Electronic Medical Record (EMR) or updating a paper chart. The process requires meticulous attention to detail to maintain data integrity and confidentiality. Once documented, the medical assistant must promptly communicate these results to the healthcare provider for further evaluation and decision-making. This task ensures continuity of care by facilitating timely access to critical information, enabling providers to make informed clinical decisions. Proper documentation and communication are essential for patient safety, legal compliance, and effective healthcare delivery.

3.5.2 Knowledge Of:
3.5.2.1   Minimizing Artifacts: Procedures & Instructions
Artifacts are unwanted alterations in data or images that can obscure accurate results. In clinical settings, minimizing artifacts is crucial for obtaining precise diagnostic information. To reduce artifacts, ensure proper skin preparation by cleaning and drying the area before electrode placement. Use high-quality electrodes and ensure they are securely attached to prevent movement. Educate patients to remain still and relaxed during procedures to avoid muscle tremors or movements that can cause interference. Regularly check equipment for faults and calibrate it as necessary. Additionally, maintain a quiet environment to minimize electrical interference from nearby devices. These steps help ensure clarity and accuracy in diagnostic readings, which are crucial for effective patient care.

3.5.2.2   Artifacts and Electrical Interference:
Artifacts in electrocardiography (ECG) refer to extraneous signals that obscure the true heart rhythm. Signal distortions occur when these artifacts alter the ECG waveform. Common causes include patient movement, loose electrodes, and external electronic devices. Electrical interference, such as fuzz or a wandering baseline, results from electromagnetic sources like nearby equipment or power lines. Fuzz appears as random noise on the ECG trace, while a wandering baseline is a slow drift of the baseline due to poor electrode contact or respiratory movements. Identifying and correcting these issues is crucial for accurate diagnosis, requiring medical assistants to ensure proper electrode placement and minimize external interference.

3.5.2.3   Patient Preparation, Positioning, and Draping:
Preparation involves ensuring that the patient understands the procedure, verifying identification, and confirming consent. Positioning is crucial for both patient comfort and procedural access, requiring an understanding of various positions such as supine, prone, or Fowler's. Proper positioning minimizes risk and optimizes procedural efficiency. Draping maintains patient dignity and privacy while exposing only the necessary areas for examination or treatment. It requires a skillful arrangement of drapes to prevent contamination and provide warmth. Medical assistants must adeptly manage these tasks to facilitate effective clinical procedures, ensuring patient safety and comfort throughout the process. Mastery of these skills is essential for successful CCMA certification.

3.5.2.4   Supplies (paper, Proper Leads):
In a clinical setting, supplies such as paper and proper leads are essential for accurate patient diagnostics and record-keeping. Paper is primarily used for printing and recording electrocardiograms (ECGs), ensuring that the tracings are clear for interpretation. High-quality ECG paper is heat-sensitive, allowing for precise recordings of cardiac activity. Proper leads refer to the electrodes and wires that connect the patient to diagnostic machines like ECGs. The correct placement of these leads is crucial for obtaining accurate readings, as misplacement can result in incorrect data and lead to misdiagnosis. Medical assistants must be proficient in using these supplies to ensure effective patient care and reliable diagnostic results.

3.5.2.5   Electrode Placement for Limbs and Chest:
The correct placement of limb and chest electrodes is crucial for accurate electrocardiogram (ECG) readings. Limb electrodes are placed on the wrists and ankles, specifically on the right arm (RA), left arm (LA), right leg (RL), and left leg (LL), ensuring that they are equidistant from the heart. Chest electrodes, also known as precordial leads, are positioned on the chest at specific intercostal spaces: V1 is placed at the fourth intercostal space to the right of the sternum, V2 at the fourth intercostal space to the left of the sternum, V3 between V2 and V4, V4 at the fifth intercostal space along the midclavicular line, V5 at the anterior axillary line level with V4, and V6 at the midaxillary line level with V4. Proper placement ensures effective monitoring of cardiac activity.

3.5.2.6   EKG Techniques and Methods:
Electrocardiograms (EKGs) are essential diagnostic tools used to assess the electrical activity of the heart. Medical assistants must be proficient in EKG techniques, including accurate electrode placement, which involves attaching electrodes to the patient's limbs and chest in a standardized 12-lead configuration. Proper skin preparation is crucial to ensure electrode adhesion and signal clarity. Understanding the operation of EKG machines, such as setting the paper speed and gain, is vital for obtaining clear tracings. Recognizing artifacts, such as muscle tremors or electrical interference, allows for corrective measures. Mastery of these techniques ensures accurate readings, aids in the diagnosis of cardiac conditions, and enhances the quality of patient care.

3.5.2.7   Adverse Reaction Indicators in Testing:
Adverse reactions during testing are critical indicators that a patient may be experiencing a negative response to a procedure or medication. Medical assistants must recognize signs such as distress, elevated blood pressure (BP), and increased respiration rate. Distress can manifest as anxiety, discomfort, or confusion. Elevated BP may indicate cardiovascular stress, while increased respiration suggests respiratory distress or anxiety. Prompt recognition and reporting of these signs are essential to prevent further complications. Medical assistants should monitor patients closely, document any changes, and communicate with the healthcare team immediately to ensure patient safety and appropriate intervention. Understanding these signs is vital for effective patient care and management.

3.5.2.8   Calibration Of Equipment:
Calibration of equipment involves the process of adjusting and verifying the accuracy of medical instruments to ensure they provide precise measurements. This process is crucial for maintaining the reliability and safety of diagnostic and therapeutic procedures. Calibration entails comparing the instrument's output with a known standard or reference, identifying any discrepancies, and making necessary adjustments to align the readings. Regular calibration is essential to prevent errors in patient care, as inaccurate equipment can lead to misdiagnosis or inappropriate treatment. Medical assistants must understand calibration protocols, adhere to manufacturer guidelines, and document calibration activities meticulously to uphold clinical standards and ensure optimal patient outcomes.

3.5.2.9   Dysrhythmias in Cardiovascular Testing:
Abnormal rhythms, or dysrhythmias, are irregular heartbeats identified during cardiovascular testing, such as electrocardiograms (ECGs). These irregularities can include tachycardia (rapid heartbeat), bradycardia (slow heartbeat), atrial fibrillation (irregular and often rapid heart rate), and ventricular fibrillation (disorganized electrical activity leading to ineffective heart contractions). Dysrhythmias may result from electrolyte imbalances, myocardial infarction, or structural changes in the heart. Recognizing these patterns is crucial for medical assistants to assist in diagnosing and managing potential cardiovascular issues. Understanding the implications of each type of dysrhythmia helps in providing appropriate patient care and ensuring timely intervention by healthcare providers.

3.5.2.10   Waveforms, Intervals, Segment:
Waveforms, intervals, and segments are essential components of an electrocardiogram (ECG or EKG), which records the electrical activity of the heart. Waveforms include the P wave, QRS complex, and T wave, representing atrial depolarization, ventricular depolarization, and ventricular repolarization, respectively. Intervals, such as the PR interval and QT interval, measure the time between waveforms and indicate the efficiency of electrical conduction through the heart. Segments, like the ST segment, represent periods when the heart's ventricles are depolarized. Understanding these components is crucial for identifying normal cardiac function and diagnosing arrhythmias or other cardiac abnormalities in clinical practice.

4   Enhancing Patient Care Coordination:

Patient care coordination and education involve the systematic organization of patient care activities and the sharing of information among all participants concerned with a patient's care to achieve safer and more effective outcomes. This process ensures that patients receive comprehensive care tailored to their individual needs, thereby improving both outcomes and satisfaction. Medical assistants play a pivotal role by facilitating communication between patients and healthcare providers, scheduling appointments, managing referrals, and providing educational resources to patients. Educating patients about their conditions, treatment plans, and preventive health measures empowers them to take an active role in their health management. Effective coordination reduces redundancies, prevents errors, and enhances the overall quality of healthcare delivery.

4.1 Tasks:

4.1.1 Pre-Visit Patient Record Review:

Reviewing a patient's record before their visit is essential for delivering thorough and personalized care. This task involves examining the patient's medical history, current medications, previous diagnoses, lab results, and any recent treatment plans. By doing so, medical assistants can identify any gaps in care or pending issues that require attention. This proactive approach ensures that the healthcare team is prepared to address all aspects of the patient's health during the visit. It also facilitates continuity of care by keeping the healthcare provider informed about the patient's past interactions and ongoing needs, ultimately enhancing patient outcomes and satisfaction.

4.1.2 Collaboration with Healthcare and Community Organizations:

Medical assistants play a crucial role in ensuring seamless patient care by collaborating with healthcare providers and community-based organizations. This involves actively participating in interdisciplinary teams to coordinate patient care plans, facilitating communication between various healthcare professionals, and ensuring that patients receive comprehensive services tailored to their needs. By engaging with community resources, medical assistants help address social determinants of health, such as housing and nutrition, contributing to improved patient outcomes. Effective collaboration requires understanding the roles of different providers, maintaining accurate records, and advocating for patient needs. This holistic approach enhances continuity of care and empowers patients through education and access to necessary support services.

4.1.3 Coordinating Care with Community Agencies:

Medical assistants play a crucial role in facilitating seamless patient care by coordinating with community agencies for both clinical and non-clinical services. This involves identifying patient needs beyond the healthcare facility, such as home health services, rehabilitation, social services, and financial assistance programs. Medical assistants must effectively communicate with various community resources to ensure that patients receive comprehensive care. They gather necessary documentation, schedule appointments, and provide patients with information on available resources. This coordination helps bridge gaps in care, enhances patient outcomes, and supports providers in delivering holistic healthcare services. By doing so, medical assistants contribute significantly to integrated healthcare delivery systems.

4.1.4 Enhancing Patient Compliance for Optimal Health:

Facilitating patient compliance involves ensuring that patients adhere to their treatment plans to enhance health outcomes. This includes promoting continuity of care by coordinating with healthcare providers to maintain a consistent treatment approach. Medical assistants play a crucial role in scheduling and reminding patients about follow-up appointments, which are essential for monitoring progress and adjusting treatments as needed. Ensuring medication compliance requires educating patients on the importance of taking medications as prescribed, addressing any concerns or barriers they may face, and verifying their understanding. By actively engaging patients in their care process, medical assistants help improve treatment efficacy and patient satisfaction.

4.1.5 Transition of Care Participation:

In the context of medical assisting, participating in the transition of care for patients involves coordinating and facilitating seamless movement between different healthcare settings, such as from hospital to home or rehabilitation center. This includes ensuring accurate communication of patient information, medication reconciliation, and follow-up appointments. Medical assistants play a crucial role by gathering and updating medical records, educating patients about their care plans, and ensuring they understand discharge instructions. Effective participation helps prevent readmissions and enhances patient outcomes. It requires collaboration with healthcare teams to address any barriers to care continuity, ensuring that patients receive comprehensive support during transitions.

4.1.6 Team-Based Patient Care Participation:

Team-based patient care involves collaboration among healthcare professionals to provide comprehensive care. In a Patient-Centered Medical Home (PCMH), medical assistants work with physicians, nurses, and other healthcare providers to ensure coordinated and continuous care tailored to the patients' needs. This model emphasizes preventive care, chronic disease management, and patient education. Similarly, in an Accountable Care Organization (ACO), medical assistants support efforts to improve quality and reduce healthcare costs by facilitating communication among team members and assisting in the implementation of care plans. Medical assistants play a crucial role in these settings by managing patient records, scheduling appointments, and ensuring effective information flow across the care team.

4.2 Knowledge Of:

4.2.1 Preventive Medicine And Wellness:

Preventive medicine and wellness focus on promoting health and preventing disease before it occurs. This approach involves routine screenings, vaccinations, lifestyle counseling, and education to reduce risk factors for chronic diseases. Medical assistants play a crucial role in this by collecting patient histories, measuring vital signs, and educating patients on healthy habits such as balanced nutrition, regular exercise, and smoking cessation. They assist in coordinating care, ensuring that patients receive timely preventive services like mammograms and colonoscopies. Emphasizing prevention over treatment not only improves individual health outcomes but also reduces healthcare costs by minimizing the need for more intensive medical interventions later on.

4.2.2 Education Delivery and Learning Styles:

Education delivery methods encompass various approaches used to convey knowledge, including lectures, hands-on practice, e-learning, and blended learning. Instructional techniques refer to strategies such as demonstrations, discussions, and simulations that enhance learning. Learning styles describe individual preferences for acquiring information, often categorized as visual, auditory, or kinesthetic. Understanding these components is crucial for tailoring education to diverse learners. For medical assistants, this means adapting teaching methods to ensure comprehension and retention of clinical skills and knowledge. Effective education delivery requires recognizing students' learning styles and implementing appropriate instructional techniques to optimize their educational experience and prepare them for the CCMA exam.

4.2.3 Coordinating Outpatient Care Resources:

Outpatient care coordination involves organizing patient care activities and sharing information among all participants involved in a patient's care to achieve safer and more effective outcomes. Resources include electronic health records (EHRs) for seamless information sharing, scheduling systems for managing appointments, and referral networks for specialist consultations. Procedures involve verifying patient insurance, obtaining prior authorizations, and coordinating follow-up appointments. Medical Assistants play a crucial role by ensuring accurate documentation, communicating effectively with healthcare providers, and educating patients about their treatment plans. Effective coordination enhances patient satisfaction, reduces wait times, and improves overall healthcare outcomes by ensuring continuity of care across different healthcare settings.

4.2.4 Clinical Services Resource Availability:

Available resources for clinical services encompass a variety of supportive options designed to enhance patient care outside traditional healthcare settings. Home health care provides medical services in a patient's residence, promoting comfort and convenience. These services include skilled nursing, physical therapy, occupational therapy, and personal care assistance. Additional resources may involve telehealth consultations, medication management programs, and community health support groups. Medical assistants must understand these resources to effectively coordinate patient care plans, ensuring continuity and quality of care. Familiarity with available services allows medical assistants to guide patients in accessing appropriate support tailored to their specific health needs and circumstances.

4.2.5 Community Resources for Non-Clinical Services:

Community resources for non-clinical services are essential supports that enhance patient well-being outside the clinical setting. These services include adult day care, which provides social and health-related services in a safe environment for adults requiring supervision during the day. Transportation vouchers offer subsidized travel options, facilitating access to healthcare appointments, grocery shopping, and community activities. Understanding these resources is crucial for medical assistants to guide patients in accessing comprehensive care that addresses both medical and social needs. By connecting patients with appropriate community services, medical assistants play a pivotal role in promoting holistic health and improving the quality of life for individuals with diverse needs.

4.2.6 Specialty Resources for Patient and Family Needs:

Specialty resources for patients and families addressing medical and mental health needs involve providing access to specialized care and support services tailored to individual health conditions. These resources include referrals to specialists, mental health professionals, and community support groups. Medical assistants play a crucial role in coordinating these services by identifying patient needs, facilitating communication between healthcare providers, and ensuring that patients receive comprehensive care. They assist in educating patients and families about available resources, helping them navigate complex healthcare systems. This holistic approach aims to address both physical and mental health challenges, enhancing overall well-being and improving patient outcomes through personalized care plans and continuous support.

4.2.7 Referral Forms And Processes:

Referral forms are standardized documents used to transfer patient care from one healthcare provider to another, ensuring continuity of care. These forms typically include essential patient information, the reason for referral, and pertinent medical history. The referral process involves the initial assessment by the primary care provider, the completion of the referral form, and communication with the receiving specialist or facility. Medical assistants play a crucial role in managing referrals by accurately completing forms, obtaining necessary authorizations, and scheduling appointments. They must ensure that all relevant information is included to facilitate effective communication between healthcare providers, ultimately enhancing patient outcomes and maintaining an efficient workflow within the healthcare system.

4.2.8 Barriers To Care:

Barriers to care are obstacles that hinder individuals from accessing or receiving adequate healthcare services. Socio-economic barriers include financial constraints that limit access to necessary treatments or preventive care. Cultural differences can lead to misunderstandings or mistrust between patients and healthcare providers, which affects the quality of care. Language barriers impede effective communication, resulting in misinterpretations of medical instructions. Educational barriers involve a lack of understanding about health conditions or the healthcare system, preventing informed decision-making. Recognizing these barriers is crucial for medical assistants to facilitate better patient-provider interactions, ensure equitable access to healthcare, and improve patient outcomes by implementing strategies that effectively address these challenges.

4.2.9 Tracking And Reporting Technologies:

Tracking and reporting technologies in healthcare refer to digital tools and systems used to monitor, record, and communicate patient information efficiently. These technologies include electronic health records (EHRs), patient management software, and data analytics platforms. They facilitate the seamless tracking of patient visits, treatments, and outcomes, ensuring that medical assistants can access up-to-date information for informed decision-making. Reporting tools generate comprehensive reports on patient data, aiding in quality assurance and compliance with healthcare regulations. Mastery of these technologies is crucial for medical assistants to maintain accurate records, enhance patient care, and improve workflow efficiency within clinical settings.

4.2.10   Team Member Roles in Patient-Centered Medical Home:

In a Patient-Centered Medical Home (PCMH), healthcare professionals work collaboratively to provide comprehensive care. The primary care physician leads the team, coordinating patient care and ensuring continuity. Nurses manage chronic conditions, educate patients, and monitor health status. Medical assistants support clinical tasks, such as taking vital signs and preparing patients for exams. Behavioral health specialists address mental health needs, while pharmacists optimize medication management. Care coordinators facilitate communication among providers and connect patients with community resources. Administrative staff manage scheduling and record-keeping. Each member's role is integral to delivering holistic, patient-focused care that enhances outcomes and patient satisfaction.

5   Administrative Assisting:

Administrative assisting in the context of a Certified Clinical Medical Assistant (CCMA) involves managing various non-clinical tasks to ensure the efficient operation of healthcare facilities. This role includes patient scheduling, managing medical records, handling billing and coding, and coordinating communication between patients and healthcare providers. Administrative assistants must maintain patient confidentiality, adhere to healthcare regulations such as HIPAA, and ensure accurate documentation. Proficiency in electronic health records (EHR) systems is essential for updating patient information and managing appointments. Additionally, they may assist in inventory management and ordering supplies. Effective administrative assistance enhances patient care by streamlining processes and allowing clinical staff to focus on direct patient interactions.

5.1 Tasks:

5.1.1 Patient Appointment Scheduling and Monitoring:

Scheduling and monitoring patient appointments involve managing both electronic and paper-based systems to ensure efficient healthcare delivery. Electronic systems, such as Electronic Health Records (EHR), allow for real-time updates, automated reminders, and easy rescheduling. These systems enhance accuracy and accessibility, reducing errors associated with manual entries. Paper-based systems, while traditional, require meticulous attention to detail for recording appointments, cancellations, and follow-ups. Medical Assistants must be adept at navigating both systems, ensuring seamless integration and communication between them. Mastery of these tasks ensures optimal patient flow, minimizes wait times, and enhances overall patient satisfaction by maintaining organized and accurate appointment schedules.

5.1.2 Verify Insurance Coverage/financial Eligibility:

Verifying insurance coverage and financial eligibility involves confirming a patient's health insurance status and determining their ability to pay for medical services. Medical assistants must accurately collect and review insurance information, including policy numbers, coverage details, and any pre-authorization requirements. This process ensures that the healthcare provider will be reimbursed for services rendered and helps identify any patient financial responsibilities, such as co-pays or deductibles. It is crucial to communicate effectively with insurance companies to verify active coverage and understand the scope of benefits. Additionally, this task may involve discussing payment options with patients who lack sufficient insurance coverage, ensuring transparency and financial preparedness.

5.1.3 Patient Check-In/Out Process:

Medical assistants play a crucial role in the patient check-in and check-out process, ensuring smooth administrative operations. During check-in, they verify patient identity by confirming personal details and appointment specifics, and they update medical records as necessary. They collect co-pays and ensure that all necessary forms are completed. At check-out, medical assistants schedule follow-up appointments, provide patients with any required referrals or documentation, and ensure that all billing information is accurately processed. This process requires attention to detail, effective communication skills, and proficiency with electronic health record systems to maintain patient confidentiality and streamline clinic workflow. Efficient check-in and check-out procedures enhance patient satisfaction and clinic efficiency.

5.1.4 Verification of Diagnostic and Procedural Codes:

Verifying diagnostic and procedural codes involves ensuring the accuracy and appropriateness of the codes assigned to patient diagnoses and procedures. This process is crucial for accurate medical billing and compliance with healthcare regulations. Medical assistants must cross-reference patient records with standardized coding systems, such as ICD-10 for diagnoses and CPT for procedures. They ensure that the codes reflect the services provided, are supported by documentation, and comply with payer requirements. This verification prevents billing errors, reduces claim denials, and ensures proper reimbursement. It also involves staying updated on coding changes and guidelines to maintain accuracy in medical records and facilitate efficient healthcare operations.

5.1.5 Prior Authorizations & Pre-certifications Process:

Prior authorizations and pre-certifications are crucial administrative tasks in healthcare. These processes involve obtaining approval from a patient's insurance provider before services are rendered to ensure coverage and reimbursement. Medical Assistants must contact the insurer with detailed patient information, including diagnosis codes and proposed treatments or procedures. Verification is essential to confirm the authorization number, validity period, and any specific conditions or limitations. This task prevents claim denials and unexpected costs for patients. By meticulously managing these authorizations, Medical Assistants facilitate smooth healthcare delivery and maintain compliance with insurance requirements, ultimately contributing to efficient practice operations and enhanced patient satisfaction.

5.1.6 Documentation and Billing: Current Coding Guidelines

Medical assistants must accurately prepare documentation and billing requests by adhering to current coding guidelines, such as ICD-10-CM for diagnoses and CPT for procedures. This involves meticulously reviewing patient records to ensure that all necessary information is included and correctly coded. Proper documentation supports accurate billing, facilitates insurance claims processing, and ensures compliance with healthcare regulations. It is essential to stay updated on coding changes and to utilize electronic health record (EHR) systems efficiently. By doing so, medical assistants play a crucial role in minimizing errors, reducing claim denials, and enhancing the financial health of the medical practice while maintaining high standards of patient care and confidentiality.

5.1.7 Compliance in Documentation Standards:

Medical assistants must ensure that all patient documentation adheres to governmental and insurance standards. This involves accurately recording patient information, treatments, and procedures, ensuring that they align with regulations such as HIPAA for privacy and confidentiality. Proper documentation supports billing processes by providing the necessary details to justify claims to insurance companies. It also involves understanding coding systems like ICD-10 and CPT to accurately document diagnoses and services. Compliance prevents legal issues, reduces claim denials, and ensures timely reimbursement. Medical assistants must stay updated on evolving regulations and guidelines to maintain compliance and support the healthcare facility's operational efficiency and financial stability.

5.1.8 Perform Charge Reconciliation:

Charge reconciliation involves verifying and ensuring the accuracy of billing information in healthcare settings. Medical assistants must proficiently use Electronic Health Record (EHR) software to enter and manage patient charges accurately. This includes inputting services rendered, applying the correct billing codes, and ensuring compliance with insurance requirements. Adjustments may be necessary to correct discrepancies or apply discounts, which require attention to detail and an understanding of billing policies. Accounts receivable procedures involve tracking outstanding payments, sending invoices, and following up on unpaid accounts to maintain financial health. Mastery of these tasks ensures accurate financial records, minimizes errors, and supports efficient revenue cycle management in medical practices.

5.1.9 Billing for Healthcare Services:
Billing patients, insurers, and third-party payers involves the accurate preparation and submission of claims for medical services rendered. Medical assistants must ensure that all patient information is correct and complete, including diagnosis and procedure codes that align with the services provided. This process requires knowledge of insurance policies, billing software, and adherence to regulations such as HIPAA. Medical assistants must also communicate effectively with insurance companies to resolve claim discrepancies or denials. Timely billing is crucial for maintaining cash flow in healthcare settings. Understanding these billing procedures is essential for efficient administrative operations and for ensuring that healthcare providers receive appropriate reimbursement for their services.

5.1.10   Billing Issues Resolution with Insurers:
Medical assistants play a crucial role in resolving billing issues with insurers and third-party payers. This involves understanding the intricacies of insurance policies and accurately interpreting Explanations of Benefits (EOBs). When claims are denied, medical assistants must investigate the cause, which can range from coding errors to missing documentation. They prepare and submit appeals by providing the necessary documentation and clear explanations to justify the claim. Effective communication skills are essential for liaising between healthcare providers and payers. Additionally, staying updated on payer policies and regulations is vital to prevent future denials and ensure timely reimbursement for services rendered.

5.1.11   Managing Electronic and Paper Medical Records:
Managing electronic and paper medical records involves systematically organizing, storing, and retrieving patient information to ensure accuracy and confidentiality. Medical assistants must maintain up-to-date electronic health records (EHRs) using specialized software, ensuring that data is entered correctly and securely. This includes updating patient demographics, medical histories, and treatment plans. For paper records, they must file documents accurately in a secure environment, adhering to privacy regulations such as HIPAA. Regular audits are necessary to verify completeness and correctness. Transitioning between electronic and paper systems requires meticulous attention to detail to prevent data loss. Efficient management supports healthcare delivery by providing reliable access to patient information for clinical decision-making.

5.1.12   Referral Facilitation in Healthcare:
Medical assistants play a crucial role in managing patient referrals to other healthcare providers and allied health professionals. This process involves coordinating with physicians to determine the necessity for specialized care or additional services, ensuring that all relevant patient information is accurately documented and shared. Medical assistants must effectively communicate with both patients and receiving offices to schedule appointments, verify insurance coverage, and confirm receipt of referral documentation. They also track the progress of referrals to ensure timely follow-up and continuity of care. Proficiency in electronic health records (EHR) systems is essential for maintaining organized records and facilitating seamless transitions between healthcare providers.

5.1.13   Customer Service and Service Recovery:
Providing customer service in a clinical setting involves ensuring patient satisfaction through effective communication and efficient service delivery. This includes following up on patient calls to address concerns or inquiries, confirming appointments to reduce no-shows, and monitoring patient flow sheets to enhance clinic efficiency. Additionally, collecting on accounts ensures that financial responsibility is maintained while addressing billing questions. Service recovery focuses on rectifying poor customer service experiences by promptly addressing complaints, offering solutions, and ensuring that patients feel valued and heard. This proactive approach not only improves patient trust and retention but also enhances the overall reputation of the healthcare facility, contributing to a positive patient experience.

5.1.14   Data Entry in Databases & Spreadsheets:
Enter Information Into Databases or Spreadsheets (for example, Excel, EHR & EMR, Billing Modules, Scheduling Systems):

Medical assistants are tasked with accurately entering patient data into various databases and spreadsheets to ensure efficient healthcare delivery and administrative operations. This involves using software such as Excel for organizing data, Electronic Health Records (EHR), and Electronic Medical Records (EMR) systems for maintaining comprehensive patient records. Billing modules require precise entry of financial information to facilitate accurate billing and insurance claims. Scheduling systems are used to manage patient appointments, ensuring optimal workflow and resource allocation. Proficiency in these tasks ensures data integrity, enhances communication among healthcare providers, and supports effective patient care management. Mastery of these skills is crucial for a successful career as a Certified Clinical Medical Assistant.

5.1.15   Safety Evaluations and Reporting Concerns:
Medical assistants play a crucial role in maintaining a safe healthcare environment by actively participating in safety evaluations and reporting safety concerns. This involves conducting regular assessments of the clinical setting to identify potential hazards, such as faulty equipment or unsafe practices. Medical assistants must be vigilant and proactive, ensuring that any identified risks are promptly reported to the appropriate personnel for corrective action. They should also be familiar with the facility's safety protocols and emergency procedures. By doing so, medical assistants help prevent accidents and ensure compliance with regulatory standards, ultimately contributing to the well-being of patients and staff within the healthcare facility.

5.1.16   Inventory Management of Clinical and Administrative Supplies:
Maintaining an inventory of clinical and administrative supplies involves systematically tracking, ordering, and managing the materials necessary for the smooth operation of a medical facility. This includes both clinical supplies, such as syringes, bandages, and medications, as well as administrative supplies like paper, pens, and forms. Medical assistants must ensure that stock levels are adequate to meet the demands of patient care without overstocking, which can lead to waste. They utilize inventory management systems to monitor usage patterns and reorder supplies in a timely manner. Effective inventory management minimizes disruptions in patient care, reduces costs, and ensures compliance with healthcare regulations. Accurate record-keeping and regular audits are essential components of this process.

5.2 Knowledge Of:
5.2.1 Filing Systems:
Filing systems are organized methods for storing, arranging, and retrieving patient records and other important documents in a healthcare setting. They ensure that information is easily accessible, secure, and efficiently managed. Common types include

alphabetical, numerical, and electronic filing systems. Alphabetical systems arrange files by patient names, while numerical systems use unique identifiers, such as medical record numbers. Electronic filing systems utilize digital platforms to store records electronically, enhancing accessibility and reducing physical storage needs. Proper filing systems are crucial for maintaining patient confidentiality, ensuring compliance with legal and regulatory standards, and facilitating a smooth workflow in clinical environments. Mastery of these systems is essential for Certified Clinical Medical Assistants (CCMA).

5.2.2 Scheduling Software:
Scheduling software is a digital tool used in healthcare settings to efficiently manage and organize patient appointments. It streamlines the scheduling process by allowing medical assistants to book, reschedule, and cancel appointments with ease. This software typically integrates with electronic health record (EHR) systems, ensuring that patient information is up-to-date and accessible. It helps prevent double-booking and reduces errors by providing real-time availability of healthcare providers. Additionally, scheduling software often includes features such as automated reminders via email or SMS, which help reduce no-show rates. Mastery of scheduling software is crucial for medical assistants to optimize patient flow and enhance overall clinic efficiency.

5.2.3 Urgent Appointment Needs Recognition:
The recognition of the urgency of appointment needs involves assessing the patient's condition to determine the immediacy required for medical attention. Medical assistants must be skilled in identifying symptoms that necessitate prompt care, such as chest pain, difficulty breathing, or severe allergic reactions. This skill ensures that patients receive timely intervention, potentially preventing complications. Medical assistants should be familiar with triage protocols and communicate effectively with healthcare providers to prioritize appointments based on urgency. Understanding these protocols helps distinguish between routine and urgent cases, ensuring efficient scheduling and optimal patient care. Accurate recognition aids in maintaining a smooth workflow within the healthcare setting while enhancing patient outcomes.

5.2.4 Duration of Visit Requirements:
The duration of a patient visit is determined by various factors, including the purpose of the visit and physician preferences. For routine check-ups, visits may be shorter, focusing on preventive care and updates on health status. Conversely, visits for chronic disease management or complex conditions require more time for thorough assessment and discussion. Physicians may also have personal preferences based on their practice style, patient load, and specific protocols. Medical assistants must adeptly schedule appointments to accommodate these variables, ensuring efficient clinic flow while allowing sufficient time for quality patient care. Understanding these requirements is crucial for optimizing both patient satisfaction and clinical productivity.

5.2.5 Telephone Etiquette:
Telephone etiquette refers to the set of guidelines and practices for professional and courteous communication over the phone. For medical assistants, it involves answering calls promptly, introducing oneself with one's name and position, and maintaining a polite tone. It is crucial to listen actively, ensure clarity in communication, and confirm understanding by summarizing key points. Handling patient inquiries with empathy and confidentiality is essential. Proper etiquette also includes knowing when to transfer calls appropriately and ensuring that messages are accurately recorded and delivered. Effective telephone etiquette enhances patient satisfaction, promotes trust, and reflects positively on the healthcare facility's professionalism.

5.2.6 Records Management Systems Overview:
Records management systems encompass both manual and electronic methods for organizing and storing patient information. Manual filing systems, such as alphabetical and numeric systems, involve the physical organization of files in cabinets or storage areas, ensuring easy retrieval and reference. Office storage for archived files requires secure and accessible solutions to maintain historical records. Electronic Medical Records (EMR) and Electronic Health Records (EHR) software applications digitize patient data, facilitating quick access, sharing, and updating across healthcare settings. These systems enhance efficiency, accuracy, and compliance with legal standards. Mastery of these systems is essential for Certified Clinical Medical Assistants to ensure the seamless integration of patient care and administrative duties.

5.2.7 Legal Compliance for Record Management:
Medical assistants must adhere to legal standards for maintaining, storing, and disposing of patient records to ensure confidentiality and compliance with regulations such as HIPAA. Records must be accurately maintained, securely stored, and accessible only to authorized personnel. Storage solutions should protect against unauthorized access, loss, or damage. Retention periods vary by state law and facility policy, often requiring records to be kept for several years. Proper disposal involves methods such as shredding or incineration to prevent unauthorized access to sensitive information. Compliance with these legal requirements safeguards patient privacy and upholds the integrity of the healthcare system.

5.2.8 Medical Record Categories:
Medical records are systematically categorized to ensure comprehensive patient care and efficient healthcare delivery. Administrative records include demographic data, insurance information, and appointment schedules, which are essential for patient identification and billing. Clinical records encompass medical history, diagnoses, treatment plans, and progress notes, providing a detailed account of the patient's healthcare journey. Billing records document financial transactions related to medical services rendered. Procedural records detail specific medical procedures performed, including outcomes and complications. Notes refer to healthcare provider observations and instructions. Consents are legally binding documents indicating patient agreement to treatments or procedures. Understanding these categories is crucial for maintaining accurate, organized, and legally compliant patient records in clinical practice.

5.2.9 Patient Review Documentation Requirements:
In clinical settings, obtaining a patient's review and signature on required documentation is crucial for legal and ethical compliance. This process involves presenting documents such as consent forms, privacy notices, and treatment plans to patients for their acknowledgment and approval. Medical Assistants must ensure that these documents are complete, accurate, and presented in a manner that patients can understand. The patient's signature signifies their informed consent and agreement to the proposed medical interventions, as well as their acknowledgment of their rights and responsibilities. Proper documentation not only safeguards patient autonomy but also protects healthcare providers from legal disputes by providing evidence of informed consent and communication.

5.2.10   Chart Review:
Chart review is a critical process in clinical settings where medical assistants systematically examine patient records to ensure accuracy, completeness, and compliance with healthcare standards. This involves verifying personal information, reviewing medical history, and ensuring that all documentation, such as physician notes, lab results, and medication lists, is up-to-date and accurately recorded. Medical assistants must be adept at identifying discrepancies or missing information that could impact patient care. The review process aids in preparing for patient visits by organizing pertinent data for the healthcare provider's assessment. Effective chart reviews enhance communication within the healthcare team and contribute to improved patient outcomes by ensuring continuity and quality of care.

5.2.11   E-referrals:
E-referrals are electronic referrals used to streamline the process of sending patient information from one healthcare provider to another. They are created using electronic health record (EHR) systems, ensuring accurate and efficient data transfer. Required information includes patient demographics, medical history, the reason for referral, and any pertinent diagnostic results. E-referrals are sent through secure, encrypted channels to protect patient confidentiality and comply with HIPAA regulations. This digital method enhances communication between providers, reduces paperwork, and expedites patient care by minimizing delays associated with traditional paper referrals. Medical assistants play a crucial role in managing e-referrals by ensuring that all necessary information is accurately entered and transmitted.

5.2.12   Financial Eligibility and Indigent Programs:
Financial eligibility refers to the criteria used to determine a patient's ability to pay for healthcare services. Sliding scales are pricing structures that adjust fees based on a patient's income and ability to pay, ensuring access to care for low-income individuals. Indigent programs are initiatives designed to provide healthcare services at reduced or no cost to patients who cannot afford them. Medical assistants must understand these concepts to assist in assessing patient eligibility for financial assistance, guide them through application processes, and ensure they receive necessary care without financial burden. This knowledge is crucial for promoting equitable healthcare access and supporting patient well-being.

5.2.13   Impact of Government Regulations on Healthcare:
Government regulations such as Meaningful Use and MACRA are essential frameworks in healthcare, aimed at improving patient care and ensuring the efficient use of technology. Meaningful Use is part of the EHR Incentive Programs, promoting the adoption of electronic health records to enhance clinical outcomes. MACRA, or the Medicare Access and CHIP Reauthorization Act, establishes a quality payment program that incentivizes high-quality care through either the Merit-based Incentive Payment System (MIPS) or Advanced Alternative Payment Models (APMs). Medical Assistants must understand these regulations to ensure compliance, optimize patient data management, and support physicians in delivering value-based care. Familiarity with these regulations enhances practice efficiency and patient satisfaction.

5.2.14   CMS Billing Requirements:
CMS Billing Requirements are the regulations and guidelines set by the Centers for Medicare & Medicaid Services (CMS) that medical assistants must adhere to when processing claims for reimbursement. These requirements ensure accurate and compliant billing practices, which include proper documentation, coding, and submission of claims. Medical assistants must be familiar with Current Procedural Terminology (CPT) codes, International Classification of Diseases (ICD) codes, and Healthcare Common Procedure Coding System (HCPCS) codes. Additionally, understanding the importance of patient eligibility verification, maintaining confidentiality according to HIPAA standards, and timely submission of claims is crucial. Compliance with CMS Billing Requirements is essential to avoid denials, reduce errors, and ensure prompt payment for healthcare services rendered.

5.2.15   Third Party Payer Billing Essentials:
Third Party Payer Billing Requirements refer to the specific guidelines and protocols established by insurance companies and other entities that provide payment for healthcare services. These requirements dictate how medical assistants must prepare, submit, and follow up on claims to ensure accurate reimbursement. Key components include understanding coding systems such as ICD-10 and CPT, verifying patient insurance coverage, obtaining necessary pre-authorizations, and ensuring compliance with payer-specific documentation standards. Adhering to these requirements minimizes claim denials and delays in payment, ensuring a smooth revenue cycle for healthcare facilities. Medical assistants must stay informed about updates in billing practices to maintain compliance and optimize reimbursement processes.

5.2.16   Advanced Beneficiary Notice (ABN):
An Advanced Beneficiary Notice (ABN) is a document that healthcare providers give to Medicare beneficiaries when there is a possibility that Medicare may not cover certain services or items. The ABN informs patients of their potential financial responsibility before receiving the service. It must include details about why the provider believes Medicare might deny coverage, along with an estimated cost for the patient. By signing the ABN, patients acknowledge that they understand they might have to pay out of pocket if Medicare denies the claim. This notice ensures transparency and allows beneficiaries to make informed decisions about their healthcare choices and financial obligations.

5.2.17   Specialty Pharmacies: Compounding & Nuclear
Specialty pharmacies focus on providing medications that are not typically available at standard retail pharmacies. Compounding pharmacies customize medications by altering ingredients or dosage forms to meet specific patient needs, such as creating allergen-free formulations or liquid versions of solid medications. Nuclear pharmacies specialize in preparing and dispensing radiopharmaceuticals used in diagnostic imaging and treatment, which requires stringent safety protocols due to the presence of radioactive materials. Both types of specialty pharmacies require specialized knowledge and equipment to ensure the safe and effective preparation and dispensing of medications. Understanding these pharmacies is crucial for medical assistants, as they may need to coordinate with them for patient-specific medication needs and ensure that proper handling and administration instructions are followed.

5.2.18   Types of Medication: Liquid, Elixir, Balm, Ointment
Medications are available in various forms to facilitate administration and absorption. Liquids are aqueous solutions or suspensions for oral or topical use, offering ease of swallowing and rapid absorption. Elixirs are clear, sweetened hydroalcoholic solutions for oral intake, often used to mask unpleasant tastes. Balms are semi-solid preparations with a waxy base, applied topically for their soothing properties and often used for pain relief. Ointments are greasy, semi-solid preparations that provide a protective barrier on

the skin and enhance medication absorption through prolonged contact. Understanding these forms is crucial for medical assistants to ensure proper administration and patient compliance.

5.2.19   Insurance Terminology:
Understanding insurance terminology is crucial for medical assistants. A co-pay is a fixed amount paid by the patient for services, while co-insurance is a percentage of costs shared with the insurer after meeting the deductible. The deductible is the amount paid out-of-pocket before insurance coverage begins. Tier levels refer to the categorization of drugs or services that affect cost-sharing; higher tiers typically mean higher costs. The Explanation of Benefits (EOB) is a document detailing which medical services were covered, the amount paid by insurance, and what the patient owes. Mastery of these terms ensures efficient patient communication and accurate billing processes.

5.2.20   Financial Aging Reports & Collections:
Aging reports are financial documents used to track outstanding patient balances over time, categorized by the duration they have been unpaid (e.g., 30, 60, or 90 days). Collections due refer to the amounts owed by patients that need to be collected to maintain cash flow. Adjustments are modifications made to patient accounts to correct billing errors or apply discounts, ensuring accurate financial records. Write-offs involve removing uncollectible debts from accounting records when deemed irrecoverable. Understanding these concepts is crucial for medical assistants to manage patient accounts effectively, minimize financial discrepancies, and ensure compliance with healthcare billing standards, ultimately aiding in the efficient operation of healthcare facilities.

5.2.21   Online Banking: Deposits & Transfers
Online banking for deposits and electronic transfers refers to the digital management of financial transactions through secure internet platforms. Medical assistants may utilize these services to handle patient co-pays, insurance reimbursements, and vendor payments efficiently. This system allows for the swift transfer of funds between accounts, reducing the need for physical checks or cash handling. It enhances accuracy in financial record-keeping and supports real-time tracking of transactions. Additionally, online banking ensures data security through encryption and authentication measures, safeguarding sensitive financial information. By understanding this technology, medical assistants can contribute to streamlined office operations and improved financial management within healthcare settings.

5.2.22   Payment Processing Approval Authorizations:
Authorizations for payment processing refer to the necessary permissions and procedures required for medical assistants to facilitate financial transactions related to patient care services. This involves verifying insurance coverage, obtaining pre-authorization for specific treatments, and ensuring compliance with healthcare regulations. Medical assistants must accurately document patient information, confirm eligibility, and communicate with insurance providers to secure approval for payments. Understanding the nuances of coding and billing is crucial to preventing errors and delays in payment. By managing these authorizations effectively, medical assistants help maintain the financial health of the healthcare facility while ensuring that patients receive timely and appropriate care without unexpected financial burdens.

5.2.23   Auditing Methods and Sign-offs:
Auditing methods involve a systematic examination of medical records and procedures to ensure compliance with healthcare standards. The processes include selecting records, reviewing documentation for accuracy and completeness, and identifying discrepancies or areas for improvement. Auditors use established protocols to evaluate adherence to clinical guidelines and regulatory requirements. Sign-offs are formal approvals by authorized personnel, confirming that audits have been conducted thoroughly and that the findings are accurate. This process ensures accountability and enhances the quality of patient care by identifying errors or inefficiencies. Medical assistants should understand these auditing procedures to contribute effectively to maintaining high standards in clinical settings, thereby ensuring patient safety and institutional integrity.

5.2.24   Data Entry and Fields Overview:
Data entry involves the accurate and efficient input of patient information into electronic health records (EHR) or other medical databases. Data fields are specific areas within these systems where distinct types of information are recorded, such as patient demographics, medical history, and treatment details. As a medical assistant, it is crucial to ensure that each data field is completed accurately to maintain the integrity of patient records. This process supports effective communication among healthcare providers and ensures continuity of care. Understanding how to navigate EHR systems and correctly enter data minimizes errors and enhances the quality of patient care, reflecting the proficiency essential for the CCMA exam.

5.2.25   Equipment Inspection Logs and Compliance:
Medical equipment inspection logs are detailed records that track the maintenance and inspection history of medical devices. These logs ensure adherence to required schedules for routine checks and servicing, which are vital for maintaining equipment functionality and safety. Compliance requirements mandate that medical facilities follow specific guidelines to ensure all equipment is regularly inspected and serviced by qualified medical equipment servicers. This process involves periodic evaluations, calibrations, and repairs as needed. Regular inspections help prevent equipment malfunctions, ensure patient safety, and meet regulatory standards set by healthcare authorities. Proper documentation in inspection logs is crucial for audits and maintaining accreditation status for healthcare facilities.

6   Communication And Customer Service:
In the healthcare setting, communication and customer service are vital for ensuring patient satisfaction and effective care delivery. Communication involves the clear and accurate exchange of information between medical assistants, patients, and other healthcare professionals. This includes verbal, non-verbal, and written forms of communication. Effective communication aids in understanding patient needs, explaining procedures, and providing instructions. Customer service in healthcare refers to the ability to provide compassionate, respectful, and responsive care to patients. It involves active listening, empathy, and the ability to address patient concerns promptly. Together, these skills enhance patient trust, improve clinical outcomes, and foster a positive healthcare environment, which is essential for the role of a Certified Clinical Medical Assistant (CCMA).

6.1 Tasks:
6.1.1 Adapting Communication for Diversity:
Adapting verbal and non-verbal communication to suit diverse audiences is crucial for medical assistants. This involves tailoring language, tone, and gestures to effectively interact with providers, coworkers, supervisors, patients, caregivers, and external providers. For example, use medical terminology with healthcare professionals while opting for simpler explanations with patients.

Non-verbal cues, such as eye contact and body language, should be adjusted to convey empathy and professionalism appropriately. Recognizing cultural differences is essential to avoid miscommunication. Active listening ensures understanding and responsiveness to each audience's needs. Mastery of these skills enhances patient care, fosters teamwork, and improves overall communication within the healthcare environment.

6.1.2 Tailoring Communication with Patients and Caregivers:
Effective communication with patients and caregivers requires adapting verbal and non-verbal cues to meet diverse needs. For pediatric patients, use simple language and maintain a comforting tone. Engage with visual aids and maintain eye level to foster trust. With geriatric patients, speak clearly, using respectful, slower-paced speech while ensuring comprehension. For hearing-impaired individuals, face them directly, use visual cues, and consider written communication. Vision-impaired patients benefit from descriptive language and tactile engagement. When interacting with individuals with intellectual disabilities, use clear, concise language and be patient, offering reassurance through positive body language. Tailoring communication enhances understanding and improves the quality of care across diverse patient populations.

6.1.3 Enhancing Patient-Provider Communication:
Medical assistants play a critical role in bridging communication between patients and healthcare providers. This involves accurately interpreting and conveying information to ensure that both parties understand medical instructions, concerns, and feedback. Medical assistants must listen actively to patients, ask clarifying questions, and document details precisely. When relaying information to providers, they must be concise yet comprehensive, ensuring that all relevant patient information is communicated without distortion. This process helps prevent misunderstandings and errors in patient care. Effective communication fosters trust, enhances patient satisfaction, and improves overall healthcare outcomes by ensuring that all parties are well-informed and aligned in the care process.

6.1.4 Telephone Communication in Healthcare:
Effective telephone communication is essential for medical assistants to ensure accurate information exchange and foster trust. When speaking with patients and caregivers, clear articulation of medical instructions, appointment details, and empathetic listening are crucial. For providers, concise transmission of patient information and coordination of care are vital. Interactions with third-party payers require precise documentation and a thorough understanding of billing procedures to resolve inquiries efficiently. Always maintain confidentiality by verifying the caller's identity before sharing sensitive information. Utilize active listening skills to clarify misunderstandings and confirm comprehension. Professionalism, patience, and adaptability are key in managing diverse calls while upholding the healthcare facility's standards.

6.1.5 Prepare Written/Electronic Communications/Business Correspondence:
Medical assistants must adeptly prepare written and electronic communications to ensure effective information exchange within healthcare settings. This involves drafting clear, concise, and professional documents such as emails, memos, reports, and letters. Attention to detail is crucial; all correspondence should be free of grammatical errors and accurately convey the intended message. Understanding the audience is essential to tailor the tone and content appropriately. Additionally, medical assistants must adhere to confidentiality regulations, such as HIPAA, when handling patient information. Proficiency in using word processing software and electronic health record systems enhances efficiency. Mastery of these skills ensures seamless communication between healthcare providers, patients, and administrative staff.

6.1.6 Navigating Tough Customer Service Situations:
Handling challenging or difficult customer service occurrences involves effectively managing interactions with patients or clients who may be upset, frustrated, or dissatisfied. As a medical assistant, it is crucial to remain calm, empathetic, and professional. Actively listen to understand the patient's concerns, acknowledge their feelings, and provide reassurance. Use clear communication to explain procedures or delays and offer solutions or alternatives when possible. Maintain a respectful demeanor and avoid becoming defensive. Document the interaction accurately and follow up if necessary to ensure resolution. By employing these strategies, medical assistants can enhance patient satisfaction and maintain a positive healthcare environment, which is essential for patient trust and continuity of care.

6.1.7 Engaging in Crucial Conversations in Healthcare:
Crucial conversations involve discussing sensitive, high-stakes topics where opinions vary and emotions run strong. Medical Assistants must navigate these discussions with empathy and clarity to ensure effective communication. With patients and caregivers, this involves explaining medical procedures or addressing concerns compassionately. When engaging with staff and providers, it requires clear articulation of patient needs or discrepancies in care plans while maintaining professionalism. Active listening, open-ended questions, and non-verbal cues are essential skills for facilitating understanding and resolution. By mastering these conversations, Medical Assistants contribute to a collaborative healthcare environment, enhancing patient outcomes and fostering a supportive workplace culture.

6.1.8 Enhancing Teamwork and Engagement:
Facilitating and promoting teamwork and team engagement involves creating an environment where collaboration is encouraged and each team member feels valued. Medical Assistants play a crucial role in fostering this atmosphere by actively participating in team discussions, respecting diverse perspectives, and communicating effectively. They should encourage open dialogue, ensure that all voices are heard, and mediate conflicts constructively. By promoting a culture of mutual respect and shared goals, Medical Assistants help enhance team efficiency and improve patient care outcomes. Engaging in regular team meetings and collaborative problem-solving sessions can also strengthen bonds and improve overall team dynamics, leading to a more cohesive healthcare delivery system.

6.2 Knowledge Of:
6.2.1 Communication Styles:
Communication styles refer to the various ways individuals express themselves and interpret others during interactions. In a medical setting, understanding communication styles is crucial for effective patient care and teamwork. The four primary styles are assertive, aggressive, passive, and passive-aggressive. Assertive communication is characterized by the clear and respectful expression of thoughts and needs, fostering mutual respect. Aggressive communication involves dominating conversations, often leading to conflict. Passive communication is marked by the avoidance of expressing true feelings, which can result in misunderstandings. Passive-aggressive communication combines elements of both passive and aggressive styles, often causing

confusion. Medical assistants should adapt their communication style to ensure clarity and empathy, thereby enhancing patient trust and collaboration with healthcare teams.

6.2.2 Patient Characteristics Impacting Communication:
Patient characteristics significantly influence communication within clinical settings. Cultural differences and language barriers can hinder understanding and rapport, necessitating the use of interpreters or culturally sensitive communication strategies. Cognitive levels, which vary among individuals, require tailored communication approaches to ensure comprehension, especially for patients with cognitive impairments. Developmental stages also play a crucial role; for instance, communicating with children demands simpler language and visual aids, while adolescents might benefit from more direct engagement. Recognizing these characteristics allows medical assistants to adapt their communication techniques, ensuring effective information exchange and fostering a supportive environment that respects each patient's unique needs and preferences.

6.2.3 Sensory And Physical Disabilities:
Sensory and physical disabilities encompass impairments that affect an individual's ability to engage with their environment. Sensory disabilities include visual and hearing impairments, which can hinder communication and interaction. Physical disabilities involve limitations in mobility or dexterity, affecting tasks such as walking, grasping, or coordinating movements. Medical assistants should be aware of these challenges to provide appropriate care and accommodations. This includes ensuring accessibility, using assistive devices, and employing effective communication techniques. Understanding the specific needs of patients with sensory and physical disabilities is crucial for delivering compassionate care and facilitating their participation in healthcare decisions, thereby enhancing their overall quality of life.

6.2.4 Age:
Age is a crucial demographic factor that influences medical care and patient interaction. It refers to the chronological number of years a person has lived. Understanding age is vital for medical assistants, as it affects physiological processes, disease risk factors, and treatment plans. Different age groups have specific health needs; for instance, pediatric patients require growth monitoring, while geriatric patients often need chronic disease management. Medical assistants must be adept at adjusting communication styles and care techniques based on age to ensure effective patient engagement and compliance. Additionally, age influences medication dosages and contraindications, necessitating precise knowledge for safe administration and patient education.

6.2.5 Decoding Medical Terminology for Laymen:
Medical terminology is a specialized language used by healthcare professionals to ensure precise communication. It comprises terms derived from Greek and Latin roots, prefixes, and suffixes that describe the human body, its functions, conditions, and procedures. Jargon refers to the technical vocabulary specific to a profession, which can be complex for those outside the field. Layman's terms are simplified versions of medical language intended for non-professional audiences to facilitate understanding. As a medical assistant, mastering medical terminology allows you to communicate effectively with colleagues, while translating jargon into layman's terms ensures that patients comprehend their diagnoses, treatments, and care instructions, thereby enhancing patient education and compliance.

6.2.6 Therapeutic Communication:
Therapeutic communication is a purposeful interaction between healthcare providers and patients aimed at improving the patient's mental, emotional, and physical well-being. It involves active listening, empathy, and both verbal and non-verbal communication skills to build a trusting relationship. Medical assistants use therapeutic communication to gather information, educate patients, and provide emotional support. Techniques include open-ended questions, reflective listening, and validation of patient feelings. This approach helps in understanding patient needs, reducing anxiety, and promoting compliance with medical advice. Effective therapeutic communication requires awareness of cultural differences and personal biases to ensure respectful and individualized care. Mastery of these skills is crucial for successful patient interactions and outcomes.

6.2.7 Effective Interviewing Techniques:
Effective interviewing and questioning techniques are crucial for gathering accurate patient information. Screening questions are initial queries designed to identify patients who need further assessment. Open-ended questions encourage detailed responses, allowing patients to express their concerns in their own words, such as, Can you describe your symptoms? Closed-ended questions elicit specific information, often answered with a 'yes' or 'no', such as, Have you experienced a fever? Probing questions delve deeper into responses to clarify or expand on information, such as, What makes the pain worse? Mastery of these techniques enables medical assistants to obtain comprehensive patient histories, ensuring accurate diagnoses and effective treatment planning.

6.2.8 Permitted Questions: Scope and Boundaries
In the context of the CCMA exam, the Scope of Permitted Questions and Boundaries for Questions refers to the range and limits of topics that can be addressed during the examination. This scope is defined by the Medical-Surgical Nursing Certification Board (MSNCB) and ensures that all questions are relevant to the competencies required for a Certified Clinical Medical Assistant. The boundaries ensure that questions pertain specifically to clinical duties, patient care, medical ethics, and administrative tasks within a medical setting. Understanding these parameters helps candidates focus their study efforts on pertinent areas and avoid extraneous information, thus enhancing their preparedness for the exam.

6.2.9 Active Listening:
Active listening is a crucial communication skill for medical assistants, involving fully concentrating, understanding, responding, and remembering what the patient says. It requires giving undivided attention to the speaker, making eye contact, and using verbal and non-verbal cues, such as nodding or brief affirmations, to show engagement. Active listening aids in accurately gathering patient information, understanding their concerns, and building trust. It involves not only hearing words but also interpreting emotions and underlying messages. By paraphrasing or summarizing what the patient has said, medical assistants can confirm their understanding and ensure clarity. This skill enhances the quality of patient care by promoting effective communication and reducing misunderstandings.

6.2.10　Effective Communication Cycle:
The communication cycle is a structured process that ensures the effective exchange of information between parties. It involves the sender encoding a message clearly and concisely, transmitting it through an appropriate channel, and the receiver decoding and interpreting it. Feedback from the receiver completes the cycle, confirming understanding or prompting clarification. In medical

settings, clear and concise communication is critical to avoid misunderstandings that could impact patient care. Medical assistants must master this cycle to relay accurate information swiftly, ensuring patient safety and efficiency in healthcare delivery. Active listening and empathy are essential components that enhance the quality of interaction and foster trust with patients and colleagues.

6.2.11   Coaching and Positive Reinforcement:
Coaching in a medical setting involves guiding and supporting medical assistants to enhance their skills and performance. Feedback is a critical component, providing specific information about their actions and outcomes. Positive reinforcement is a strategy used to encourage effective behavior by acknowledging and rewarding desirable actions. This reinforcement can take the form of verbal praise, recognition, or tangible rewards, which help to reinforce the behavior, making it more likely to be repeated. In practice, when medical assistants receive constructive feedback paired with positive reinforcement, it boosts their confidence, motivation, and job satisfaction. This approach not only improves individual performance but also contributes to a positive work environment and better patient care.

6.2.12   Professional Presence:
Professional presence encompasses the image and behavior that a medical assistant projects in a clinical setting. Appearance involves maintaining a clean, neat, and appropriate uniform, reflecting professionalism and respect for patients and colleagues. Demeanor refers to the attitude and behavior displayed, emphasizing empathy, patience, and attentiveness, which are crucial for building trust and rapport with patients. Tone involves the manner of speaking, ensuring it is clear, respectful, and considerate, thereby facilitating effective communication. Together, these elements of professional presence contribute to creating a positive environment that enhances patient care and upholds the standards expected in healthcare settings, which are essential for success in the CCMA role.

6.2.13   Patient Satisfaction Surveys:
Patient satisfaction surveys are tools used to gauge patients' perceptions of their care experience within a healthcare facility. These surveys assess various aspects, such as communication with healthcare providers, the efficiency of service delivery, and the overall environment of the facility. They are crucial for identifying areas needing improvement and ensuring that patient-centered care is delivered. For medical assistants, understanding these surveys is vital, as they often interact directly with patients and can impact their satisfaction levels. By analyzing survey results, medical assistants can contribute to enhancing service quality, thereby improving patient outcomes and loyalty. Additionally, these surveys help facilities maintain compliance with healthcare standards and accreditation requirements.

6.2.14   Timing for Problem Escalation:
Recognizing when to escalate problem situations is crucial for medical assistants to ensure patient safety and efficient healthcare delivery. Escalation is necessary when a patient's condition deteriorates or when an issue exceeds the assistant's scope of practice or expertise. For instance, if a patient exhibits acute symptoms such as chest pain or difficulty breathing, immediate escalation to a physician or nurse is required. Similarly, if there are discrepancies in medication orders or diagnostic results, these must be promptly reported to supervising healthcare providers. Effective communication and documentation during escalation ensure continuity of care and help mitigate potential risks, maintaining a high standard of patient care.

6.2.15   Patient Management Techniques:
Effectively managing patient interactions requires a blend of communication skills and emotional intelligence. For irate clients, remain calm, listen actively, and acknowledge their concerns to defuse tension. Employ empathy and clarify misunderstandings without escalating the situation. In custody issues between parents, maintain neutrality and adhere to legal guidelines while ensuring patient privacy. Follow the chain of command by reporting complex situations to supervisors or legal advisors when necessary. Document interactions meticulously for accountability. Utilize these techniques to foster a professional environment, prioritize patient safety, and ensure compliance with medical protocols, ultimately contributing to a harmonious clinical setting.

6.2.16   Incident/event/unusual Occurrence Reports:
Incident, event, or unusual occurrence reports are formal documents used in healthcare settings to record any unexpected or adverse events that occur within a medical facility. These reports are crucial for identifying potential risks, ensuring patient safety, and improving healthcare practices. The report includes detailed information about the incident, such as the date, time, location, individuals involved, and a thorough description of the event. It also outlines any immediate actions taken to address the situation. Medical assistants must accurately document these occurrences to facilitate effective communication among healthcare teams and contribute to quality improvement initiatives. Proper reporting helps in analyzing trends, preventing future incidents, and maintaining compliance with regulatory standards.

6.2.17   Documentation Of Event:
Documentation of events refers to the accurate and detailed recording of any significant occurrences or interventions during patient care. This includes documenting the date, time, nature of the event, and any actions taken by healthcare providers. Proper documentation is crucial for ensuring continuity of care, legal protection, and quality assurance. It serves as a communication tool among healthcare team members, providing a clear and comprehensive account of patient interactions and clinical decisions. Medical Assistants must ensure that documentation is complete, legible, and follows institutional protocols. Accurate documentation supports patient safety and enhances the overall efficiency of healthcare delivery by providing a reliable record for future reference.

6.2.18   Cause-and-effect Analysis:
Cause-and-effect analysis is a critical thinking process used to identify and understand the relationship between an action (cause) and its outcome (effect). In medical contexts, this analysis helps determine how physiological or psychological factors influence health outcomes. For instance, anxiety, a psychological condition, can trigger physiological responses such as increased blood pressure or heart rate. This occurs because anxiety activates the body's fight-or-flight response, releasing stress hormones like adrenaline, which constrict blood vessels and increase cardiac output. Understanding these relationships allows medical assistants to anticipate potential health issues and provide appropriate care or interventions. Mastery of cause-and-effect analysis is essential for effective patient assessment and management.

6.2.19   Risk Management in Patient and Employee Safety:
Risk management in healthcare involves identifying, assessing, and mitigating risks to ensure the safety of patients and employees. It requires a thorough review of the facility's design to ensure it supports safe practices, considering the specific setting

and population served. Protocols must be established to guide safe operations and prevent harm. Regular measurements and assessments are essential to monitor compliance and effectiveness. This includes evaluating equipment safety, infection control procedures, emergency preparedness, and staff training. By implementing robust risk management strategies, healthcare facilities can minimize potential hazards, enhance the quality of patient care, and maintain a safe working environment for employees, thereby reducing liability and improving overall operational efficiency.

6.2.20   Email Etiquette:
Email etiquette refers to the set of guidelines and best practices for composing, sending, and responding to emails in a professional manner. For medical assistants, this includes using a clear and concise subject line, addressing recipients respectfully, and maintaining patient confidentiality by avoiding the sharing of sensitive information. Emails should be well-structured, featuring a polite greeting, a coherent body, and an appropriate closing. It is crucial to use professional language, avoid slang or emoticons, and proofread for spelling and grammatical errors. Timely responses are important, as they reflect reliability and respect for colleagues' time. Adhering to email etiquette ensures effective communication, upholds professionalism, and enhances the efficiency of healthcare operations.

6.2.21   Business Letter Formats:
Business letter formats are standardized structures used for formal communication within the medical field. The most common formats include block, modified block, and semi-block. In the block format, all text is left-aligned, and paragraphs are not indented, making it clean and straightforward. The modified block format aligns the date, closing, and signature to the right, offering a more balanced appearance. The semi-block format combines elements of both block and modified block, with indented paragraphs providing a traditional look. Understanding these formats is crucial for medical assistants, as they often draft professional correspondence such as patient referrals or inter-office memos, ensuring clarity and professionalism in written communication.

6.2.22   Telephone Etiquette:
Telephone etiquette refers to the professional and courteous manner in which medical assistants communicate over the phone. It involves using a polite tone, clear articulation, and active listening to ensure effective communication. Key aspects include promptly answering calls, identifying oneself and the facility, and verifying the caller's identity to maintain confidentiality. Medical assistants should take accurate messages, repeat key information for confirmation, and provide concise responses to inquiries. Maintaining patient privacy is crucial; therefore, discretion is necessary when discussing sensitive information. Proper telephone etiquette reflects professionalism, enhances patient satisfaction, and ensures efficient practice operations, which are essential competencies for Certified Clinical Medical Assistants (CCMA).

7   Medical Law And Ethics:
Medical law and ethics encompass the legal and moral principles that guide healthcare practices. Medical law refers to the regulations and statutes that govern the responsibilities and rights of medical professionals and patients. It includes issues such as patient confidentiality, informed consent, and malpractice. Ethics in medicine deals with moral principles, such as autonomy, beneficence, non-maleficence, and justice, which guide decision-making in patient care. Understanding these concepts ensures that medical assistants uphold legal standards while maintaining ethical integrity in their duties. Adhering to medical law and ethics protects patient rights, promotes trust in healthcare relationships, and ensures professional accountability, which is critical for competent clinical practice.

7.1 Tasks:
7.1.1 Legal and Regulatory Compliance:
Medical assistants must adhere to legal and regulatory standards to ensure patient safety and uphold the integrity of the healthcare system. This involves understanding and following laws such as the Health Insurance Portability and Accountability Act (HIPAA), which protects patient confidentiality, and the Occupational Safety and Health Administration (OSHA) regulations, which ensure workplace safety. Compliance also includes proper documentation, accurate coding and billing practices, and adherence to clinical guidelines. Medical assistants must stay informed about changes in healthcare laws and regulations, participate in ongoing education, and collaborate with healthcare teams to maintain compliance, thereby minimizing legal risks and enhancing the quality of care.

7.1.2 Upholding Professional Ethics:
Adhering to professional codes of ethics involves following established guidelines that dictate the moral and ethical conduct expected of medical assistants. These codes serve as a framework to ensure that patient care is delivered with integrity, confidentiality, and respect. Medical assistants must maintain professionalism by safeguarding patient information, obtaining informed consent, and providing unbiased care regardless of personal beliefs. Ethical codes also require practitioners to report any misconduct or unethical behavior observed in the healthcare setting. By adhering to these standards, medical assistants uphold the trust placed in them by patients and colleagues, promoting a culture of ethical practice and accountability within the healthcare environment.

7.1.3 Medical Directives Compliance:
Medical directives are legally binding instructions regarding a patient's medical care preferences. Obtaining these directives involves collecting written or verbal instructions from patients or their authorized representatives. Reviewing these directives requires a thorough understanding to ensure clarity and accuracy regarding the patient's wishes. Compliance involves strictly adhering to these directives during patient care, ensuring that all actions align with the documented preferences. This process is crucial for respecting patient autonomy and meeting legal requirements while minimizing liability risks. Medical assistants must be diligent in documenting and communicating these directives to the healthcare team, ensuring that patient care aligns with their expressed desires and legal standards.

7.1.4 Healthcare Proxies and Agents Documentation:
Healthcare proxies and agents are designated individuals authorized to make medical decisions on behalf of a patient who is unable to do so. Medical assistants must understand the importance of obtaining and accurately documenting these legal designations in the patient's medical records. This involves verifying the validity of the proxy or agent, which typically requires a legal document such as a power of attorney for healthcare. Proper documentation ensures that healthcare providers are aware of who can legally make decisions, thereby safeguarding patient autonomy and ensuring compliance with legal standards. Accurate record-keeping is crucial to prevent disputes and to ensure that patient care aligns with their wishes.

7.1.5 MOLST Forms Management:
MOLST forms are critical documents that outline a patient's preferences for life-sustaining treatments. Medical Assistants play a vital role in managing these forms by ensuring they are provided to patients or their representatives during consultations. They must accurately collect completed MOLST forms, verifying that all sections are filled out correctly and signed by both the patient and the healthcare provider. Proper storage is essential; MOLST forms should be kept in a secure, easily accessible location within the patient's medical records. This ensures that healthcare providers can quickly reference them during emergencies, honoring the patient's treatment preferences and ensuring legal compliance.

7.1.6 Safeguarding Patient Privacy and Medical Records:
Patient privacy and confidentiality are fundamental principles in healthcare, ensuring that personal health information is safeguarded. Medical Assistants must adhere to the Health Insurance Portability and Accountability Act (HIPAA) regulations, which mandate the protection of patient data. This involves securing medical records, limiting access to authorized personnel only, and ensuring that discussions about patient information occur in private settings. It is crucial to obtain patient consent before sharing their information with third parties. Breaches of confidentiality can lead to legal repercussions and a loss of trust. By diligently maintaining these standards, Medical Assistants uphold ethical practices and contribute to a secure healthcare environment.

7.1.7 Compliance with Reportable Violations:
Medical assistants must understand and comply with legal mandates for reporting violations or incidents, such as abuse, neglect, or communicable diseases. Adherence involves recognizing reportable events and following protocols to promptly notify the appropriate authorities. This ensures patient safety and legal compliance, protecting both the patient and the healthcare provider from legal repercussions. Medical assistants should be familiar with federal, state, and local regulations, which may vary. Documentation of incidents must be thorough and accurate, maintaining confidentiality while fulfilling legal obligations. Understanding these requirements is crucial for ethical practice and contributes to the integrity of healthcare delivery.

7.1.8 Unbiased Care: Recognizing Beliefs and Values
Medical assistants must recognize their own personal or religious beliefs and values to ensure they do not interfere with the provision of unbiased care. This involves self-reflection and awareness of potential biases that could affect patient interactions or treatment decisions. It is crucial to maintain professionalism by respecting the diverse beliefs and values of patients, ensuring that personal views do not influence medical advice or care delivery. Providing unbiased care means treating every patient with equal respect, dignity, and without discrimination. Medical assistants should focus on patient-centered care, adhering to ethical principles and standards that prioritize the health and well-being of all patients, regardless of their background.

7.2 Knowledge Of:
7.2.1 Informed Consent:
Informed consent is a fundamental ethical and legal requirement in healthcare, ensuring that patients are fully aware of and understand the nature, benefits, risks, and alternatives of proposed medical procedures or treatments. It involves a clear communication process in which the healthcare provider discloses all relevant information, allowing the patient to make a voluntary and informed decision regarding their care. For informed consent to be valid, the patient must be competent to make decisions, provided with adequate information, and not subjected to coercion. Medical assistants play a crucial role in facilitating this process, ensuring that documentation is complete and verifying that patients' questions are addressed before obtaining their consent.

7.2.2 Understanding Advanced Directives:
Advanced directives are legal documents that outline a patient's preferences for medical treatment in situations where they may be unable to communicate their decisions. A Living Will specifies the types of medical care a person wishes or does not wish to receive, such as life-sustaining measures. A Do Not Resuscitate (DNR) order instructs healthcare providers not to perform cardiopulmonary resuscitation (CPR) if the patient's breathing or heart stops. Do Not Intubate (DNI) orders indicate that the patient does not want intubation for mechanical ventilation. These directives ensure that medical care aligns with the patient's values and desires, providing clarity and guidance to healthcare professionals and family members.

7.2.3 Power Of Attorney:
A Power of Attorney (POA) is a legal document that grants an individual, known as the agent or attorney-in-fact, the authority to act on behalf of another person, referred to as the principal. In a medical context, a POA allows the agent to make healthcare decisions for the principal if they become incapacitated or unable to communicate their wishes. This ensures that medical treatments align with the principal's preferences and best interests. Medical assistants should understand that a POA is crucial for patient autonomy and must be respected in clinical settings, ensuring that any decisions made by the agent are documented and followed according to legal and ethical standards.

7.2.4 Storage Of Medical Records:
Medical records storage involves the systematic organization and safekeeping of patient information to ensure confidentiality, accessibility, and compliance with legal standards. Records can be stored electronically or in physical form, with each requiring secure environments to protect against unauthorized access and data breaches. Electronic Health Records (EHRs) offer efficient retrieval and sharing capabilities, while physical records must be filed in locked cabinets within secure areas. Compliance with regulations such as HIPAA is essential for safeguarding patient privacy. Proper indexing and labeling facilitate quick access, while retention policies dictate the duration for which records are kept before secure disposal. Regular audits ensure adherence to storage protocols and maintain data integrity.

7.2.5 Information Sharing Conditions:
The release of patient information is governed by strict legal and ethical guidelines to ensure confidentiality and privacy. Medical Assistants must adhere to the Health Insurance Portability and Accountability Act (HIPAA), which mandates that patient information can only be shared with authorized individuals or entities for purposes such as treatment, payment, or healthcare operations. Consent from the patient is usually required unless disclosure is mandated by law, such as in cases of reporting infectious diseases or abuse. Additionally, only the minimum necessary information should be disclosed to fulfill the intended purpose. Understanding these conditions is crucial for maintaining trust and compliance within the healthcare setting.

7.2.6 Criminal vs. Civil Acts in Medical Malpractice:
Criminal acts in healthcare involve violations of laws that can result in imprisonment or fines, such as fraud or abuse. Civil acts pertain to disputes between parties where compensation may be awarded, often involving breaches of contract or negligence. Medical malpractice is a specific type of civil act in which a healthcare professional deviates from the standard of care, resulting in

harm to the patient. It requires proving duty, breach, causation, and damages. Understanding these concepts is crucial for medical assistants to ensure compliance with legal standards and to protect patient rights while minimizing liability risks for healthcare providers.

7.2.7 Mandatory Reporting Laws and Triggers:

Mandatory reporting laws require healthcare professionals, including medical assistants, to report certain conditions or incidents, such as child abuse, elder abuse, domestic violence, and communicable diseases. These laws are designed to protect vulnerable populations and ensure public safety. Triggers for reporting include observable signs of abuse or neglect, patient disclosures, and diagnoses of reportable diseases. Medical assistants must be vigilant in identifying these triggers and understanding the specific criteria that necessitate a report. Reporting agencies vary by jurisdiction but typically include child protective services, adult protective services, and local health departments. Timely and accurate reporting is crucial to comply with legal obligations and safeguard affected individuals.

7.2.8 Hippocratic Oath:

The Hippocratic Oath is a foundational ethical guideline in medicine, originating from ancient Greece and attributed to Hippocrates. It emphasizes principles such as non-maleficence, confidentiality, and respect for patients. Medical professionals pledge to practice medicine ethically, prioritize patient welfare, and uphold professional integrity. While the original oath has evolved, its core tenets remain integral to modern medical ethics. For Certified Clinical Medical Assistants, understanding the Hippocratic Oath underscores the importance of ethical conduct in clinical settings. It reinforces the commitment to providing compassionate care, maintaining patient confidentiality, and collaborating with healthcare teams to ensure optimal patient outcomes while adhering to legal and ethical standards.

CCMA Practice Questions [SET 1]

Question 1: Which of the following medication pairs is most likely to be confused due to their similar-sounding names, potentially leading to medication errors?
A) Celebrex and Celexa
B) Zantac and Xanax
C) Lamictal and Lamisil
D) Plavix and Paxil

Question 2: Sarah, a 45-year-old woman with a history of hypertension, has been prescribed Lisinopril. After a week of taking the medication, she reports experiencing a persistent dry cough. What is the most likely explanation for her symptom?
A) Allergic reaction to Lisinopril
B) Common side effect of Lisinopril
C) Adverse effect of Lisinopril
D) Contraindication for using Lisinopril

Question 3: Mrs. Johnson, a 78-year-old patient with chronic obstructive pulmonary disease (COPD), has been recently discharged from the hospital. The primary care physician recommends home health care services to manage her condition effectively. Which of the following resources would be most appropriate for ensuring continuity of care and preventing readmission?
A) A visiting nurse service for daily medication administration.
B) A physical therapist for weekly rehabilitation sessions.
C) A telehealth service for remote monitoring and consultations.
D) A social worker to assist with community resources and support.

Question 4: A 68-year-old patient named Mr. Johnson is admitted to the hospital with a urinary tract infection (UTI) caused by Escherichia coli (E. coli). During his stay, he develops symptoms of pneumonia. Which of the following breaks in the chain of infection most likely led to Mr. Johnson's secondary infection?
A) Improper hand hygiene by healthcare workers
B) Contaminated urinary catheter
C) Lack of isolation precautions for respiratory infections
D) Improper sterilization of medical equipment

Question 5: During a procedure, you notice that the autoclave used to sterilize surgical instruments malfunctioned. What is the most appropriate immediate action to ensure the instruments are properly sterilized before use?
A) Re-run the instruments through the autoclave after fixing it.
B) Use chemical sterilization as an alternative method.
C) Switch to using pre-sterilized disposable instruments.
D) Perform manual cleaning followed by high-level disinfection.

Question 6: What is the primary purpose of generating an aging report in a medical practice?
A) To identify overdue patient accounts for follow-up
B) To determine the total amount of revenue generated
C) To track daily patient appointments
D) To monitor staff performance

Question 7: Which filing system is most suitable for a medical practice that needs to quickly retrieve patient records based on their last names?
A) Numerical
B) Subject
C) Alphabetical
D) Geographical

Question 8: Which of the following is a critical step in ensuring the accuracy of Point Of Care Testing (POCT) results?
A) Regularly updating the software of POCT devices.
B) Performing daily quality control checks on POCT devices.
C) Ensuring that POCT devices are used by certified personnel only.
D) Calibrating POCT devices annually.

Question 9: During a gynecological examination, what is the most crucial step a medical assistant must take to ensure accurate results?
A) Ensure the patient has an empty bladder.
B) Position the patient in the lithotomy position.
C) Prepare and label specimen containers accurately.
D) Verify the patient's medical history.

Question 10: When engaging in a crucial conversation with a patient's caregiver who is upset about the patient's care plan, which strategy is most effective in de-escalating the situation?
A) Assertively stating the medical facts and emphasizing the caregiver's need to trust the healthcare team's expertise.
B) Actively listening to the caregiver's concerns and validating their feelings before discussing potential solutions.
C) Redirecting the conversation to focus on positive aspects of the patient's progress to alleviate the caregiver's anxiety.
D) Providing detailed explanations of medical procedures and outcomes to reassure the caregiver with comprehensive information.

Question 11: During a routine audit, you discover that patient Jane Doe's medical records contain duplicate entries for her recent lab results. What is the most appropriate action to take in order to maintain accurate and compliant medical records?
A) Delete one of the duplicate entries without further documentation.
B) Merge the duplicate entries into a single record and document the correction.
C) Leave both entries as they are but make a note about the duplication in the patient's file.
D) Consult with your supervisor before making any changes to ensure compliance with office policies.

Question 12: Maria, a CCMA at Dr. Smith's clinic, needs to obtain prior authorization for a patient named John who requires an MRI scan. She has already checked the patient's insurance coverage and filled out the necessary forms. What should Maria do next to ensure the authorization process is completed correctly?
A) Submit the forms directly to the MRI facility.
B) Contact John's insurance provider to confirm receipt of the forms.
C) Schedule the MRI scan before receiving authorization confirmation.
D) Inform John that he can proceed with scheduling his MRI scan.

Question 13: When documenting a healthcare proxy, which of the following is essential to ensure its validity?
A) The document must be signed by the patient and two witnesses.
B) The document must be notarized by a licensed notary public.
C) The document must include the patient's medical history.
D) The document must specify the patient's primary care physician.

Question 14: Patient Sarah has been prescribed a

medication that needs to be applied topically to her skin for localized pain relief. The medication should remain on the surface without being absorbed deeply into the skin layers. Which form of medication is most appropriate for Sarah?
A) Liquid
B) Elixir
C) Balm
D) Ointment

Question 15: Emily is a 4-year-old child who is beginning to assert her independence and engage in more interactive play with her peers. According to Erikson's stages of psychosocial development, which developmental stage is Emily most likely experiencing?
A) Trust vs. Mistrust
B) Autonomy vs. Shame and Doubt
C) Initiative vs. Guilt
D) Industry vs. Inferiority

Question 16: What is the most critical step a medical assistant should take when preparing a patient for a minor surgical procedure?
A) Ensure the patient has fasted for at least 8 hours before the procedure.
B) Obtain and verify the patient's informed consent before starting the procedure.
C) Position the patient comfortably on the examination table.
D) Provide detailed post-procedure care instructions before starting the procedure.

Question 17: Which diagnostic measure is most appropriate for confirming a diagnosis of deep vein thrombosis (DVT) in a patient presenting with unilateral leg swelling and pain?
A) D-dimer test
B) Venous duplex ultrasound
C) Magnetic resonance imaging (MRI)
D) Computed tomography (CT) angiography

Question 18: Which drug classification under the Controlled Substances Act is characterized by having a high potential for abuse, with use potentially leading to severe psychological or physical dependence, but also has accepted medical uses?
A) Schedule I
B) Schedule II
C) Schedule III
D) Schedule IV

Question 19: Mrs. Johnson, an elderly patient with dementia, has been prescribed a new medication. Her daughter, who is her primary caregiver, expresses concern about potential side effects. As a medical assistant, how should you handle this crucial conversation to ensure both Mrs. Johnson and her daughter feel heard and informed?
A) Reassure them that the medication is safe and has been prescribed by a knowledgeable physician.
B) Explain the potential side effects clearly and provide written information for their reference.
C) Listen to their concerns empathetically, explain the potential side effects clearly, and provide written information.
D) Suggest they discuss their concerns directly with the prescribing physician.

Question 20: When documenting an event in a patient's medical record, which of the following is the most crucial aspect to ensure the integrity and reliability of the documentation?
A) Documenting events immediately after they occur
B) Using medical jargon to ensure precision
C) Including only relevant information

D) Using abbreviations for efficiency

Question 21: When performing a CLIA-waived glucose test, which of the following is the most critical step to ensure accurate results?
A) Ensuring the test strip is not expired
B) Calibrating the glucometer before each use
C) Wearing gloves to prevent contamination
D) Recording patient information accurately

Question 22: During an audit at a medical clinic, it was discovered that patient records were not being disposed of properly. As a Certified Clinical Medical Assistant (CCMA), what is the most appropriate action to ensure compliance with legal requirements for the disposal of patient records?
A) Shred all patient records immediately after five years.
B) Transfer all records to an offsite storage facility after two years.
C) Follow state-specific regulations and guidelines for record retention and disposal.
D) Dispose of records by incineration regardless of their age.

Question 23: Which of the following questions is most appropriate for a Certified Clinical Medical Assistant (CCMA) to ask a patient during an initial consultation?
A) "Can you describe any allergies you have to medications?"
B) "What do you think caused your current symptoms?"
C) "Do you have any family history of chronic illnesses?"
D) "How often do you exercise and what type of exercise do you do?"

Question 24: Which instrument is specifically designed for the removal of skin staples?
A) Hemostat
B) Suture scissors
C) Staple remover
D) Needle holder

Question 25: During a routine blood draw for patient Mr. Johnson, you are required to collect samples for a complete blood count (CBC) and coagulation studies. Which of the following actions is correct regarding the type of tubes, their positions in the draw order, number of inversions, and fill level/ratios?
A) Collect the light blue top tube first for coagulation studies, invert it 3-4 times, and ensure it is filled to at least 50% capacity.
B) Collect the lavender top tube first for CBC, invert it 8-10 times, and ensure it is filled to at least 75% capacity.
C) Collect the light blue top tube first for coagulation studies, invert it 3-4 times, and ensure it is filled to at least 90% capacity.
D) Collect the lavender top tube first for CBC, invert it 5-6 times, and ensure it is filled to at least 50% capacity.

Question 26: John, a 45-year-old patient with a history of chronic obstructive pulmonary disease (COPD), presents with fever, productive cough, and shortness of breath. A sputum culture reveals the presence of Gram-negative rods. Based on this information, which infectious agent is most likely responsible for John's symptoms?
A) Streptococcus pneumoniae
B) Haemophilus influenzae
C) Mycoplasma pneumoniae
D) Staphylococcus aureus

Question 27: Maria, a 45-year-old patient with chronic back pain, requires a referral to see an orthopedic specialist. As a Certified Clinical Medical Assistant (CCMA), what is your primary responsibility in ensuring

Maria's referral authorization is processed correctly?
A) Verify that Maria's insurance plan covers visits to the orthopedic specialist and obtain prior authorization if required.
B) Schedule the appointment with the orthopedic specialist and inform Maria about any out-of-pocket costs.
C) Contact the orthopedic specialist directly to discuss Maria's case and ensure they accept her insurance.
D) Ensure that all of Maria's medical records are sent to the orthopedic specialist before her appointment.

Question 28: Mr. Johnson, a 65-year-old patient with a history of hypertension, is prescribed medication to manage his blood pressure. The prescription reads "Metoprolol 50 mg PO BID." As a Certified Clinical Medical Assistant, how should you interpret this prescription?
A) Metoprolol 50 mg by mouth twice daily
B) Metoprolol 50 mg by mouth once daily
C) Metoprolol 50 mg intravenously twice daily
D) Metoprolol 50 mg subcutaneously twice daily

Question 29: Which type of infectious agent is primarily responsible for causing tuberculosis in humans?
A) Virus
B) Bacterium
C) Fungus
D) Protozoan

Question 30: Which of the following is the most crucial element to include in a patient's medication log to ensure compliance with legal and clinical standards?
A) Patient's full name and date of birth
B) Medication name and dosage
C) Date and time of administration
D) Prescribing physician's contact information

Question 31: Sarah, a medical assistant, is verifying insurance coverage for a new patient, Mr. Thompson. She needs to confirm whether specific procedures are covered under his current plan. What is the most critical step Sarah should take to ensure accurate verification?
A) Contact the insurance company directly to confirm coverage details.
B) Review the patient's insurance card for policy numbers and group numbers.
C) Check the clinic's electronic health record (EHR) system for previous coverage information.
D) Ask the patient for detailed information about their past medical procedures.

Question 32: Which instrument is specifically used during a gynecological examination to visualize the cervix?
A) Otoscope
B) Colposcope
C) Laryngoscope
D) Ophthalmoscope

Question 33: A 45-year-old patient has a fasting blood glucose level measured at 130 mg/dL. How should this result be interpreted?
A) Normal fasting blood glucose
B) Impaired fasting glucose
C) Diabetes mellitus
D) Hypoglycemia

Question 34: When administering a subcutaneous injection, which of the following is the most appropriate angle of needle insertion?
A) 45 degrees
B) 90 degrees
C) 15 degrees
D) 30 degrees

Question 35: Patient Maria, a 58-year-old female, presents with sudden onset of severe headache, nausea, and visual disturbances. Her blood pressure is 190/120 mmHg. Which of the following actions should the medical assistant take first?
A) Document the symptoms and schedule an urgent follow-up appointment.
B) Advise Maria to rest and monitor her symptoms at home.
C) Report the symptoms immediately to the supervising physician.
D) Administer over-the-counter pain medication and reassess in an hour.

Question 36: Emily, a CCMA, is preparing to collect multiple blood samples from a patient for various tests. Which of the following tubes should she use first to ensure accurate test results?
A) Light blue top (sodium citrate)
B) Red top (serum)
C) Lavender top (EDTA)
D) Yellow top (SPS)

Question 37: Which of the following is a critical requirement for submitting claims to third-party payers to ensure compliance and prompt reimbursement?
A) Including the patient's social security number on every claim
B) Using standardized codes from the ICD-10-CM and CPT manuals
C) Providing a detailed narrative description of each service rendered
D) Submitting claims only after receiving prior authorization for all services

Question 38: Which abbreviation correctly indicates that a medication should be administered subcutaneously?
A) IM
B) SC
C) IV
D) SL

Question 39: Which abnormal rhythm is characterized by an irregularly irregular rhythm with no distinct P waves on an ECG?
A) Atrial Fibrillation
B) Atrial Flutter
C) Ventricular Tachycardia
D) Sinus Arrhythmia

Question 40: Which instrument is essential for examining the internal structures of the ear during a general physical examination?
A) Ophthalmoscope
B) Otoscope
C) Stethoscope
D) Sphygmomanometer

Question 41: What does the abbreviation "PRN" stand for in medical terminology?
A) As Needed
B) By Mouth
C) Every Night
D) Before Meals

Question 42: Sarah, a 35-year-old patient, is scheduled for a minor surgical procedure. The medical assistant informs her about the procedure, risks, benefits, and alternatives. Sarah verbally agrees to proceed. What is the most appropriate next step to ensure compliance with consent requirements?
A) Proceed with the surgery since Sarah has verbally

agreed.
B) Document Sarah's verbal consent in her medical record.
C) Obtain Sarah's written consent before proceeding with the surgery.
D) Have Sarah sign a waiver form acknowledging her verbal agreement.

Question 43: During a minor surgical procedure, Maria, a CCMA, is preparing to assist Dr. Smith in suturing a laceration on a patient's arm. After donning sterile gloves, she accidentally touches the edge of the sterile field with her gloved hand. What should Maria do next to maintain surgical asepsis?
A) Continue with the procedure as long as her gloves appear clean.
B) Remove her gloves, perform hand hygiene, and don new sterile gloves.
C) Use an antiseptic wipe on her gloves before continuing.
D) Ask Dr. Smith to inspect her gloves for contamination.

Question 44: A 35-year-old patient named John presents with symptoms of sneezing, itchy eyes, and a runny nose. He mentions that these symptoms worsen during springtime when he spends time outdoors. Based on this information, which common allergen is most likely causing John's symptoms?
A) Dust mites
B) Pet dander
C) Tree pollen
D) Mold spores

Question 45: Which of the following steps is most critical for a Clinical Medical Assistant to ensure a successful prior authorization for a medication?
A) Verifying patient eligibility and benefits
B) Collecting relevant clinical documentation
C) Communicating directly with the prescribing physician
D) Submitting the prior authorization request promptly

Question 46: When determining the most appropriate venipuncture site for an elderly patient with fragile veins, which site is generally considered optimal?
A) Dorsal hand veins
B) Cephalic vein
C) Basilic vein
D) Median cubital vein

Question 47: You are preparing to administer a subcutaneous injection of insulin to Mr. Johnson, a 55-year-old diabetic patient. Which of the following steps is essential to ensure proper technique and absorption?
A) Pinch the skin at the injection site before inserting the needle at a 45-degree angle.
B) Insert the needle at a 90-degree angle without pinching the skin.
C) Administer the injection into the deltoid muscle.
D) Massage the injection site immediately after administering the insulin.

Question 48: Sarah, a newly graduated medical assistant, is preparing to apply for her CCMA certification. She needs to ensure she meets all the necessary requirements before submitting her application. Which of the following is a mandatory requirement for obtaining CCMA certification through the Medical-Surgical Nursing Certification Board (MSNCB)?
A) Completion of an accredited medical assisting program
B) A minimum of two years of work experience in a clinical setting
C) Passing a background check and drug screening
D) Obtaining a letter of recommendation from a licensed physician

Question 49: During a dermatological examination for Sarah, a 45-year-old patient with suspected melanoma, which of the following actions should the medical assistant prioritize to assist the provider effectively?
A) Prepare the biopsy kit and ensure proper labeling of specimens.
B) Educate Sarah about post-biopsy wound care.
C) Document Sarah's family history of skin cancer.
D) Position Sarah under adequate lighting for optimal visualization.

Question 50: Emma, a clinical medical assistant, is responsible for distributing laboratory results. After verifying that the results belong to the correct patient, John Doe, what should she do next to ensure compliance with guidelines?
A) Immediately call the ordering provider's office and verbally communicate the results.
B) Send an encrypted email with the lab results to the ordering provider.
C) Document in John Doe's medical record that the results have been distributed and then fax them to the provider.
D) Use the electronic health record (EHR) system to securely send the lab results to the ordering provider.

Question 51: Which type of suture is most appropriate for closing a subcutaneous layer due to its absorbable nature and minimal tissue reaction?
A) Polyglactin 910 (Vicryl)
B) Silk
C) Polypropylene (Prolene)
D) Nylon

Question 52: Dr. Smith is preparing an electronic prescription for his patient, John Doe. Which of the following is a legal requirement for the content and transmission of this electronic prescription?
A) The prescription must include the patient's full name and date of birth.
B) The prescription must be transmitted through a secure, encrypted system.
C) The prescription must include the prescriber's National Provider Identifier (NPI).
D) The prescription must be printed and signed before being sent electronically.

Question 53: When collecting and storing a MOLST form, which of the following steps is essential to ensure its validity and proper documentation?
A) Ensure the form is signed by both the patient and a witness.
B) Verify that the form is reviewed annually by a healthcare provider.
C) Confirm that the form is stored in the patient's electronic health record (EHR).
D) Check that the form includes specific instructions for emergency medical services (EMS).

Question 54: When communicating with elderly patients, which approach is most effective in ensuring they understand medical instructions?
A) Use medical jargon to explain conditions clearly.
B) Speak slowly and use simple language.
C) Assume they are hard of hearing and raise your voice.
D) Provide written instructions only.

Question 55: John, a 55-year-old male patient with a history of chronic obstructive pulmonary disease (COPD), presents with shortness of breath and fatigue. His vital signs are as follows: Temperature: 99.1°F, Pulse: 110 bpm, Respiration Rate: 28 breaths per minute, and Pulse Oximetry: 89%. Based on these

findings, what is the most appropriate immediate action for the medical assistant to take?
A) Administer supplemental oxygen and notify the physician.
B) Recheck the vital signs in 15 minutes.
C) Encourage deep breathing exercises and reassess in an hour.
D) Administer an antipyretic for the elevated temperature.

Question 56: Which of the following is the most accurate method for measuring a patient's blood pressure?
A) Positioning the patient's arm at heart level and using an appropriately sized cuff.
B) Using an automated blood pressure monitor while the patient is standing.
C) Measuring blood pressure immediately after the patient has exercised.
D) Taking multiple readings in quick succession without allowing rest periods.

Question 57: Which route of administration is most appropriate for a medication that requires rapid onset of action and complete absorption?
A) Intramuscular (IM)
B) Subcutaneous (SC)
C) Intravenous (IV)
D) Oral (PO)

Question 58: A patient named Mr. Thompson requires a specialized medication that is not commercially available and must be tailored to his specific needs. Which type of pharmacy is best suited to prepare this medication?
A) Retail Pharmacy
B) Hospital Pharmacy
C) Compounding Pharmacy
D) Nuclear Pharmacy

Question 59: Emily, a 45-year-old patient, comes in for staple removal following an abdominal surgery. During the procedure, you notice slight redness and swelling around the incision site. What is the most appropriate next step?
A) Proceed with removing all staples as planned.
B) Remove only half of the staples and schedule a follow-up visit.
C) Delay staple removal and consult with the physician.
D) Apply an antibiotic ointment and then proceed with staple removal.

Question 60: John, a 45-year-old male, presents with severe epigastric pain radiating to his back. Considering his symptoms and anatomical structures involved, which organ is most likely affected?
A) Liver
B) Stomach
C) Pancreas
D) Gallbladder

Question 61: During a routine EKG, a 55-year-old patient named Mr. Johnson presents with chest pain and shortness of breath. The EKG shows ST-segment elevation in leads II, III, and aVF. Which condition is most likely indicated by these findings?
A) Anterior myocardial infarction
B) Inferior myocardial infarction
C) Lateral myocardial infarction
D) Posterior myocardial infarction

Question 62: Maria, a Certified Clinical Medical Assistant (CCMA), is assisting a provider in coordinating care for a patient who requires both clinical and non-clinical services. The patient, John, has been diagnosed with diabetes and needs nutritional counseling, transportation to medical appointments, and assistance with medication management. Which of the following actions should Maria prioritize to effectively coordinate John's care with community agencies?
A) Arrange for a home health nurse to visit John for medication management.
B) Schedule an appointment with a registered dietitian for nutritional counseling.
C) Coordinate with a local transportation service to ensure John can attend his medical appointments.
D) Refer John to a social worker who can assist with accessing all required services.

Question 63: Which structure in the respiratory system is primarily responsible for gas exchange?
A) Trachea
B) Bronchi
C) Alveoli
D) Bronchioles

Question 64: Patient John Doe has been prescribed an injectable medication at a dosage of 0.5 mg/kg. John weighs 70 kg. The medication is available in vials of 50 mg/10 mL. How many milliliters should be administered to John?
A) 3 mL
B) 7 mL
C) 5 mL
D) 2.5 mL

Question 65: When developing a patient care plan, which of the following is the most critical factor to ensure effective patient outcomes?
A) Standardized treatment protocols
B) Patient's individual needs and preferences
C) Primary physician's recommendations
D) Latest clinical guidelines

Question 66: Sarah, a Certified Clinical Medical Assistant, is responsible for maintaining the inventory of clinical supplies at her clinic. She notices that several items are nearing their expiration dates. What is the most appropriate action she should take to ensure optimal inventory management?
A) Increase the reorder quantity of these items to avoid future shortages.
B) Immediately dispose of all items nearing expiration to maintain safety standards.
C) Rotate the stock by placing items with nearer expiration dates in front and using them first.
D) Delay ordering new stock until the current items are used up to minimize waste.

Question 67: During a busy shift, Medical Assistant Sarah is preparing to assist Dr. Johnson with a minor surgical procedure. She needs to ensure her hands are thoroughly clean to prevent infection. Which of the following steps is most critical in ensuring effective hand hygiene?
A) Rinsing hands thoroughly under running water before applying soap.
B) Scrubbing all surfaces of the hands, including under nails, for at least 20 seconds.
C) Using an alcohol-based hand sanitizer immediately after washing with soap and water.
D) Drying hands completely with a sterile towel after washing.

Question 68: When documenting an unusual occurrence in a healthcare setting, which of the following is the most crucial detail to include in the report?
A) The names of all staff members present during the incident.

B) A detailed description of the event, including time, location, and actions taken.
C) Personal opinions on what caused the incident.
D) The medical history of the patient involved.

Question 69: Which principle is most explicitly stated in the original Hippocratic Oath?
A) Non-maleficence
B) Beneficence
C) Autonomy
D) Justice

Question 70: A medical assistant is using scheduling software to manage appointments for Dr. Smith's clinic. One of the features they need is automated appointment reminders to reduce no-shows. Which of the following features should they prioritize in the scheduling software to achieve this goal?
A) Integration with patient electronic health records (EHR)
B) Automated SMS and email reminders
C) Real-time appointment booking updates
D) Customizable calendar views

Question 71: Emily, a 45-year-old patient with chronic illness and depression, requires coordinated care involving multiple specialties. Which resource is most appropriate for ensuring that both her medical and mental health needs are met comprehensively?
A) Social Worker
B) Psychiatrist
C) Case Manager
D) Primary Care Physician

Question 72: You are a Certified Clinical Medical Assistant tasked with collecting a blood sample from Mr. John Doe for a complete blood count (CBC) test. After drawing the blood, what is the most critical step to ensure the specimen is correctly matched and labeled?
A) Label the specimen tube immediately after drawing blood, using the patient's verbal confirmation of their name.
B) Label the specimen tube immediately after drawing blood, using information from the patient's wristband and the requisition form.
C) Label the specimen tube before drawing blood, using information from the patient's medical chart.
D) Label the specimen tube immediately after drawing blood, using information from another patient's wristband.

Question 73: Sarah, a medical assistant, is preparing to draw blood from a patient with known hepatitis B. Which of the following actions is most crucial to prevent transmission of blood-borne pathogens?
A) Wearing a surgical mask during the procedure
B) Using gloves and changing them between patients
C) Disinfecting the puncture site with alcohol before inserting the needle
D) Immediately disposing of used needles in a sharps container

Question 74: Which of the following is the most critical step in ensuring the integrity of a blood specimen for glucose testing?
A) Storing the specimen at room temperature immediately after collection
B) Mixing the blood with an anticoagulant immediately after collection
C) Transporting the specimen in a light-protected container
D) Centrifuging the specimen within 2 hours of collection

Question 75: Sarah, a Certified Clinical Medical Assistant, receives a prescription for a patient that reads "Metoprolol 50 mg PO BID." What does this abbreviation indicate?

A) Metoprolol 50 mg orally once daily
B) Metoprolol 50 mg orally twice daily
C) Metoprolol 50 mg intravenously twice daily
D) Metoprolol 50 mg subcutaneously once daily

Question 76: During a routine check-up, you are communicating with Mrs. Johnson, an elderly patient with hearing impairment. Which approach is most effective in ensuring she understands the instructions?
A) Speak loudly and slowly while maintaining eye contact.
B) Use written instructions along with verbal communication.
C) Face her directly and use clear, simple language.
D) Rely on gestures and facial expressions to convey information.

Question 77: Sarah, a medical assistant, receives a complaint from a patient named Mr. Johnson about his recent visit. He was unhappy with the long wait time and felt his concerns were not adequately addressed. What is the most appropriate action Sarah should take to facilitate service recovery?
A) Apologize to Mr. Johnson and ensure his next appointment is scheduled at a less busy time.
B) Apologize and offer Mr. Johnson a discount on his next visit.
C) Apologize, document the complaint, and follow up with Mr. Johnson after discussing it with the clinic manager.
D) Apologize and immediately schedule an appointment for Mr. Johnson with another provider.

Question 78: Emily, a 30-year-old patient, is in your clinic for a routine check-up. Suddenly, she develops hives, facial swelling, and begins to experience difficulty breathing. As a Certified Clinical Medical Assistant (CCMA), what is the most appropriate immediate response?
A) Administer oral antihistamines and observe for any changes.
B) Provide an intramuscular injection of epinephrine and call emergency services.
C) Apply a cold compress to reduce swelling and monitor her vital signs.
D) Offer the patient water and instruct her to lie down while you contact her primary care physician.

Question 79: Which lifestyle modification is most effective in reducing the risk of cardiovascular disease according to contemporary research?
A) Increasing physical activity
B) Reducing dietary sodium intake
C) Quitting smoking
D) Managing stress levels

Question 80: Which of the following scenarios requires mandatory reporting by a Certified Clinical Medical Assistant (CCMA) under legal requirements?
A) A patient discloses they have been using illegal drugs recreationally.
B) A patient reveals they have been experiencing domestic violence.
C) A patient admits to having consensual sexual relations with multiple partners.
D) A patient confesses to frequently missing doses of prescribed medication.

Question 81: Which cellular organelle is primarily responsible for the synthesis of lipids and detoxification of drugs?
A) Mitochondria
B) Rough Endoplasmic Reticulum
C) Smooth Endoplasmic Reticulum
D) Golgi Apparatus

Question 82: Which credential is specifically designated for a medical assistant who has successfully passed the certification exam administered by the National Healthcareer Association (NHA)?
A) CMA (Certified Medical Assistant)
B) CCMA (Certified Clinical Medical Assistant)
C) RMA (Registered Medical Assistant)
D) CMAC (Clinical Medical Assistant Certified)

Question 83: Mr. Smith, a 68-year-old male with a history of hypertension and diabetes, presents with shortness of breath, fatigue, and peripheral edema. His echocardiogram reveals an ejection fraction of 35%. Which pathophysiological mechanism is primarily responsible for his symptoms?
A) Increased preload due to renal sodium retention
B) Decreased cardiac output due to systolic dysfunction
C) Increased afterload due to systemic hypertension
D) Decreased myocardial oxygen supply due to coronary artery disease

Question 84: Patient John Doe visits the clinic for a follow-up on his Type 2 Diabetes Mellitus management. During the visit, he also mentions experiencing mild chest pain. As a Certified Clinical Medical Assistant (CCMA), how should you prepare the documentation and billing request using current coding guidelines?
A) Document and code only the follow-up visit for Type 2 Diabetes Mellitus.
B) Document and code both the follow-up visit for Type 2 Diabetes Mellitus and the new symptom of chest pain.
C) Document only the new symptom of chest pain and code it as a primary diagnosis.
D) Document and code only the most severe condition, which is chest pain.

Question 85: When performing venipuncture, which of the following is the most appropriate angle for needle insertion to ensure successful access to the vein while minimizing patient discomfort and risk of complications?
A) 15-30 degrees
B) 5-10 degrees
C) 45-60 degrees
D) 75-90 degrees

Question 86: When answering a call in a medical office, which of the following practices best demonstrates professional telephone etiquette?
A) Answering with a cheerful tone and stating your name and department.
B) Answering promptly within three rings and asking, "How can I help you today?"
C) Answering with a neutral tone and stating the clinic's name followed by your name.
D) Answering promptly within three rings and stating the clinic's name followed by "How may I assist you?"

Question 87: Which of the following is a key requirement for COLA accreditation regarding quality control in laboratory testing?
A) Laboratories must perform quality control tests daily on all instruments.
B) Laboratories must document all quality control results and review them monthly.
C) Laboratories must ensure that quality control samples are run with each batch of patient specimens.
D) Laboratories must calibrate their instruments annually.

Question 88: What is the most crucial instruction to give a patient preparing for a colonoscopy?
A) Consume a high-fiber diet 48 hours before the procedure.
B) Avoid eating solid foods the day before the procedure.

C) Take all prescribed medications, including blood thinners, as usual.
D) Drink plenty of water up until the time of the procedure.

Question 89: Which scenario would require a Certified Clinical Medical Assistant (CCMA) to make a mandatory report to child protective services?
A) A 16-year-old patient discloses consensual sexual activity with a peer.
B) A 14-year-old patient presents with unexplained bruises and reports fear of going home.
C) An 18-year-old patient mentions past physical abuse that occurred when they were 10 years old.
D) A 17-year-old patient reports substance use at a party.

Question 90: Which of the following tasks is primarily associated with maintaining patient confidentiality in a clinical setting?
A) Filing patient records accurately
B) Ensuring secure communication channels
C) Scheduling patient appointments
D) Verifying patient insurance information

Question 91: During a routine check-up, Maria, a medical assistant, needs to draw blood from a patient with a suspected respiratory infection. Which sequence of Personal Protective Equipment (PPE) should Maria follow when donning and doffing to ensure maximum infection control?
A) Donning: Gown, Mask, Gloves; Doffing: Gloves, Gown, Mask
B) Donning: Gloves, Mask, Gown; Doffing: Mask, Gloves, Gown
C) Donning: Mask, Gown, Gloves; Doffing: Gloves, Gown, Mask
D) Donning: Gown, Gloves, Mask; Doffing: Gown, Mask, Gloves

Question 92: During a routine vision screening, you use the Snellen eye chart to test Mr. Johnson's visual acuity. He can read the 20/40 line with his right eye but struggles with the 20/30 line. What is the correct documentation of Mr. Johnson's visual acuity for his right eye?
A) 20/40
B) 20/30
C) 20/50
D) 20/20

Question 93: A 45-year-old male presents with confusion, rapid breathing, fruity-smelling breath, and abdominal pain. What is the most likely diagnosis?
A) Diabetic ketoacidosis (DKA)
B) Heat stroke
C) Anaphylactic shock
D) Seizure

Question 94: Mrs. Johnson, a diabetic patient, is scheduled for minor surgery involving reusable surgical instruments. As a certified clinical medical assistant, which sterilization technique should you use to ensure the instruments are free from all forms of microbial life, including spores?
A) Autoclave
B) Instrument Cleaner
C) Germicidal Disinfectants
D) Disposables

Question 95: Emily, a 5-year-old girl, visits the clinic for her annual check-up. Her height and weight are plotted on the CDC growth chart. Her height is at the 25th percentile, and her weight is at the 75th percentile. Based on this information, what is the most appropriate

interpretation of Emily's growth pattern?
A) Emily's height and weight are both within normal limits.
B) Emily may be at risk for being overweight.
C) Emily's height is concerningly low for her age.
D) Emily's weight is concerningly high for her age.

Question 96: During her shift, Medical Assistant Sarah is documenting patient care for Mr. Johnson, who was admitted with severe dehydration. Which of the following actions is MOST appropriate for Sarah to ensure accurate and compliant documentation in Mr. Johnson's patient record?
A) Documenting Mr. Johnson's symptoms and interventions immediately after each interaction.
B) Summarizing all care provided at the end of her shift.
C) Using abbreviations that are commonly understood by all medical staff.
D) Including subjective opinions about Mr. Johnson's condition.

Question 97: During her shift, Medical Assistant Sarah witnesses a patient, Mr. Johnson, slip and fall in the hallway. What is the most appropriate immediate action Sarah should take according to incident/event/unusual occurrence report protocols?
A) Assist Mr. Johnson and immediately notify the attending physician.
B) Complete an incident report after ensuring Mr. Johnson's safety.
C) Call for help and document the incident in Mr. Johnson's medical record.
D) Ensure Mr. Johnson is safe and then notify the nurse manager before completing an incident report.

Question 98: Which route of administration is characterized by rapid absorption through the mucous membranes under the tongue?
A) Sublingual
B) Buccal
C) Intranasal
D) Transdermal

Question 99: During a routine check-up, Sarah, a medical assistant, notices bruises on Mrs. Thompson's arms that resemble handprints. When asked about them, Mrs. Thompson hesitates and then mentions she fell down the stairs. Sarah suspects domestic abuse but is unsure whether this incident is legally reportable. What should Sarah do according to legal requirements regarding reportable violations or incidents?
A) Document the observation in Mrs. Thompson's medical record and monitor for further signs.
B) Report the suspicion of abuse to the appropriate authorities immediately.
C) Discuss her concerns with a colleague to seek their opinion before taking any action.
D) Wait until Mrs. Thompson confirms abuse before making any report.

Question 100: Patient John is prescribed a medication that needs to be absorbed through the skin for localized treatment of inflammation. Which form of medication is most appropriate for this purpose?
A) Pill
B) Capsule
C) Ointment
D) Liquid

Question 101: Which cytochrome P450 enzyme is primarily responsible for the metabolism of approximately 50% of all clinically used drugs?
A) CYP1A2
B) CYP2C9

C) CYP2D6
D) CYP3A4

Question 102: When performing a capillary puncture on an adult patient, which site is most appropriate to obtain an accurate blood sample while minimizing discomfort and risk of complications?
A) The tip of the index finger
B) The lateral side of the heel
C) The palmar surface of the ring finger
D) The earlobe

Question 103: What is the primary reason for allowing a blood sample to clot completely before centrifugation when preparing serum?
A) To prevent hemolysis
B) To ensure complete separation of serum from cells
C) To avoid contamination of the sample
D) To enhance the accuracy of biochemical tests

Question 104: Maria has scheduled an appointment with Dr. Smith for a routine follow-up visit. Dr. Smith prefers follow-up visits to be scheduled for 20 minutes to allow adequate time for patient interaction and review of medical history. However, Maria also needs a flu shot during this visit. How should the medical assistant adjust the duration of Maria's visit?
A) Schedule the visit for 20 minutes as per Dr. Smith's preference.
B) Schedule the visit for 30 minutes to accommodate both the follow-up and flu shot.
C) Schedule two separate visits: one for the follow-up and one for the flu shot.
D) Schedule the visit for 25 minutes, combining both purposes in a single session.

Question 105: What is the recommended storage condition for a multi-dose vial of insulin after it has been opened?
A) Store at room temperature for up to 28 days.
B) Store in the refrigerator at 2-8°C (36-46°F) for up to 14 days.
C) Store at room temperature for up to 14 days.
D) Store in the refrigerator at 2-8°C (36-46°F) for up to 28 days.

Question 106: Under which condition is it legally permissible for a medical assistant to release patient information without explicit consent from the patient?
A) When the information is requested by an insurance company for billing purposes.
B) When the information is necessary to prevent a serious threat to public health or safety.
C) When another healthcare provider requests it for continuity of care.
D) When a family member inquires about the patient's condition.

Question 107: During an EKG procedure for Mr. Johnson, you notice that the tracing is erratic and inconsistent. Which of the following actions is most likely to correct this issue?
A) Replace the EKG paper with a new roll.
B) Ensure all leads are properly attached and making good contact with the skin.
C) Increase the sensitivity setting on the EKG machine.
D) Adjust the speed setting of the EKG paper.

Question 108: Which of the following is a common side effect of Metformin?
A) Lactic acidosis
B) Hypoglycemia
C) Gastrointestinal upset

D) Weight gain

Question 109: Which of the following is the most effective precaution to prevent the transmission of blood-borne pathogens in a clinical setting?
A) Wearing gloves during patient contact
B) Using alcohol-based hand sanitizer after patient contact
C) Proper disposal of used needles and sharps
D) Wearing a surgical mask during procedures

Question 110: Which of the following online resources is most commonly used by clinical medical assistants to verify drug interactions and obtain comprehensive drug information?
A) MedlinePlus
B) Epocrates
C) WebMD
D) Mayo Clinic

Question 111: Sarah, a 68-year-old Medicare beneficiary, is scheduled for a routine screening mammogram. However, her physician also recommends an additional diagnostic mammogram due to a recent concern. What should the medical assistant do to ensure compliance with Medicare regulations regarding the ABN?
A) Provide Sarah with an ABN before performing the routine screening mammogram.
B) Provide Sarah with an ABN before performing the diagnostic mammogram.
C) Provide Sarah with an ABN after performing both the screening and diagnostic mammograms.
D) Do not provide Sarah with an ABN as it is not required for either procedure.

Question 112: During a routine blood draw, Maria notices that her patient, Mr. Johnson, is exhibiting signs of anxiety. Which of the following actions should Maria take first to accurately assess Mr. Johnson's comfort and anxiety level?
A) Ask Mr. Johnson directly if he is feeling anxious about the procedure.
B) Observe Mr. Johnson's body language and facial expressions for signs of discomfort.
C) Review Mr. Johnson's medical history for any previous issues with phlebotomy.
D) Explain the procedure in detail to Mr. Johnson to alleviate his anxiety.

Question 113: Sarah, a Certified Clinical Medical Assistant (CCMA), is preparing a claim for Medicare reimbursement. She must ensure that all services provided are documented correctly to comply with CMS billing requirements. Which of the following actions is crucial for Sarah to avoid claim denial?
A) Including the patient's demographic information only.
B) Ensuring all provided services are medically necessary and documented.
C) Listing only the primary diagnosis code.
D) Submitting claims without verifying insurance coverage.

Question 114: A patient presents with shortness of breath, chest pain, and sweating. Which of the following should be documented and reported immediately as a potential sign of a myocardial infarction (heart attack)?
A) Shortness of breath
B) Chest pain
C) Sweating
D) All of the above

Question 115: You are a medical assistant tasked with drafting an email to inform Mrs. Johnson about her upcoming appointment and necessary pre-appointment instructions. Which of the following is the most appropriate way to ensure clarity and professionalism in your email?
A) "Hi Mrs. Johnson, Your appointment is on Friday at 10 AM. Please come fasting."
B) "Dear Mrs. Johnson, Your appointment is scheduled for Friday at 10 AM. Please ensure you fast for 12 hours prior."
C) "Hello Mrs. Johnson, Just a reminder about your appointment on Friday at 10 AM. Don't eat anything before coming."
D) "Mrs. Johnson, Appointment on Friday at 10 AM. Fast before."

Question 116: Sarah, a 30-year-old woman, has recently been experiencing significant stress at work. Instead of acknowledging her anxiety, she begins to excessively clean her house and organize her belongings. Which defense mechanism is Sarah most likely exhibiting?
A) Displacement
B) Projection
C) Sublimation
D) Reaction Formation

Question 117: Patient John Doe requires an MRI scan for a suspected spinal injury. As a Certified Clinical Medical Assistant (CCMA), you need to obtain insurance authorization before scheduling the procedure. What is the most critical step in this process?
A) Submitting a detailed clinical report from the physician to the insurance company.
B) Verifying the patient's insurance coverage and benefits before contacting the insurance company.
C) Scheduling the MRI scan and informing the patient about potential out-of-pocket costs.
D) Contacting the insurance company directly to request pre-authorization without verifying coverage first.

Question 118: A 45-year-old patient presents with fatigue, weight loss, and hyperpigmentation of the skin. Which condition is most likely responsible for these symptoms?
A) Addison's disease
B) Cushing's syndrome
C) Hyperthyroidism
D) Hypothyroidism

Question 119: Sarah is scheduled for a colonoscopy next week. As her medical assistant, you need to provide her with pre-procedural instructions. Which of the following instructions is most accurate?
A) "You should avoid all solid foods and drink only clear liquids starting 24 hours before the procedure."
B) "You can have a light breakfast on the morning of the procedure, but avoid dairy products."
C) "You should stop eating solid foods and switch to clear liquids starting 48 hours before the procedure."
D) "You can continue your regular diet until 12 hours before the procedure."

Question 120: Which of the following tasks is within the scope of practice for a Certified Clinical Medical Assistant (CCMA)?
A) Administering intramuscular injections
B) Prescribing medications
C) Interpreting diagnostic test results
D) Performing minor surgical procedures

Question 121: Which interval on an EKG represents the time from the onset of atrial depolarization to the onset of ventricular depolarization?
A) PR Interval
B) QT Interval
C) ST Segment
D) QRS Complex

Question 122: When preparing a patient for a Holter monitor test, which of the following steps is crucial to ensure accurate data collection?
A) Instructing the patient to avoid bathing during the monitoring period
B) Advising the patient to maintain their usual daily activities
C) Ensuring the patient fasts for at least 8 hours before application
D) Recommending the patient avoids caffeine on the day of application

Question 123: Which of the following tasks is primarily the responsibility of a Clinical Medical Assistant when managing patient care?
A) Administering intravenous medications
B) Preparing patients for minor surgical procedures
C) Diagnosing medical conditions
D) Developing patient treatment plans

Question 124: John, a 45-year-old male, presents with acute chest pain radiating to his left arm and shortness of breath. The attending physician orders an electrocardiogram (ECG) and cardiac enzyme tests. Which of the following is the most appropriate initial treatment modality if the results indicate an acute myocardial infarction?
A) Administering aspirin
B) Starting intravenous nitroglycerin
C) Initiating thrombolytic therapy
D) Providing supplemental oxygen

Question 125: When obtaining a manual blood pressure reading, which of the following is crucial for ensuring an accurate measurement?
A) Ensuring the patient's arm is at heart level
B) Using a cuff that is too small for the patient's arm
C) Placing the stethoscope directly over the radial artery
D) Deflating the cuff rapidly to avoid discomfort

Question 126: When assisting a provider with a patient presenting with a minor laceration, what is the most appropriate initial step to ensure proper wound management?
A) Apply an antibiotic ointment immediately.
B) Irrigate the wound thoroughly with sterile saline.
C) Cover the wound with a sterile gauze pad.
D) Administer a tetanus shot immediately.

Question 127: John, a 45-year-old male with a history of cardiovascular disease, is advised to modify his diet to manage his condition better. Which of the following dietary changes is most beneficial for reducing his risk of further cardiovascular complications?
A) Increase intake of saturated fats.
B) Increase intake of omega-3 fatty acids.
C) Increase intake of trans fats.
D) Increase intake of refined carbohydrates.

Question 128: What is the most appropriate first step a Certified Clinical Medical Assistant (CCMA) should take when preparing a patient for a routine venipuncture?
A) Identify the patient using two identifiers.
B) Apply a tourniquet above the venipuncture site.
C) Assemble all necessary equipment.
D) Cleanse the venipuncture site with an antiseptic swab.

Question 129: Sarah, a medical assistant, receives a call from a patient's family member requesting information about the patient's recent surgery. Which action should Sarah take to comply with legal and regulatory requirements?
A) Provide the information only if the caller is an immediate family member.
B) Confirm the patient's identity before providing any information.
C) Refer the caller to the physician for more detailed information.
D) Verify that the patient has given explicit consent before sharing any information.

Question 130: Which of the following services is most likely to be provided by a specialist rather than a general practitioner?
A) Routine physical examinations
B) Management of chronic conditions like diabetes
C) Advanced cardiac care and interventions
D) Immunizations and vaccinations

Question 131: John, a 45-year-old male patient, presents with complaints of hearing difficulties and frequent ear infections. As part of his assessment, you perform tympanometry to evaluate his middle ear function. Which tympanometric finding would most likely indicate Eustachian tube dysfunction?
A) Type A tympanogram
B) Type B tympanogram
C) Type C tympanogram
D) Type Ad tympanogram

Question 132: Which of the following procedures is most effective in minimizing artifacts during an EKG recording?
A) Ensuring the patient is lying still and relaxed
B) Cleaning the skin with alcohol before electrode placement
C) Using a higher sensitivity setting on the EKG machine
D) Placing electrodes over bony prominences for better adherence

Question 133: According to Kübler-Ross's model, which stage of grief is characterized by a person's attempt to make deals or promises in hopes of reversing or delaying the loss?
A) Denial
B) Bargaining
C) Depression
D) Acceptance

Question 134: Sarah, a 30-year-old patient, presents with symptoms of seasonal allergies. As a Certified Clinical Medical Assistant, you are tasked with performing an allergy test to determine the specific allergens causing her symptoms. Which of the following is the most appropriate initial test to perform?
A) Intradermal skin test
B) Patch test
C) Serum-specific IgE test
D) Skin prick test

Question 135: Jane, a 28-year-old patient with a history of seasonal allergies, is undergoing allergy testing. The physician decides to use both scratch and intradermal tests. After performing the scratch test, the physician observes no reaction and proceeds with the intradermal test. Within 15 minutes, Jane develops a wheal and flare reaction at one of the intradermal test sites. What does this indicate?
A) Jane is allergic to the allergen tested in the scratch test.
B) Jane is allergic to the allergen tested in the intradermal test.
C) Jane has no allergies since there was no reaction in the scratch test.
D) Jane's reaction indicates a false positive result.

Question 136: Patient Maria presents with symptoms of a urinary tract infection (UTI). As a medical assistant,

you are required to perform a CLIA-waived urinalysis test. After obtaining the sample, what is the most crucial next step to ensure accurate results?
A) Immediately refrigerate the urine sample until testing can be performed.
B) Label the sample with the patient's name and date of collection before proceeding.
C) Mix the urine sample thoroughly before dipping the test strip.
D) Ensure that the test strip is fully immersed in the urine for at least 30 seconds.

Question 137: What is the correct order of cleaning surfaces in a clinical setting to ensure optimal infection control?
A) Clean with detergent, then disinfect with bleach, followed by sterilization.
B) Disinfect with bleach, clean with detergent, followed by sterilization.
C) Clean with detergent, disinfect with alcohol-based solution, followed by sterilization.
D) Sterilize first, then clean with detergent, followed by disinfection.

Question 138: Mr. Johnson, a 75-year-old patient with terminal cancer, has an advanced directive specifying that he does not want any life-prolonging treatments if his condition becomes irreversible. During a routine check-up, he mentions to his medical assistant that he has changed his mind and wants all possible measures taken to prolong his life. What should the medical assistant do next?
A) Update the advanced directive immediately as per Mr. Johnson's verbal request.
B) Inform Mr. Johnson that changes can only be made by his primary physician.
C) Advise Mr. Johnson to discuss his wishes with his healthcare proxy.
D) Suggest Mr. Johnson complete a new advanced directive form and have it witnessed.

Question 139: Mr. Johnson, a 65-year-old patient with diabetes, is admitted for a minor surgical procedure. As a Certified Clinical Medical Assistant (CCMA), you are responsible for his preoperative care. After helping him use the restroom, what is the most appropriate hand hygiene practice before assisting another patient?
A) Use an alcohol-based hand sanitizer for at least 20 seconds.
B) Wash hands with soap and water for at least 15 seconds.
C) Use an alcohol-based hand sanitizer for at least 15 seconds.
D) Wash hands with soap and water for at least 20 seconds.

Question 140: Emily, a Certified Clinical Medical Assistant (CCMA), is preparing to fax a patient's medical records to a specialist for further consultation. What is the most appropriate action Emily should take to ensure compliance with patient privacy and confidentiality regulations?
A) Fax the records directly without additional steps since it is for medical purposes.
B) Call the specialist's office to confirm the fax number before sending the records.
C) Send an email to the specialist confirming that she has sent the fax.
D) Include a cover sheet with a confidentiality statement when faxing the records.

Question 141: Sarah, a 45-year-old woman with a history of hypertension and diabetes, presents with chest pain and shortness of breath. The physician orders an echocardiogram to assess her heart function. As a

Certified Clinical Medical Assistant, how would you determine if this procedure meets medical necessity guidelines?
A) Review Sarah's symptoms and medical history to ensure they align with the indications for an echocardiogram.
B) Check if Sarah has insurance coverage for echocardiograms as per her policy.
C) Confirm that the physician's order includes detailed documentation of Sarah's symptoms and clinical findings.
D) Ensure that the echocardiogram is listed as a standard diagnostic tool for hypertension in clinical guidelines.

Question 142: Which of the following is the most critical step in ensuring accurate calibration of clinical laboratory equipment?
A) Regularly scheduling calibration checks
B) Using certified reference materials
C) Documenting calibration procedures
D) Training staff on calibration techniques

Question 143: Sarah, a Certified Clinical Medical Assistant, is responsible for managing the medication storage at her clinic. She notices that a bottle of insulin has been left out of the refrigerator overnight. What should Sarah do according to proper storage and disposal protocols?
A) Return the insulin to the refrigerator immediately.
B) Discard the insulin as it may have lost its potency.
C) Store the insulin at room temperature for up to 28 days.
D) Consult with a pharmacist before deciding on further action.

Question 144: When dealing with a highly agitated patient who is upset about a long wait time, what is the most effective initial step a medical assistant should take?
A) Apologize for the wait and assure them it won't happen again.
B) Listen actively to the patient's concerns without interrupting.
C) Explain the reasons for the delay in detail.
D) Offer to reschedule their appointment at a more convenient time.

Question 145: Which form of medication is designed to dissolve slowly in the mouth to provide a localized effect?
A) Capsule
B) Pill
C) Lozenge
D) Ointment

Question 146: A patient named Sarah is seeking primary care services and requires a referral for a specialist consultation. In which type of health care setting would Sarah most likely start her journey?
A) Urgent Care Center
B) Hospital Emergency Department
C) Primary Care Physician's Office
D) Specialty Clinic

Question 147: Which EKG finding is most indicative of an acute myocardial infarction (AMI)?
A) ST-segment elevation
B) T-wave inversion
C) Prolonged PR interval
D) QRS complex widening

Question 148: Maria, a 5-year-old child from a non-English speaking family, is scheduled for a routine vaccination. Which communication strategy should the medical assistant prioritize to ensure Maria understands the procedure?

A) Use simple medical terminology and speak slowly.
B) Employ visual aids and gestures to demonstrate the procedure.
C) Provide written instructions translated into the family's language.
D) Rely on a family member to translate complex information.

Question 149: When verifying diagnostic and procedural codes, which step is essential to ensure the accuracy and appropriateness of the codes used?
A) Cross-referencing the codes with the patient's medical history.
B) Using only the most recent version of the coding manual.
C) Ensuring that the codes are consistent with the physician's documentation.
D) Double-checking that all codes are within the same category.

Question 150: When performing a standard 12-lead EKG, where should the V1 electrode be placed?
A) Fourth intercostal space at the left sternal border
B) Fourth intercostal space at the right sternal border
C) Fifth intercostal space at the left midclavicular line
D) Fifth intercostal space at the right midclavicular line

ANSWER WITH DETAILED EXPLANATION SET [1]

Question 1: Correct Answer: A) Celebrex and Celexa
Rationale: Celebrex (celecoxib) is a nonsteroidal anti-inflammatory drug (NSAID), while Celexa (citalopram) is an antidepressant. Their similar-sounding names can lead to confusion, particularly in busy clinical settings. Zantac (ranitidine) and Xanax (alprazolam), Lamictal (lamotrigine) and Lamisil (terbinafine), and Plavix (clopidogrel) and Paxil (paroxetine) also have similar-sounding names but are less commonly confused compared to Celebrex and Celexa. Understanding these distinctions is crucial for preventing medication errors. - Celebrex vs. Celexa: Both have similar-sounding names but very different uses—one for pain/inflammation, the other for depression. - Zantac vs. Xanax: Though they sound alike, their indications (acid reflux vs. anxiety) make them less likely to be confused. - Lamictal vs. Lamisil: These sound similar but treat vastly different conditions (seizures vs. fungal infections). - Plavix vs. Paxil: Despite their phonetic resemblance, their purposes (blood thinner vs. antidepressant) reduce confusion risk. The correct option highlights the importance of distinguishing medications with similar names but different uses, emphasizing patient safety in pharmacology.

Question 2: Correct Answer: B) Common side effect of Lisinopril
Rationale: The persistent dry cough is a well-documented common side effect of Lisinopril, an ACE inhibitor. While an allergic reaction (Option A) could cause respiratory symptoms, it typically presents with more severe reactions such as rash or swelling. An adverse effect (Option C) implies a more severe or harmful reaction than what is commonly expected; however, the dry cough is not considered harmful. A contraindication (Option D) would prevent the use of Lisinopril altogether, which does not apply in this case since the patient was already prescribed and started on the medication.

Question 3: Correct Answer: C) A telehealth service for remote monitoring and consultations.
Rationale: Telehealth services provide continuous remote monitoring and consultations, which are crucial for managing chronic conditions like COPD. This resource allows healthcare providers to track Mrs. Johnson's health status in real-time, adjust treatments promptly, and prevent potential complications that could lead to readmission. - Option A is incorrect because while visiting nurses can help with medication administration, they do not offer the comprehensive monitoring needed for chronic conditions. - Option B is incorrect as physical therapy alone does not address the overall management of COPD. - Option D is incorrect because although social workers provide valuable support, they do not offer medical oversight necessary for preventing readmission. Thus, telehealth services are optimal for ensuring continuity of care in this scenario.

Question 4: Correct Answer: A) Improper hand hygiene by healthcare workers
Rationale: Improper hand hygiene by healthcare workers is a primary factor in breaking the chain of infection and leading to secondary infections like pneumonia. While contaminated catheters (B), lack of isolation precautions (C), and improper sterilization (D) are significant, they do not directly address how E. coli from a UTI could lead to pneumonia. Proper hand hygiene prevents cross-contamination and transmission from one body site or patient to another, making it critical in this scenario.

Question 5: Correct Answer: C) Switch to using pre-sterilized disposable instruments.
Rationale: The most appropriate immediate action is to switch to using pre-sterilized disposable instruments (Option C). This ensures sterility without delay. Re-running through the autoclave (Option A) is not feasible due to time constraints and uncertainty about complete repair. Chemical sterilization (Option B) might not be suitable for all instruments and takes longer. Manual cleaning followed by high-level disinfection (Option D) does not guarantee complete sterility required for surgical procedures. Using pre-sterilized disposable instruments ensures compliance with infection control standards immediately.

Question 6: Correct Answer: A) To identify overdue patient accounts for follow-up
Rationale: The primary purpose of an aging report is to identify overdue patient accounts for follow-up. This helps in managing collections and ensuring timely payments. Option B is incorrect because revenue generation is not the main focus of aging reports. Option C is misleading as it pertains to scheduling, not financial tracking. Option D, while important, relates to performance metrics rather than financial oversight through aging reports. Understanding these distinctions is crucial for effective administrative assisting in a medical setting.

Question 7: Correct Answer: C) Alphabetical
Rationale: The alphabetical filing system is ideal for organizing patient records by last name, allowing for quick and efficient retrieval. This system is straightforward and commonly used in medical practices where patient names are the primary identifier. In contrast, numerical filing (A) is better suited for large volumes of records requiring unique identifiers; subject filing (B) categorizes information by topic rather than individual; and geographical filing (D) organizes records by location, which is less practical for patient records. Each option has its merits but does not match the efficiency of alphabetical filing for this specific need.

Question 8: Correct Answer: B) Performing daily quality control checks on POCT devices.
Rationale: Daily quality control checks are essential for maintaining the accuracy and reliability of POCT results. These checks ensure that the device is functioning correctly and producing valid results. While regularly updating software (A), using certified personnel (C), and annual calibration (D) are important, they do not provide the immediate assurance of accuracy that daily quality control checks offer. Regular updates may improve functionality but don't directly verify current performance. Certified personnel ensure proper use but can't guarantee device accuracy without QC checks. Annual calibration is too infrequent to catch daily variations or issues.

Question 9: Correct Answer: B) Position the patient in the lithotomy position.
Rationale: Positioning the patient in the lithotomy position is crucial for a gynecological examination as it allows optimal access for the provider to perform an accurate assessment. While ensuring an empty bladder (Option A), preparing specimen containers (Option C), and verifying medical history (Option D) are all important steps, they are secondary to proper patient positioning. Correct positioning directly impacts the provider's ability to conduct a thorough examination and obtain accurate results.

Question 10: Correct Answer: B) Actively listening to the caregiver's concerns and validating their feelings before discussing potential solutions.
Rationale: Active listening and validation are essential in de-escalating emotionally charged situations. This approach demonstrates empathy and builds trust, making caregivers feel heard and respected. Option A may come across as dismissive; Option C can seem like avoidance; Option D might overwhelm or confuse rather than reassure. Active listening addresses emotional needs first, laying a foundation for effective problem-solving.

Question 11: Correct Answer: D) Consult with your supervisor before making any changes to ensure compliance with office policies.
Rationale: Consulting with your supervisor ensures adherence to office policies and legal requirements. Simply deleting (Option A) or merging (Option B) entries without proper documentation could violate compliance standards. Leaving both entries (Option C) can lead to confusion and inaccuracies in patient care. Supervisory consultation aligns with best practices for maintaining compliant and accurate medical records.

Question 12: Correct Answer: B) Contact John's insurance provider to confirm receipt of the forms.
Rationale: After filling out and submitting the necessary forms, it is crucial for Maria to contact John's insurance provider to confirm they have received the forms and to check on the status of the authorization. This step ensures there are no delays or issues with obtaining approval. Options A, C, and D are incorrect because submitting forms directly to the MRI facility or proceeding without confirmation can lead to denial of coverage or delays in care. - Option A is incorrect because submitting forms directly to the MRI facility bypasses necessary verification by the insurance provider. - Option C is incorrect as scheduling before confirmation risks unauthorized services. - Option D is incorrect since informing John prematurely could lead to misunderstandings about his coverage status.

Question 13: Correct Answer: A) The document must be signed by the patient and two witnesses.
Rationale: For a healthcare proxy to be valid, it typically requires the signature of the patient and two witnesses. This ensures that the patient's wishes are clearly documented and legally recognized. While notarization (Option B) can add an extra layer of verification, it is not always required. Including medical history (Option C) or specifying a primary care physician (Option D) are not necessary for the validity of a healthcare proxy but may provide additional context for care decisions.

Question 14: Correct Answer: C) Balm
Rationale: A balm is designed for topical application and provides localized relief by staying on the surface of the skin. Unlike ointments, which may penetrate deeper, balms are thicker and remain on the skin's surface. Liquids and elixirs are not suitable as they are typically ingested or used for systemic effects rather than topical application. Therefore, a balm is the most appropriate choice for Sarah's condition. - Option A (Liquid): Incorrect because liquids are generally intended for oral ingestion or other systemic uses, not for topical application. - Option B (Elixir): Incorrect as elixirs are also meant for oral consumption and contain alcohol, which is unsuitable for topical pain relief. - Option D (Ointment): Incorrect because ointments can penetrate deeper into the skin layers, whereas Sarah needs a medication that stays on the surface. This comprehensive analysis ensures that each option is closely related but distinct in its purpose and application method, making the question challenging yet fair.

Question 15: Correct Answer: C) Initiative vs. Guilt
Rationale: According to Erikson, children aged 3-6 years are in the "Initiative vs. Guilt" stage, where they begin to assert control and power over their environment through directing play and social interactions. "Trust vs. Mistrust" (A) occurs from birth to 18 months, focusing on developing trust when caregivers provide reliability. "Autonomy vs. Shame and Doubt" (B) occurs from 18 months to 3 years, where children develop personal control over physical skills and independence. "Industry vs. Inferiority" (D) occurs from ages 6-12, focusing on mastering knowledge and intellectual skills.

Question 16: Correct Answer: B) Obtain and verify the patient's informed consent before starting the procedure.
Rationale: Obtaining and verifying informed consent is crucial as it ensures that the patient understands the procedure, risks, benefits, and alternatives, thus respecting

their autonomy. Option A is incorrect because fasting is not always required for minor procedures. Option C, while important for comfort and access, is secondary to obtaining consent. Option D is also important but typically occurs after explaining and obtaining consent. Therefore, B is essential to proceed ethically and legally with any medical procedure.

Question 17: Correct Answer: B) Venous duplex ultrasound
Rationale: Venous duplex ultrasound is the gold standard for diagnosing deep vein thrombosis (DVT) due to its high sensitivity and specificity. The D-dimer test (A) can indicate clot presence but is not definitive. MRI (C) is used for more detailed imaging but is not first-line for DVT. CT angiography (D) is primarily used for pulmonary embolism, not DVT. Thus, venous duplex ultrasound (B) remains the most accurate initial diagnostic tool for confirming DVT in patients with symptoms like unilateral leg swelling and pain.

Question 18: Correct Answer: B) Schedule II
Rationale: Schedule II drugs have a high potential for abuse, which may lead to severe psychological or physical dependence, but they also have accepted medical uses. In contrast: - Schedule I drugs (Option A) have no accepted medical use and a high potential for abuse. - Schedule III drugs (Option C) have a moderate to low potential for physical and psychological dependence. - Schedule IV drugs (Option D) have a low potential for abuse relative to substances in Schedule III. Understanding these distinctions is crucial for medical assistants managing medications under controlled substances regulations.

Question 19: Correct Answer: C) Listen to their concerns empathetically, explain the potential side effects clearly, and provide written information.
Rationale: Option C is correct because it combines empathy (listening to concerns), clarity (explaining side effects), and providing additional resources (written information). This approach aligns with contemporary communication theories emphasizing active listening and comprehensive information sharing. Option A lacks empathy and detailed information. Option B provides clarity but misses empathetic listening. Option D deflects responsibility without addressing immediate concerns.

Question 20: Correct Answer: A) Documenting events immediately after they occur
Rationale: Documenting events immediately after they occur is crucial for maintaining accuracy and reliability in medical records. This practice helps ensure that details are fresh in the provider's memory, reducing the risk of errors or omissions. While using medical jargon (B), including only relevant information (C), and using abbreviations (D) have their places in documentation, none are as critical as timely documentation. Medical jargon can be confusing, abbreviations can lead to misinterpretation, and deciding relevance can be subjective. Timeliness ensures that all other aspects of documentation are built on accurate and complete information.

Question 21: Correct Answer: A) Ensuring the test strip is not expired
Rationale: Ensuring that the test strip is not expired is crucial because expired strips can give inaccurate results due to degradation of reactive chemicals. While calibration (B) is important, it is typically done periodically rather than before each use. Wearing gloves (C) prevents contamination but does not directly affect test accuracy. Accurate recording of patient information (D) is essential for documentation but does not impact the test's immediate accuracy. Thus, option A is the most critical for ensuring accurate results in a CLIA-waived glucose test.

Question 22: Correct Answer: C) Follow state-specific regulations and guidelines for record retention and disposal.
Rationale: Following state-specific regulations ensures compliance with legal requirements, as different states have varying rules regarding the retention period and disposal methods for patient records. Option A is incorrect because the retention period may vary by state and type of record.

Option B is incorrect as transferring records does not address proper disposal. Option D is incorrect because incineration may not be an approved method in all states or situations. Understanding state-specific guidelines is crucial for legal compliance in maintaining, storing, and disposing of medical records.

Question 23: Correct Answer: A) "Can you describe any allergies you have to medications?"

Rationale: Option A is correct because it directly pertains to patient safety and is essential for preventing adverse reactions. Option B, while relevant, could lead to speculative answers that may not be medically useful. Option C, although important, is typically part of a more comprehensive health history taken by a physician. Option D focuses on lifestyle habits but is less critical in an initial consultation compared to identifying potential medication allergies. Understanding these distinctions helps ensure that medical assistants ask pertinent questions within their scope.

Question 24: Correct Answer: C) Staple remover

Rationale: The staple remover is specifically designed for the safe and efficient removal of skin staples. Unlike hemostats (A), which are used to clamp blood vessels, suture scissors (B), which are designed for cutting sutures, and needle holders (D), which are used for holding needles during suturing, the staple remover has a unique design that allows it to lift and remove staples without causing damage to the surrounding tissue. This distinction makes option C the correct answer.

Question 25: Correct Answer: C) Collect the light blue top tube first for coagulation studies, invert it 3-4 times, and ensure it is filled to at least 90% capacity.

Rationale: The correct order of draw requires that the light blue top tube for coagulation studies be collected first to avoid contamination with additives from other tubes. It must be inverted 3-4 times to mix the anticoagulant properly. The fill level should be at least 90% to maintain the correct blood-to-additive ratio crucial for accurate test results. Option A is incorrect because a fill level of at least 50% is insufficient. Option B incorrectly suggests collecting the lavender top tube first. Option D has an incorrect number of inversions and fill level requirement for a lavender top tube.

Question 26: Correct Answer: B) Haemophilus influenzae

Rationale: Haemophilus influenzae is a Gram-negative rod commonly associated with respiratory infections, particularly in patients with COPD. Streptococcus pneumoniae (A) is a Gram-positive coccus, making it an incorrect option despite its prevalence in respiratory infections. Mycoplasma pneumoniae (C) lacks a cell wall and does not appear as Gram-negative rods on culture. Staphylococcus aureus (D) is a Gram-positive coccus, not fitting the Gram-negative rod description. Hence, Haemophilus influenzae is the most accurate choice based on the provided clinical scenario and microbiological findings.

Question 27: Correct Answer: A) Verify that Maria's insurance plan covers visits to the orthopedic specialist and obtain prior authorization if required.

Rationale: The primary responsibility of a CCMA in this scenario is to verify that Maria's insurance plan covers the visit to the orthopedic specialist and obtain prior authorization if necessary. This step ensures that the visit will be covered by insurance, preventing unexpected costs for Maria. Scheduling appointments (Option B) and sending medical records (Option D) are also important but secondary tasks. Contacting the specialist directly (Option C) is less common practice as it falls more under administrative coordination rather than direct CCMA duties.

Question 28: Correct Answer: A) Metoprolol 50 mg by mouth twice daily

Rationale: The abbreviation "PO" stands for "by mouth," and "BID" means "twice daily." Therefore, the correct interpretation is "Metoprolol 50 mg by mouth twice daily." Option B is incorrect because it misinterprets "BID" as once daily. Option C is incorrect as it suggests intravenous

administration, which does not match the "PO" abbreviation. Option D is incorrect because it suggests subcutaneous administration, which also does not align with "PO." Understanding these abbreviations is crucial for proper medication administration.

Question 29: Correct Answer: B) Bacterium

Rationale: Tuberculosis (TB) is caused by the bacterium Mycobacterium tuberculosis. Viruses (Option A) are not responsible for TB; they cause diseases like influenza and HIV. Fungi (Option C) can cause infections such as athlete's foot but not TB. Protozoans (Option D) are responsible for diseases like malaria but not TB. Understanding the specific pathogens associated with particular diseases is crucial for accurate diagnosis and treatment in medical practice.

Question 30: Correct Answer: C) Date and time of administration

Rationale: The date and time of administration are critical for ensuring accurate records, monitoring patient compliance, and avoiding medication errors. While the patient's full name and date of birth (A), medication name and dosage (B), and prescribing physician's contact information (D) are also important, they do not directly impact the timing of doses, which is essential for clinical accuracy and legal documentation. Option A (Patient's full name and date of birth): Important for patient identification but does not track when medications are administered. Option B (Medication name and dosage): Crucial for knowing what was given but lacks temporal context. Option D (Prescribing physician's contact information): Useful for follow-up questions but irrelevant to the timing of dose administration.

Question 31: Correct Answer: A) Contact the insurance company directly to confirm coverage details.

Rationale: The most critical step in verifying insurance coverage is contacting the insurance company directly to confirm coverage details (Option A). This ensures up-to-date and accurate information. While reviewing the patient's insurance card (Option B) provides necessary identifiers, it doesn't verify current coverage specifics. Checking the EHR system (Option C) may offer historical data but not current validity. Asking the patient (Option D) might yield incomplete or inaccurate information. Direct confirmation with the insurer ensures that Sarah has precise details about what procedures are covered under Mr. Thompson's plan.

Question 32: Correct Answer: B) Colposcope

Rationale: The colposcope is specifically designed for gynecological examinations to provide a magnified view of the cervix, aiding in the detection of abnormalities. The otoscope (A) is used for ear examinations, the laryngoscope (C) is used to visualize the larynx, and the ophthalmoscope (D) is used for eye examinations. These instruments may appear similar due to their optical nature but serve distinct purposes in different specialties. Understanding these differences is crucial for accurate clinical practice.

Question 33: Correct Answer: C) Diabetes mellitus

Rationale: A fasting blood glucose level of 130 mg/dL is indicative of diabetes mellitus. The normal range for fasting blood glucose is typically between 70-99 mg/dL. Impaired fasting glucose is defined as a level between 100-125 mg/dL. Hypoglycemia is characterized by levels below 70 mg/dL. Therefore, a reading of 130 mg/dL falls into the diabetic range, making option C correct. Options A and B are incorrect because they fall within different ranges, and D is incorrect as it indicates low blood sugar levels.

Question 34: Correct Answer: A) 45 degrees

Rationale: The correct angle for a subcutaneous injection is typically 45 degrees to ensure proper delivery into the subcutaneous tissue. Option B (90 degrees) is often used for intramuscular injections, while Options C (15 degrees) and D (30 degrees) are generally used for intradermal injections. Understanding these distinctions is crucial for ensuring medication efficacy and patient safety.

Question 35: Correct Answer: C) Report the symptoms

immediately to the supervising physician.

Rationale: The severe headache, nausea, visual disturbances, and significantly elevated blood pressure are potential signs of a hypertensive crisis, which is a medical emergency. Reporting these symptoms immediately to the supervising physician ensures prompt intervention. Option A is incorrect because scheduling an appointment delays necessary immediate action. Option B is inappropriate as it downplays the urgency of Maria's condition. Option D is incorrect because over-the-counter pain medication will not address the underlying cause and may delay proper treatment. Prompt reporting aligns with best practices for managing potential hypertensive emergencies.

Question 36: Correct Answer: A) Light blue top (sodium citrate)

Rationale: The correct order of draw for blood collection starts with the light blue top tube containing sodium citrate. This is crucial to prevent contamination from additives in other tubes that could interfere with coagulation tests. The red top tube is used for serum tests but should follow coagulation tubes. The lavender top contains EDTA and is used for hematology tests, while the yellow top contains SPS and is typically used for blood cultures but should not precede coagulation tubes. - Option A is correct because sodium citrate tubes are drawn first to avoid cross-contamination. - Option B is incorrect as serum tubes come after coagulation tubes. - Option C is incorrect because EDTA can contaminate coagulation tests if drawn first. - Option D is incorrect since SPS tubes are used for blood cultures and should not precede coagulation tubes.

Question 37: Correct Answer: B) Using standardized codes from the ICD-10-CM and CPT manuals

Rationale: The use of standardized codes from the ICD-10-CM (International Classification of Diseases, 10th Revision, Clinical Modification) and CPT (Current Procedural Terminology) manuals is essential for submitting claims to third-party payers. These codes ensure uniformity, accuracy, and compliance with payer requirements. Option A is incorrect as including the patient's social security number is not universally required and can pose privacy risks. Option C is incorrect because narrative descriptions are not typically required if standardized codes are used correctly. Option D is incorrect because prior authorization is necessary only for specific services, not all services.

Question 38: Correct Answer: B) SC

Rationale: The abbreviation "SC" stands for subcutaneous, indicating that the medication should be administered under the skin. "IM" (A) stands for intramuscular, which involves injecting into muscle tissue. "IV" (C) means intravenous, referring to administration into a vein. "SL" (D) stands for sublingual, indicating placement under the tongue. Each incorrect option is closely related but represents different administration routes, making this question challenging and testing detailed knowledge of medical abbreviations.

Question 39: Correct Answer: A) Atrial Fibrillation

Rationale: Atrial fibrillation (AF) is identified by an irregularly irregular rhythm and absence of distinct P waves on an ECG. In contrast, atrial flutter (B) shows sawtooth flutter waves, ventricular tachycardia (C) presents with wide QRS complexes and a regular rhythm, and sinus arrhythmia (D) has a regularly irregular pattern linked to respiration. AF's hallmark features differentiate it from these other rhythms.

Question 40: Correct Answer: B) Otoscope

Rationale: An otoscope is specifically designed to examine the internal structures of the ear, making it essential for otoscopic examinations. The ophthalmoscope (A) is used for eye examinations, which is different from ear examination. A stethoscope (C) is used to listen to heart and lung sounds, not for visual inspection of the ear. A sphygmomanometer (D) measures blood pressure and does not serve any function in examining ear structures. Each incorrect option is closely related but serves different diagnostic purposes, making them tricky yet distinguishable upon careful

consideration.

Question 41: Correct Answer: A) As Needed

Rationale: The abbreviation "PRN" stands for "pro re nata," which translates to "as needed" in English. Option B (By Mouth) is represented by "PO," option C (Every Night) is represented by "QHS," and option D (Before Meals) is represented by "AC." The similarity in these abbreviations makes this question challenging, but understanding the specific Latin origin of "PRN" clarifies why "As Needed" is correct.

Question 42: Correct Answer: C) Obtain Sarah's written consent before proceeding with the surgery.

Rationale: Written consent is necessary for surgical procedures to ensure legal compliance and patient understanding. Verbal consent (Option A) or documentation alone (Option B) does not suffice for surgical interventions. A waiver form (Option D) is not appropriate here as it does not replace written informed consent. Written consent provides a clear record that the patient was informed and agreed to the procedure, protecting both patient rights and healthcare providers legally.

Question 43: Correct Answer: B) Remove her gloves, perform hand hygiene, and don new sterile gloves.

Rationale: To maintain surgical asepsis after contaminating the sterile field, Maria must remove her contaminated gloves, perform proper hand hygiene, and don new sterile gloves. Option A is incorrect because visual cleanliness does not ensure sterility. Option C is incorrect as antiseptic wipes cannot guarantee sterility of the gloves. Option D is incorrect because inspection alone cannot confirm sterility; proper protocol must be followed to avoid infection risk. This ensures adherence to strict aseptic techniques critical in preventing infection during surgical procedures.

Question 44: Correct Answer: C) Tree pollen

Rationale: Tree pollen is a common allergen that peaks during springtime and can cause symptoms such as sneezing, itchy eyes, and a runny nose. Dust mites (A) are more prevalent indoors and year-round. Pet dander (B) is associated with exposure to animals rather than seasonal changes. Mold spores (D) can cause similar symptoms but are more common in damp environments rather than specifically peaking in spring. Therefore, tree pollen is the most likely allergen affecting John based on his symptom pattern and timing.

Question 45: Correct Answer: B) Collecting relevant clinical documentation

Rationale: Collecting relevant clinical documentation is most critical because it provides the necessary medical justification required by insurance companies for approving a medication. While verifying patient eligibility (A), communicating with the physician (C), and submitting requests promptly (D) are important steps, they depend on having accurate and complete clinical information. Without thorough documentation, prior authorization requests are likely to be denied or delayed. Thus, collecting detailed clinical data ensures that all other steps can proceed effectively.

Question 46: Correct Answer: D) Median cubital vein

Rationale: The median cubital vein is typically the preferred site for venipuncture in elderly patients due to its larger size and stability compared to other veins. This minimizes the risk of complications such as vein collapse or hematoma. The dorsal hand veins (Option A) are more prone to rolling and collapsing. The cephalic vein (Option B) can be difficult to locate in some elderly patients due to reduced subcutaneous fat. The basilic vein (Option C) is less stable and closer to arteries and nerves, increasing the risk of injury.

Question 47: Correct Answer: A) Pinch the skin at the injection site before inserting the needle at a 45-degree angle.

Rationale: For subcutaneous injections, pinching the skin helps lift the fatty tissue away from muscle, ensuring proper medication delivery. Inserting at a 45-degree angle minimizes risk of injecting into muscle. Option B is incorrect because not pinching can lead to intramuscular injection. Option C describes an intramuscular injection site, not suitable for subcutaneous injections. Option D is incorrect as massaging can alter insulin absorption rates.

Question 48: Correct Answer: A) Completion of an accredited medical assisting program

Rationale: The completion of an accredited medical assisting program is mandatory for obtaining CCMA certification. This ensures that candidates have received standardized education and training. Options B, C, and D are plausible but not required; two years of work experience can enhance qualifications but isn't mandatory, while background checks and letters of recommendation may be part of employment requirements rather than certification prerequisites. Therefore, understanding specific certification requirements is crucial.

Question 49: Correct Answer: A) Prepare the biopsy kit and ensure proper labeling of specimens.

Rationale: Preparing the biopsy kit and ensuring proper labeling of specimens is crucial as it directly impacts the diagnostic process. While educating Sarah about post-biopsy wound care (B), documenting her family history (C), and positioning her under adequate lighting (D) are important, they are secondary to preparing for the biopsy itself. Proper specimen handling is essential for accurate diagnosis, making option A the priority action.

Question 50: Correct Answer: D) Use the electronic health record (EHR) system to securely send the lab results to the ordering provider.

Rationale: The correct procedure involves using an EHR system for secure transmission of lab results, ensuring confidentiality and traceability. Option A is incorrect because verbal communication lacks documentation. Option B is close but less secure than EHR. Option C involves documentation but faxing can be less secure and outdated compared to EHR.

Question 51: Correct Answer: A) Polyglactin 910 (Vicryl)

Rationale: Polyglactin 910 (Vicryl) is an absorbable suture known for causing minimal tissue reaction, making it ideal for subcutaneous closures. Silk is non-absorbable and elicits a more significant tissue reaction. Polypropylene (Prolene) is also non-absorbable and used primarily for skin closures due to its high tensile strength. Nylon, while causing minimal tissue reaction, is non-absorbable and typically used for skin or vascular anastomosis. Thus, Vicryl's absorbability and compatibility with subcutaneous tissues make it the most suitable choice.

Question 52: Correct Answer: B) The prescription must be transmitted through a secure, encrypted system.

Rationale: Federal law mandates that electronic prescriptions must be transmitted through secure, encrypted systems to protect patient information and ensure privacy. While including the patient's full name and date of birth (Option A) and the prescriber's NPI (Option C) are important details, they are not specifically required by law for transmission security. Option D is incorrect because printing and signing an electronic prescription before sending it electronically defeats the purpose of e-prescribing and is not a legal requirement.

Question 53: Correct Answer: C) Confirm that the form is stored in the patient's electronic health record (EHR).

Rationale: The correct answer is C) Confirm that the form is stored in the patient's electronic health record (EHR). This ensures immediate accessibility to all healthcare providers involved in patient care. Option A, while important, does not guarantee validity without proper storage. Option B pertains to review frequency but not storage. Option D is relevant for clarity of instructions but does not address storage. Proper storage in EHR ensures compliance with legal and clinical standards.

Question 54: Correct Answer: B) Speak slowly and use simple language.

Rationale: Speaking slowly and using simple language ensures that elderly patients can follow along without feeling overwhelmed or confused by complex terminology. Medical jargon (Option A) can be confusing; raising your voice (Option C) can be perceived as patronizing; providing written instructions only (Option D) ignores the importance of verbal communication and immediate clarification. This approach aligns with contemporary research emphasizing clear, respectful communication tailored to the cognitive processing abilities of elderly individuals.

Question 55: Correct Answer: A) Administer supplemental oxygen and notify the physician.

Rationale: Administering supplemental oxygen is crucial due to John's low pulse oximetry reading (89%), indicating hypoxemia. Immediate intervention is necessary to improve oxygenation and prevent further complications. Notifying the physician ensures prompt medical evaluation and treatment. Rechecking vital signs or reassessing later (options B and C) delays essential care. Administering an antipyretic (option D) addresses only the mild fever but not the critical issue of hypoxemia.

Question 56: Correct Answer: A) Positioning the patient's arm at heart level and using an appropriately sized cuff.

Rationale: The most accurate method for measuring blood pressure involves positioning the patient's arm at heart level and using an appropriately sized cuff. This ensures that readings are not influenced by gravity or incorrect cuff size, which can lead to inaccurate measurements. Option B is incorrect because standing can affect blood pressure readings due to postural changes. Option C is incorrect as exercise temporarily elevates blood pressure, leading to false readings. Option D is incorrect because not allowing rest between readings can result in higher measurements due to lack of stabilization.

Question 57: Correct Answer: C) Intravenous (IV)

Rationale: The intravenous (IV) route is most appropriate for medications requiring rapid onset and complete absorption because it delivers the drug directly into the bloodstream, bypassing absorption barriers. Intramuscular (IM) injections also provide relatively fast absorption but are slower than IV. Subcutaneous (SC) injections have slower absorption rates due to limited blood flow in subcutaneous tissue. Oral (PO) administration involves first-pass metabolism in the liver, leading to slower onset and incomplete absorption compared to IV.

Question 58: Correct Answer: C) Compounding Pharmacy

Rationale: A compounding pharmacy specializes in creating customized medications that are not commercially available, tailored to individual patient needs. Retail pharmacies typically dispense commercially available medications. Hospital pharmacies manage medications within hospital settings but do not specialize in custom formulations. Nuclear pharmacies prepare radiopharmaceuticals for diagnostic imaging and treatment, which is different from custom medication compounding. - Option A (Retail Pharmacy): Incorrect because retail pharmacies dispense standard medications rather than custom formulations. - Option B (Hospital Pharmacy): Incorrect as they focus on inpatient care and standard medications. - Option D (Nuclear Pharmacy): Incorrect since they specialize in radiopharmaceuticals, not custom non-radioactive medications. The correct choice (C) is validated by its specific role in tailoring medications per individual patient requirements, a practice grounded in contemporary pharmaceutical guidelines and recognized standards.

Question 59: Correct Answer: C) Delay staple removal and consult with the physician.

Rationale: The presence of redness and swelling around the incision site suggests possible infection or inflammation. Delaying staple removal and consulting with a physician ensures proper assessment and treatment to prevent complications. Removing all staples (Option A) could exacerbate the issue. Removing only half (Option B) might not address underlying concerns adequately. Applying antibiotic ointment (Option D) without delaying removal may not suffice if there's an infection.

Question 60: Correct Answer: C) Pancreas

Rationale: The pancreas is located in the epigastric region and can cause pain radiating to the back when inflamed (pancreatitis). The liver (A) is in the right upper quadrant and typically causes right-sided pain. The stomach (B) also resides in the epigastric area but usually causes localized pain without radiation to the back. The gallbladder (D) is under the liver and generally causes right upper quadrant pain that may radiate to the shoulder, not typically to the back.

Question 61: Correct Answer: B) Inferior myocardial infarction

Rationale: ST-segment elevation in leads II, III, and aVF typically indicates an inferior myocardial infarction due to occlusion of the right coronary artery. Anterior MI (option A) would show changes in V1-V4 leads. Lateral MI (option C) affects leads I, aVL, V5-V6. Posterior MI (option D) can be inferred from reciprocal changes in V1-V3 but not directly from II, III, and aVF. Hence, option B is correct as it accurately matches the presented EKG findings.

Question 62: Correct Answer: D) Refer John to a social worker who can assist with accessing all required services.

Rationale: Referring John to a social worker is the most comprehensive approach because social workers are trained to coordinate multiple aspects of care, including clinical and non-clinical services. While arranging for a home health nurse (Option A), scheduling an appointment with a dietitian (Option B), and coordinating transportation (Option C) are important tasks, they address individual needs rather than providing holistic support. Social workers can integrate these services, ensuring that all of John's needs are met efficiently. - Option A is incorrect because it focuses solely on medication management without addressing other needs. - Option B is incorrect because it addresses only nutritional counseling. - Option C is incorrect because it only solves the transportation issue. - Option D is correct as it ensures comprehensive coordination through the expertise of a social worker.

Question 63: Correct Answer: C) Alveoli

Rationale: The alveoli are tiny air sacs in the lungs where gas exchange occurs. Oxygen from inhaled air diffuses through the alveolar walls into the blood, while carbon dioxide diffuses from the blood into the alveoli to be exhaled. The trachea (A) and bronchi (B) are part of the airway conducting system but do not participate directly in gas exchange. Bronchioles (D) are smaller branches of the bronchi leading to alveoli but are not themselves responsible for gas exchange.

Question 64: Correct Answer: B) 7 mL

Rationale: The correct dosage for John is calculated as follows: - Dosage required: 0.5 mg/kg * 70 kg = 35 mg. - Concentration of medication: 50 mg/10 mL = 5 mg/mL. - Volume needed: 35 mg / (5 mg/mL) = 7 mL. Option A (3 mL) and Option D (2.5 mL) are incorrect as they result from miscalculations of the volume needed based on incorrect dosages or concentration interpretations. Option C (5 mL) is close but results from using an incorrect concentration or weight factor in calculations. The correct volume to administer, based on accurate calculations, is B) 7 mL, ensuring precise adherence to the prescribed dosage requirements.

Question 65: Correct Answer: B) Patient's individual needs and preferences

Rationale: While standardized treatment protocols (Option A), primary physician's recommendations (Option C), and latest clinical guidelines (Option D) are all important components of patient care, the most critical factor is the patient's individual needs and preferences (Option B). This ensures that care is tailored specifically to the patient's unique situation, promoting better adherence and outcomes.

Standardized protocols may not account for individual variations, primary physician's recommendations might not consider multidisciplinary input, and clinical guidelines provide general directions but lack personalization. Therefore, focusing on individualized care is paramount in achieving optimal patient outcomes.

Question 66: Correct Answer: C) Rotate the stock by placing items with nearer expiration dates in front and using them first.

Rationale: Rotating stock by placing items with nearer expiration dates in front ensures that older supplies are used before newer ones, reducing waste and maintaining safety standards. Option A is incorrect because increasing reorder quantity may lead to overstocking and more expired items. Option B is not cost-effective as it discards usable supplies prematurely. Option D risks running out of essential supplies if current stock depletes faster than anticipated. Thus, option C is the best practice in inventory management.

Question 67: Correct Answer: B) Scrubbing all surfaces of the hands, including under nails, for at least 20 seconds.

Rationale: Scrubbing all surfaces of the hands, including under nails, for at least 20 seconds is critical for effective hand hygiene as it ensures removal of pathogens. While rinsing (Option A), using hand sanitizer (Option C), and drying (Option D) are important, they do not replace the need for thorough scrubbing, which is essential for reducing microbial load according to CDC guidelines. Option A is incorrect because rinsing before applying soap does not ensure thorough cleaning. Option C is incorrect because while alcohol-based sanitizers are effective, they do not replace proper scrubbing with soap and water. Option D is important but secondary to thorough scrubbing.

Question 68: Correct Answer: B) A detailed description of the event, including time, location, and actions taken.

Rationale: The most crucial detail to include in an unusual occurrence report is a detailed description of the event, including time, location, and actions taken (Option B). This ensures that all relevant facts are documented for review and analysis. Option A is incorrect because while knowing who was present can be helpful, it is not as critical as detailing what happened. Option C is incorrect because personal opinions can bias the report; objective facts are necessary. Option D is incorrect because while patient history may be relevant, it does not directly describe the incident itself.

Question 69: Correct Answer: A) Non-maleficence

Rationale: The original Hippocratic Oath explicitly emphasizes "non-maleficence," often summarized by the phrase "do no harm." While beneficence (doing good), autonomy (respecting patient choice), and justice (fairness) are crucial ethical principles in contemporary medical practice, they are not explicitly stated in the original text. Non-maleficence is directly mentioned, focusing on avoiding harm to patients. Beneficence is implied but not as explicitly stated. Autonomy and justice are more modern additions to medical ethics frameworks.

Question 70: Correct Answer: B) Automated SMS and email reminders

Rationale: Automated SMS and email reminders directly address reducing no-shows by reminding patients of their upcoming appointments. While integration with EHR (Option A) is important for comprehensive patient management, it does not specifically target appointment reminders. Real-time booking updates (Option C) improve scheduling efficiency but do not directly impact reminder functionality. Customizable calendar views (Option D) enhance user experience but do not provide reminder capabilities. Therefore, Option B is the most relevant feature for reducing no-shows through automated reminders.

Question 71: Correct Answer: C) Case Manager

Rationale: A Case Manager is trained to coordinate comprehensive care, addressing both medical and mental health needs by collaborating with various healthcare providers. While a Social Worker (A) can provide support and resources, they may not manage all aspects of medical care. A Psychiatrist (B) focuses on mental health but not necessarily on coordinating overall care. A Primary Care Physician (D) can manage general health but may not have the capacity to coordinate specialized services comprehensively.

Question 72: Correct Answer: B) Label the specimen tube immediately after drawing blood, using information from the patient's wristband and the requisition form.
Rationale: The correct procedure involves labeling the specimen tube immediately after collection using information from both the patient's wristband and the requisition form. This ensures accuracy by cross-verifying two reliable sources. Option A is incorrect because relying solely on verbal confirmation can lead to errors if the patient provides incorrect information. Option C is incorrect as labeling before collection increases risk of mix-ups. Option D is entirely wrong as it involves another patient's details, leading to serious misidentification issues.

Question 73: Correct Answer: D) Immediately disposing of used needles in a sharps container
Rationale: Proper disposal of needles in a sharps container is critical to prevent needlestick injuries and subsequent transmission of blood-borne pathogens such as hepatitis B. While wearing gloves (Option B) and disinfecting the puncture site (Option C) are important, they do not address the risk posed by improper needle disposal. Wearing a surgical mask (Option A) is less relevant for blood-borne pathogen transmission compared to needlestick prevention.

Question 74: Correct Answer: B) Mixing the blood with an anticoagulant immediately after collection
Rationale: Mixing the blood with an anticoagulant immediately after collection is crucial to prevent clotting and ensure accurate glucose measurement. Storing at room temperature (A) can lead to glycolysis and altered results. Light protection (C) is essential for certain tests like bilirubin but not glucose. Centrifuging within 2 hours (D) is important but secondary to preventing clotting initially.

Question 75: Correct Answer: B) Metoprolol 50 mg orally twice daily
Rationale: The abbreviation "PO" stands for "by mouth" (orally), and "BID" means "twice daily." Therefore, the prescription indicates that the patient should take Metoprolol 50 mg orally twice a day. Option A is incorrect because it specifies once daily instead of twice. Option C is incorrect as it involves intravenous administration, not oral. Option D is also incorrect as it refers to subcutaneous administration and once daily frequency, which does not match the prescription instructions.

Question 76: Correct Answer: C) Face her directly and use clear, simple language.
Rationale: Facing Mrs. Johnson directly ensures she can read your lips and see your facial expressions, which aids in understanding. Using clear, simple language reduces confusion. Speaking loudly (Option A) can distort sounds, while written instructions (Option B) may not be immediately accessible. Relying solely on gestures (Option D) may lead to misinterpretation without verbal context.

Question 77: Correct Answer: C) Apologize, document the complaint, and follow up with Mr. Johnson after discussing it with the clinic manager.
Rationale: Option C is correct because it addresses multiple facets of effective service recovery: apologizing to acknowledge the issue, documenting it for quality improvement purposes, and ensuring follow-up after consulting with management to provide a comprehensive resolution. Option A is incorrect because scheduling at a less busy time doesn't address systemic issues or ensure follow-up. Option B is incorrect as offering discounts may not address underlying concerns effectively. Option D is incorrect because simply rescheduling without addressing the root cause does not ensure service improvement or

patient satisfaction.

Question 78: Correct Answer: B) Provide an intramuscular injection of epinephrine and call emergency services.
Rationale: Administering an intramuscular injection of epinephrine is critical in treating anaphylactic shock, which Emily's symptoms suggest. This response can prevent further progression of the reaction. Option A is incorrect because oral antihistamines are insufficient for severe reactions. Option C is inadequate as it doesn't address airway compromise. Option D delays necessary intervention. Thus, immediate administration of epinephrine and calling emergency services is vital.

Question 79: Correct Answer: C) Quitting smoking
Rationale: Quitting smoking is most effective in reducing cardiovascular disease risk because it directly impacts vascular health by reducing inflammation, improving lipid profiles, and enhancing endothelial function. While increasing physical activity (Option A), reducing dietary sodium intake (Option B), and managing stress levels (Option D) are beneficial, they do not have as immediate and profound an effect on cardiovascular health as quitting smoking. Contemporary research emphasizes the significant reduction in cardiovascular events following smoking cessation compared to other lifestyle modifications.

Question 80: Correct Answer: B) A patient reveals they have been experiencing domestic violence.
Rationale: Mandatory reporting laws require healthcare professionals to report cases of suspected abuse, including domestic violence, to appropriate authorities. While drug use (Option A), consensual sexual activity (Option C), and medication non-compliance (Option D) may require intervention or counseling, they do not typically mandate reporting under legal statutes. This distinction is crucial for CCMA compliance with legal requirements.

Question 81: Correct Answer: C) Smooth Endoplasmic Reticulum
Rationale: The Smooth Endoplasmic Reticulum (SER) is primarily responsible for lipid synthesis and detoxification processes. Unlike the Rough Endoplasmic Reticulum (RER), which is studded with ribosomes and specializes in protein synthesis, the SER lacks ribosomes, enabling it to focus on lipid metabolism and detoxification. Mitochondria are involved in energy production through ATP synthesis, while the Golgi Apparatus modifies, sorts, and packages proteins for secretion. The close relation between RER and SER makes this a challenging question, but understanding their distinct functions clarifies why SER is correct.

Question 82: Correct Answer: B) CCMA (Certified Clinical Medical Assistant)
Rationale: The CCMA credential is awarded by the National Healthcareer Association (NHA) to medical assistants who pass their certification exam. CMA, while also a valid credential for medical assistants, is typically granted by the American Association of Medical Assistants (AAMA). RMA is a credential from American Medical Technologists (AMT), and CMAC, although it sounds plausible, is not a recognized credential from any major certifying body. This distinction highlights the importance of understanding specific certifying organizations and their respective credentials in healthcare settings.

Question 83: Correct Answer: B) Decreased cardiac output due to systolic dysfunction
Rationale: The primary pathophysiological mechanism in Mr. Smith's case is decreased cardiac output due to systolic dysfunction, indicated by his low ejection fraction (35%). This leads to inadequate blood flow and oxygen delivery to tissues, causing symptoms like shortness of breath and fatigue. Option A is incorrect because while increased preload can contribute to CHF symptoms, it is not the primary mechanism here. Option C refers to increased afterload from hypertension but does not directly explain the reduced ejection fraction. Option D involves decreased myocardial oxygen supply but does not address the central

issue of systolic dysfunction.

Question 84: Correct Answer: B) Document and code both the follow-up visit for Type 2 Diabetes Mellitus and the new symptom of chest pain.

Rationale: According to current coding guidelines, all relevant patient information must be documented and coded. This includes both pre-existing conditions being managed (Type 2 Diabetes Mellitus) and any new symptoms presented during the visit (chest pain). This ensures comprehensive patient care and accurate billing. Option A is incorrect because it ignores the new symptom. Option C is incorrect because it disregards ongoing diabetes management. Option D is incorrect as it does not provide a complete picture of patient health by omitting diabetes management.

Question 85: Correct Answer: A) 15-30 degrees

Rationale: The optimal angle for needle insertion during venipuncture is between 15-30 degrees. This angle allows for successful vein access while minimizing patient discomfort and reducing the risk of complications such as hematoma formation. Inserting at a lower angle (5-10 degrees) may result in insufficient penetration, while higher angles (45-60 degrees or 75-90 degrees) increase the risk of puncturing through the vein or causing more significant injury. Understanding these angles is crucial for effective and safe phlebotomy procedures.

Question 86: Correct Answer: D) Answering promptly within three rings and stating the clinic's name followed by "How may I assist you?"

Rationale: Option D is correct because it combines promptness (answering within three rings), clear identification (stating the clinic's name), and offering assistance ("How may I assist you?"), which are key components of professional telephone etiquette. Option A lacks the identification of the clinic, which is crucial for clarity. Option B does not identify who is speaking or where they are calling, which can be confusing for callers. Option C uses a neutral tone, which might not convey warmth or readiness to help, unlike D's approach that balances professionalism with helpfulness.

Question 87: Correct Answer: C) Laboratories must ensure that quality control samples are run with each batch of patient specimens.

Rationale: Option C is correct because COLA standards require that quality control samples be run with each batch of patient specimens to ensure accuracy and reliability in test results. Option A is incorrect because while daily quality control is essential, it is not required for all instruments every day. Option B is incorrect as documentation and review should be more frequent than monthly. Option D is misleading because calibration often needs to be done more frequently than annually depending on the instrument and usage. Thus, C aligns precisely with COLA's stringent requirements for ongoing quality assurance in laboratory testing.

Question 88: Correct Answer: B) Avoid eating solid foods the day before the procedure.

Rationale: The correct answer is B) Avoid eating solid foods the day before the procedure. This is critical to ensure that the colon is clear for optimal visualization during the colonoscopy. - Option A is incorrect because a high-fiber diet should be avoided as it can leave residue in the colon. - Option C is incorrect because patients are typically advised to stop taking blood thinners to prevent excessive bleeding during the procedure. - Option D is incorrect because while hydration is important, patients are usually instructed to stop drinking liquids several hours before the procedure to avoid complications with anesthesia. Each option targets different aspects of pre-procedural preparation but only B correctly addresses what should be avoided immediately prior to a colonoscopy.

Question 89: Correct Answer: B) A 14-year-old patient presents with unexplained bruises and reports fear of going home.

Rationale: Option B is correct because it involves current potential abuse or neglect, which triggers mandatory reporting laws. Option A is incorrect because consensual activity between peers may not always require reporting unless there are other signs of abuse or coercion. Option C is incorrect as it involves past abuse without current risk, which may not trigger immediate mandatory reporting. Option D is incorrect because substance use alone does not necessarily mandate a report unless there are additional signs of neglect or abuse.

Question 90: Correct Answer: B) Ensuring secure communication channels

Rationale: Ensuring secure communication channels is crucial for maintaining patient confidentiality, as it prevents unauthorized access to sensitive information. While filing patient records accurately (Option A), scheduling appointments (Option C), and verifying insurance information (Option D) are important administrative tasks, they do not directly address the security of communication channels, which is essential for protecting patient privacy. Accurate filing helps organize records but doesn't inherently secure them. Scheduling and verifying insurance involve handling information but not necessarily securing it. Thus, Option B is the most comprehensive task related to maintaining confidentiality.

Question 91: Correct Answer: C) Donning: Mask, Gown, Gloves; Doffing: Gloves, Gown, Mask

Rationale: The correct sequence for donning PPE starts with the mask to prevent contamination during gowning and gloving. The gown follows to protect clothing and skin. Finally, gloves are donned last to maintain sterility. For doffing PPE safely to avoid self-contamination, gloves are removed first as they are most contaminated. The gown is removed next without touching the outside surface. Lastly, the mask is removed by handling only the ties or elastics. Options A), B), and D) contain incorrect sequences that could lead to contamination during either donning or doffing steps.

Question 92: Correct Answer: A) 20/40

Rationale: The correct documentation is 20/40 because Mr. Johnson can read the 20/40 line but not the 20/30 line, indicating his visual acuity is at the 20/40 level. Option B (20/30) is incorrect as he struggled with that line. Option C (20/50) is also incorrect since he could read better than that level. Option D (20/20) is incorrect as it represents normal vision, which he did not demonstrate.

Question 93: Correct Answer: A) Diabetic ketoacidosis (DKA)

Rationale: Diabetic ketoacidosis (DKA) is characterized by confusion, rapid breathing (Kussmaul respirations), fruity-smelling breath due to acetone, and abdominal pain. Heat stroke typically presents with high body temperature and altered mental status but not fruity breath. Anaphylactic shock involves severe allergic reactions with symptoms like hives and difficulty breathing. Seizures involve sudden electrical disturbances in the brain leading to convulsions or altered consciousness but not the specific metabolic signs seen in DKA. The key distinguishing factor here is the fruity-smelling breath indicative of ketosis.

Question 94: Correct Answer: A) Autoclave

Rationale: The autoclave is the most effective method for sterilizing surgical instruments as it uses pressurized steam to kill all forms of microbial life, including spores. Instrument cleaners only remove debris but do not sterilize. Germicidal disinfectants reduce microbial load but may not eliminate all spores. Disposables refer to single-use items and do not apply to reusable instruments in this context.

Question 95: Correct Answer: B) Emily may be at risk for being overweight.

Rationale: The correct interpretation of Emily's growth pattern involves recognizing that while her height is within normal limits (25th percentile), her weight at the 75th percentile suggests she may be at risk for being overweight. This discrepancy indicates a potential imbalance in her growth pattern. Option A is incorrect because it fails to address the disparity between height and weight percentiles. Option C incorrectly implies concern solely based on height, which is not warranted here. Option D focuses only on weight without considering the context provided by height percentile, making B the most accurate interpretation.

Question 96: Correct Answer: A) Documenting Mr. Johnson's symptoms and interventions immediately after each interaction.

Rationale: Immediate documentation ensures accuracy and completeness, reducing the risk of forgetting critical details. Summarizing at the end of the shift (Option B) can lead to missed or inaccurate entries due to memory lapses. Using abbreviations (Option C), unless standardized, can cause misunderstandings. Including subjective opinions (Option D) is inappropriate as documentation should be objective and factual.

Question 97: Correct Answer: D) Ensure Mr. Johnson is safe and then notify the nurse manager before completing an incident report.

Rationale: Ensuring patient safety is paramount; Sarah must first ensure Mr. Johnson is safe to prevent further injury (D). Notifying the nurse manager aligns with protocol for immediate supervision involvement before documentation (D). While A) focuses on notifying a physician, it misses involving immediate supervisory staff first. B) skips notifying a supervisor before documentation, which can lead to procedural gaps. C) involves documenting in medical records rather than initiating an incident report first, which is not standard practice for such events.

Question 98: Correct Answer: A) Sublingual

Rationale: The sublingual route involves placing medication under the tongue, where it rapidly dissolves and is absorbed through the mucous membranes into the bloodstream. This method bypasses the digestive system, leading to quicker onset of action. Buccal administration (B) involves placing medication between the gums and cheek, which also uses mucous membranes but is slower than sublingual. Intranasal (C) refers to spraying medication into the nasal cavity, which targets mucous membranes but in a different location. Transdermal (D) involves absorption through the skin over time, making it much slower compared to sublingual administration.

Question 99: Correct Answer: B) Report the suspicion of abuse to the appropriate authorities immediately.

Rationale: According to legal requirements, healthcare professionals must report any suspicion of abuse to appropriate authorities immediately, even without confirmation from the patient. This ensures patient safety and adherence to mandatory reporting laws. Option A is incorrect because merely documenting and monitoring does not fulfill legal obligations. Option C is incorrect as seeking a colleague's opinion may delay necessary action. Option D is incorrect because waiting for confirmation can endanger the patient and violates mandatory reporting laws.

Question 100: Correct Answer: C) Ointment

Rationale: Ointments are specifically designed for topical application and are effective for localized treatment as they allow the medication to be absorbed directly through the skin. Pills and capsules are intended for systemic absorption through the digestive tract, making them unsuitable for localized treatment. Liquid medications can be used topically but are generally less effective than ointments for sustained localized treatment due to their runny consistency and potential for rapid evaporation or runoff. Therefore, ointments are the most appropriate choice for localized absorption through the skin.

Question 101: Correct Answer: D) CYP3A4

Rationale: CYP3A4 is responsible for metabolizing around 50% of all clinically used drugs, making it the most significant enzyme in drug metabolism. While CYP1A2, CYP2C9, and CYP2D6 also play substantial roles in metabolizing various drugs, none are as predominant as CYP3A4. This distinction is crucial for understanding drug interactions and individual variability in drug responses due to differences in enzyme activity. - Option A (CYP1A2): Although important in metabolizing certain drugs like caffeine and some antidepressants, it does not cover as broad a spectrum as CYP3A4. - Option B (CYP2C9): Plays a key role in metabolizing nonsteroidal anti-inflammatory drugs (NSAIDs) and warfarin but is not as widespread as CYP3A4. - Option C (CYP2D6): Significant for metabolizing opioids and beta-blockers but covers fewer drugs compared to CYP3A4. - Option D (CYP3A4): Correct because it handles about half of all clinically used drugs, highlighting its extensive involvement in pharmacokinetics. This comprehensive understanding underscores the importance of recognizing the primary enzyme involved in drug metabolism to anticipate potential drug interactions and individual patient responses.

Question 102: Correct Answer: C) The palmar surface of the ring finger

Rationale: The palmar surface of the ring finger is preferred due to its accessibility and reduced likelihood of calluses compared to other fingers. The index finger (Option A) is often used but can be more sensitive. The heel (Option B) is typically reserved for infants. The earlobe (Option D), though used in specific cases, is less common due to discomfort and difficulty in handling. Thus, Option C minimizes discomfort and complications while ensuring an accurate sample.

Question 103: Correct Answer: B) To ensure complete separation of serum from cells

Rationale: Allowing a blood sample to clot completely before centrifugation ensures that the serum separates properly from the blood cells. This step is crucial for obtaining a clear serum sample. While preventing hemolysis (Option A) and avoiding contamination (Option C) are important, they are not directly related to the clotting process. Enhancing the accuracy of biochemical tests (Option D) is an outcome of proper separation but not the primary reason for allowing clotting.

Question 104: Correct Answer: B) Schedule the visit for 30 minutes to accommodate both the follow-up and flu shot.

Rationale: The correct answer is B) because it ensures that there is sufficient time to address both Maria's follow-up consultation and administer her flu shot without rushing. Option A) is incorrect as it does not account for additional time needed for the flu shot. Option C) is unnecessary as combining both purposes in one visit is more efficient. Option D) might seem reasonable but typically falls short of ensuring adequate time based on standard medical practice durations.

Question 105: Correct Answer: A) Store at room temperature for up to 28 days.

Rationale: After opening, a multi-dose vial of insulin should be stored at room temperature (up to 28 days), as refrigeration is not necessary and can cause discomfort during injection. Option B is incorrect because insulin can be stored in the refrigerator before opening, but not after. Option C is incorrect due to the shorter duration. Option D is incorrect because storing opened insulin in the refrigerator is not recommended and can lead to inaccuracies in dosing due to viscosity changes.

Question 106: Correct Answer: B) When the information is necessary to prevent a serious threat to public health or safety.

Rationale: The Health Insurance Portability and Accountability Act (HIPAA) allows for the release of patient information without explicit consent if it is necessary to prevent a serious threat to public health or safety. Option A is incorrect because insurance requests typically require patient authorization. Option C is close but usually requires patient consent for continuity of care. Option D is incorrect as family inquiries generally need patient authorization unless under specific circumstances like power of attorney. Thus, option B correctly aligns with legal exceptions under HIPAA regulations.

Question 107: Correct Answer: B) Ensure all leads are properly attached and making good contact with the skin.
Rationale: Erratic and inconsistent EKG tracings are most often due to improper lead attachment or poor contact with the skin. Ensuring all leads are properly attached can resolve this issue by improving signal quality. Option A is incorrect because replacing the paper would not address lead attachment issues. Option C is incorrect as increasing sensitivity might amplify noise rather than fix it. Option D is incorrect because adjusting speed affects how fast the paper moves, not signal quality. Each option targets different aspects of EKG operation, making it challenging for test-takers to discern without deep knowledge of EKG procedures.

Question 108: Correct Answer: C) Gastrointestinal upset
Rationale: Gastrointestinal upset, including nausea, vomiting, and diarrhea, is a well-documented and common side effect of Metformin. Lactic acidosis (Option A) is a rare but serious adverse effect. Hypoglycemia (Option B) is less common with Metformin alone as it does not typically cause low blood sugar. Weight gain (Option D) is not associated with Metformin; in fact, it may help with weight loss or be weight-neutral. Thus, the correct answer is C because it reflects the most frequent and expected side effect of Metformin.

Question 109: Correct Answer: C) Proper disposal of used needles and sharps
Rationale: Proper disposal of used needles and sharps is crucial in preventing needlestick injuries, which are a primary mode of transmission for blood-borne pathogens like HIV, HBV, and HCV. While wearing gloves (Option A) and using hand sanitizer (Option B) are important for general infection control, they do not specifically address the risk posed by contaminated sharps. Wearing a surgical mask (Option D) is essential for droplet precautions but not directly relevant to blood-borne pathogen transmission. Therefore, Option C is the most effective precaution in this context.

Question 110: Correct Answer: B) Epocrates
Rationale: Epocrates is a widely used online resource among clinical medical assistants for verifying drug interactions and obtaining comprehensive drug information. While MedlinePlus, WebMD, and Mayo Clinic provide valuable health information, they are not as specifically focused on detailed pharmacological data and drug interaction verification as Epocrates. MedlinePlus offers general health information, WebMD is more patient-oriented, and Mayo Clinic provides reliable health advice but lacks the specific pharmacological tools available in Epocrates. Therefore, Epocrates is the most appropriate choice for this context.

Question 111: Correct Answer: B) Provide Sarah with an ABN before performing the diagnostic mammogram.
Rationale: An ABN is required when Medicare may not cover a service or item that is usually covered but may not be in this specific instance. Since routine screening mammograms are typically covered by Medicare without cost-sharing, an ABN is not necessary. However, for the additional diagnostic mammogram, which may not be covered under certain conditions or frequency limits, providing an ABN before performing this procedure ensures that Sarah is informed about potential out-of-pocket costs. Options A and C are incorrect because they do not align with Medicare's requirements for timing and necessity of issuing an ABN. Option D is incorrect as it fails to recognize the conditional requirement for an ABN in specific situations like additional diagnostics beyond routine screenings.

Question 112: Correct Answer: B) Observe Mr. Johnson's body language and facial expressions for signs of discomfort.

Rationale: Observing non-verbal cues such as body language and facial expressions is crucial in accurately assessing a patient's comfort and anxiety levels because these cues often reveal more than verbal responses. Directly asking (Option A) can be useful but may not always yield honest responses due to social desirability bias. Reviewing medical history (Option C) provides context but does not reflect current state. Explaining the procedure (Option D) is a good practice for reducing anxiety but comes after initial assessment through observation.

Question 113: Correct Answer: B) Ensuring all provided services are medically necessary and documented.
Rationale: The Centers for Medicare & Medicaid Services (CMS) requires that all services billed must be medically necessary and properly documented to avoid claim denial. Option A is incorrect because demographic information alone is insufficient. Option C is incorrect as listing only the primary diagnosis code does not provide a complete picture of the patient's condition. Option D is incorrect because submitting claims without verifying insurance coverage can lead to denials or rejections. Therefore, ensuring medical necessity and thorough documentation is crucial for compliance with CMS billing requirements.

Question 114: Correct Answer: D) All of the above
Rationale: All three symptoms—shortness of breath, chest pain, and sweating—are classic signs of a myocardial infarction and should be documented and reported immediately. While each symptom alone could indicate other conditions, their combination strongly suggests a heart attack. Option A (Shortness of breath) alone can be due to various causes like asthma or anxiety. Option B (Chest pain) alone might indicate angina or musculoskeletal issues. Option C (Sweating) alone could result from fever or hypoglycemia. Only option D correctly identifies that all these symptoms together are indicative of a potentially life-threatening condition requiring urgent attention.

Question 115: Correct Answer: B) "Dear Mrs. Johnson, Your appointment is scheduled for Friday at 10 AM. Please ensure you fast for 12 hours prior."
Rationale: Option B is correct as it maintains a professional tone ("Dear Mrs. Johnson"), provides specific details about the appointment time ("Friday at 10 AM"), and gives clear pre-appointment instructions ("fast for 12 hours prior"). Option A lacks formality and specificity about fasting duration. Option C uses informal language ("Just a reminder") and does not specify fasting duration. Option D is too brief and lacks proper salutation and detailed instructions, making it less professional and clear.

Question 116: Correct Answer: C) Sublimation
Rationale: Sublimation involves channeling unacceptable impulses into socially acceptable activities, such as cleaning or organizing. Displacement (Option A) involves redirecting emotions to a safer outlet but not necessarily in a socially acceptable manner. Projection (Option B) involves attributing one's own unacceptable feelings to others. Reaction Formation (Option D) involves behaving in a way that is opposite to one's true feelings. Therefore, while all options are defense mechanisms, sublimation best describes Sarah's behavior of turning stress into productive activity.
Tone: Professional and Knowledgeable

Question 117: Correct Answer: B) Verifying the patient's insurance coverage and benefits before contacting the insurance company.
Rationale: The most critical step is verifying the patient's insurance coverage and benefits before contacting the insurance company. This ensures that you are aware of what is covered under the patient's plan and can provide accurate information when requesting pre-authorization. Submitting a clinical report (Option A) is important but secondary to verifying coverage. Scheduling without verification (Option C) could lead to unexpected costs for the patient. Contacting without verification (Option D) may result in denial of authorization if coverage details are incorrect.

Question 118: Correct Answer: A) Addison's disease
Rationale: Addison's disease is characterized by fatigue, weight loss, and hyperpigmentation due to adrenal insufficiency. Cushing's syndrome also involves adrenal glands but typically presents with weight gain and purple striae. Hyperthyroidism can cause weight loss and fatigue but lacks hyperpigmentation. Hypothyroidism generally leads to weight gain and does not cause hyperpigmentation. Understanding these distinctions is crucial for accurate diagnosis. - Addison's Disease: Fatigue, weight loss, and hyperpigmentation are hallmark signs due to insufficient cortisol production. - Cushing's Syndrome: Involves excess cortisol; symptoms include weight gain and purple striae rather than hyperpigmentation. - Hyperthyroidism: Causes weight loss and fatigue but lacks skin hyperpigmentation. - Hypothyroidism: Typically causes weight gain and does not involve hyperpigmentation. This analysis ensures each option is plausible yet distinct enough to challenge the examinee's knowledge of pathophysiology and symptomatology.

Question 119: Correct Answer: A) "You should avoid all solid foods and drink only clear liquids starting 24 hours before the procedure."
Rationale: The correct answer is A. For a colonoscopy, patients are generally instructed to avoid all solid foods and consume only clear liquids starting 24 hours before the procedure to ensure the colon is empty. Option B is incorrect because it incorrectly allows a light breakfast on the day of the procedure. Option C is close but extends the clear liquid diet unnecessarily to 48 hours. Option D incorrectly suggests that patients can eat normally until just 12 hours prior, which does not provide adequate time for bowel preparation.

Question 120: Correct Answer: A) Administering intramuscular injections
Rationale: Administering intramuscular injections is within the scope of practice for CCMAs as they are trained and certified to perform such tasks under the supervision of a licensed healthcare provider. Prescribing medications (Option B) and interpreting diagnostic test results (Option C) are outside their scope as these require advanced medical training and licensure. Performing minor surgical procedures (Option D) is also beyond their capabilities as it requires specialized surgical training. Thus, Option A is correct because it aligns with the typical duties and legal boundaries set for CCMAs.

Question 121: Correct Answer: A) PR Interval
Rationale: The PR interval measures the time from the onset of atrial depolarization (P wave) to the onset of ventricular depolarization (QRS complex). It reflects AV node conduction time. The QT interval spans from ventricular depolarization to repolarization, thus not fitting this definition. The ST segment represents the period between ventricular depolarization and repolarization, while the QRS complex indicates only ventricular depolarization. Hence, only option A accurately describes this interval.

Question 122: Correct Answer: B) Advising the patient to maintain their usual daily activities
Rationale: Maintaining usual daily activities ensures that the Holter monitor captures a representative sample of cardiac activity under normal conditions. Option A is incorrect because while avoiding bathing is recommended, it does not impact data accuracy directly. Option C is incorrect as fasting is unnecessary for Holter monitoring. Option D, although relevant in some cardiovascular tests, is not specific to Holter monitoring's accuracy.

Question 123: Correct Answer: B) Preparing patients for minor surgical procedures
Rationale: Clinical Medical Assistants are trained to prepare patients for minor surgical procedures, which includes tasks like setting up sterile fields, explaining the procedure to patients, and ensuring all necessary equipment is available. They are not typically responsible for administering intravenous medications (A), diagnosing medical conditions (C), or developing patient treatment plans (D). These tasks fall under the purview of nurses or physicians. Thus, option B is correct because it accurately reflects a CMA's role in patient care.

Question 124: Correct Answer: C) Initiating thrombolytic therapy
Rationale: Thrombolytic therapy is crucial for dissolving blood clots in acute myocardial infarction (AMI), significantly improving patient outcomes. While aspirin (Option A) is essential for its antiplatelet effect, it does not dissolve clots like thrombolytics. Intravenous nitroglycerin (Option B) helps relieve chest pain but does not address the underlying clot. Supplemental oxygen (Option D) supports oxygenation but does not treat the cause of AMI directly. Thus, initiating thrombolytic therapy is the most appropriate initial treatment in this scenario.

Question 125: Correct Answer: A) Ensuring the patient's arm is at heart level
Rationale: Ensuring the patient's arm is at heart level is crucial for an accurate blood pressure measurement because it aligns with hydrostatic pressure principles. Options B and C are incorrect because using an improperly sized cuff or placing the stethoscope over the radial artery can lead to inaccurate readings. Option D is incorrect because deflating the cuff too rapidly can miss important Korotkoff sounds, leading to inaccurate results. Proper technique ensures reliable measurements, aligning with contemporary research and recognized theories in clinical practice.

Question 126: Correct Answer: B) Irrigate the wound thoroughly with sterile saline.
Rationale: The most appropriate initial step in managing a minor laceration is to irrigate the wound thoroughly with sterile saline. This helps to remove debris and reduce the risk of infection. Applying antibiotic ointment (Option A) and covering with sterile gauze (Option C) are important but come after irrigation. Administering a tetanus shot (Option D) is crucial if indicated but not the immediate first step. Proper irrigation ensures that subsequent treatments are more effective and reduces complications.

Question 127: Correct Answer: B) Increase intake of omega-3 fatty acids.
Rationale: Increasing the intake of omega-3 fatty acids is most beneficial for reducing cardiovascular risk as they help lower triglyceride levels, reduce inflammation, and improve heart health. Saturated fats (Option A) and trans fats (Option C) can increase cholesterol levels and risk of heart disease. Refined carbohydrates (Option D) can lead to weight gain and increased blood sugar levels, which also negatively affect heart health. Therefore, Option B is the correct choice due to its positive impact on cardiovascular health supported by contemporary research.

Question 128: Correct Answer: A) Identify the patient using two identifiers.
Rationale: Identifying the patient using two identifiers is crucial to ensure patient safety and prevent errors. While applying a tourniquet, assembling equipment, and cleansing the site are all important steps in performing venipuncture, they should occur after confirming the patient's identity. This protocol aligns with contemporary safety standards and reduces risks associated with misidentification. - Option A (Correct): Ensures correct patient identification, which is critical to avoid errors. - Option B (Incorrect): Applying a tourniquet is essential but should follow proper identification. - Option C (Incorrect): Assembling equipment is necessary but secondary to confirming patient identity. - Option D (Incorrect): Cleansing the site is important but must come after ensuring correct identification.

Question 129: Correct Answer: D) Verify that the patient has given explicit consent before sharing any information.
Rationale: HIPAA regulations require that patient information can only be shared if explicit consent has been provided by the patient. Option A is incorrect because being

an immediate family member does not automatically grant access to patient information without consent. Option B is incorrect as confirming identity alone does not suffice without patient consent. Option C is incorrect because referring to a physician without verifying consent still breaches confidentiality laws. Therefore, D is correct as it ensures compliance with HIPAA by requiring explicit patient consent.

Question 130: Correct Answer: C) Advanced cardiac care and interventions

Rationale: Specialists, such as cardiologists, provide advanced cardiac care and interventions that require specific expertise beyond the scope of general practitioners. While general practitioners can manage chronic conditions (Option B), perform routine physical exams (Option A), and administer immunizations (Option D), advanced cardiac procedures necessitate specialized training. This distinction underscores the differences in services offered by generalists versus specialists.

Question 131: Correct Answer: C) Type C tympanogram

Rationale: Type C tympanogram indicates negative middle ear pressure, often due to Eustachian tube dysfunction. This is characterized by a peak that occurs at negative pressure values. Type A represents normal middle ear function, Type B suggests fluid in the middle ear or perforation, and Type Ad indicates hypermobility of the tympanic membrane. Therefore, only Type C directly correlates with Eustachian tube dysfunction.

Rationale: - Type A Tympanogram (Incorrect): Represents normal middle ear pressure and compliance. - Type B Tympanogram (Incorrect): Indicates middle ear effusion or perforation. - Type Ad Tympanogram (Incorrect): Suggests an abnormally compliant tympanic membrane, often due to ossicular chain discontinuity or scarring. - Type C Tympanogram (Correct): Shows negative middle ear pressure indicative of Eustachian tube dysfunction. The key difference is that only Type C shows negative pressure which is directly linked to Eustachian tube issues, whereas other types indicate different middle ear pathologies.

Question 132: Correct Answer: B) Cleaning the skin with alcohol before electrode placement

Rationale: Cleaning the skin with alcohol before electrode placement is crucial as it removes oils and debris, enhancing electrode contact and reducing artifacts. While ensuring the patient is still (Option A) helps, it is not as directly impactful as proper skin preparation. Using a higher sensitivity setting (Option C) can actually increase artifact detection rather than minimize it. Placing electrodes over bony prominences (Option D) is incorrect because it can lead to poor contact and increased artifacts. Proper skin preparation remains key in minimizing EKG artifacts.

Question 133: Correct Answer: B) Bargaining

Rationale: In Kübler-Ross's model, the bargaining stage involves individuals making deals or promises in hopes of reversing or delaying their loss. This is distinct from denial (A), where individuals refuse to accept reality; depression (C), characterized by deep sadness and hopelessness; and acceptance (D), where individuals come to terms with the loss. Understanding these subtle differences is crucial for correctly identifying the bargaining stage.

Question 134: Correct Answer: D) Skin prick test

Rationale: The skin prick test is generally the initial test performed for diagnosing immediate allergic reactions to various allergens, as it is quick, cost-effective, and has high sensitivity. The intradermal skin test (A) is more sensitive but used after a negative skin prick test due to higher risk of false positives. The patch test (B) is used for diagnosing contact dermatitis, not immediate allergic reactions. The serum-specific IgE test (C) is useful when skin testing cannot be performed but is typically not the first-line diagnostic tool.

Question 135: Correct Answer: B) Jane is allergic to the allergen tested in the intradermal test.

Rationale: The development of a wheal and flare reaction within 15 minutes at an intradermal test site indicates an immediate hypersensitivity reaction, confirming an allergy to that specific allergen. Option A is incorrect because no reaction was observed in the scratch test. Option C is incorrect as it ignores the positive result from the intradermal test. Option D is misleading because immediate reactions are typically reliable indicators of true allergies.

Question 136: Correct Answer: B) Label the sample with the patient's name and date of collection before proceeding.

Rationale: Proper labeling of the sample with patient identification and collection time is crucial for traceability and accuracy in clinical testing. While refrigerating (A), mixing (C), and immersing (D) are important steps, they are subsequent procedures that follow accurate labeling to avoid misidentification or errors in result interpretation. - Option A is incorrect because refrigeration is essential but secondary to labeling. - Option C is incorrect as mixing ensures even distribution of analytes but follows labeling. - Option D is incorrect because immersion time impacts test accuracy but comes after proper labeling. Labeling first ensures that all subsequent steps are correctly attributed to Maria's sample, which is critical for patient safety and result accuracy.

Question 137: Correct Answer: C) Clean with detergent, disinfect with alcohol-based solution, followed by sterilization.

Rationale: The correct order is to first clean surfaces with a detergent to remove organic material and debris. This is followed by disinfection using an alcohol-based solution to kill most pathogens. Finally, sterilization ensures that all microbial life is eliminated. Option A incorrectly places disinfection before cleaning. Option B reverses the necessary steps of cleaning and disinfection. Option D incorrectly suggests sterilizing before cleaning. Thus, option C correctly reflects the standard protocol for infection control in clinical settings.

Question 138: Correct Answer: D) Suggest Mr. Johnson complete a new advanced directive form and have it witnessed.

Rationale: The correct answer is D) Suggest Mr. Johnson complete a new advanced directive form and have it witnessed. Advanced directives are legal documents that must be updated formally; verbal requests are not legally binding (Option A). While informing the primary physician is important (Option B), it does not address updating the document itself. Discussing with a healthcare proxy (Option C) is advisable but secondary to formal documentation. Completing a new form ensures legal validity and clarity of Mr. Johnson's current wishes.

Question 139: Correct Answer: D) Wash hands with soap and water for at least 20 seconds.

Rationale: Hand hygiene after potential contact with bodily fluids requires washing hands with soap and water for at least 20 seconds to ensure thorough removal of pathogens. While alcohol-based sanitizers are effective in many situations, they are not sufficient when hands are visibly soiled or contaminated with bodily fluids. Option A is incorrect because it suggests using sanitizer instead of washing. Option B is incorrect due to insufficient duration. Option C is incorrect as it recommends an inappropriate method and duration.

Question 140: Correct Answer: B) Call the specialist's office to confirm the fax number before sending the records.

Rationale: The correct answer is B) Call the specialist's office to confirm the fax number before sending the records. This step ensures that sensitive information is sent to the correct recipient, minimizing risks of unauthorized access. Option A is incorrect because it disregards verification steps that prevent misdirected faxes. Option C is incorrect as it does not address verifying recipient details before sending sensitive information. Option D, while important for maintaining confidentiality, does not address verifying recipient details and thus doesn't fully mitigate risks of unauthorized access.

Question 141: Correct Answer: A) Review Sarah's

symptoms and medical history to ensure they align with the indications for an echocardiogram.

Rationale: Reviewing Sarah's symptoms and medical history ensures that the procedure aligns with established indications, which is crucial for meeting medical necessity guidelines. Option B is incorrect because insurance coverage does not determine medical necessity. Option C is close but focuses on documentation rather than alignment with guidelines. Option D is incorrect as it generalizes the use of echocardiograms without considering specific patient symptoms and history. Medical necessity requires matching patient-specific factors with clinical indications.

Question 142: Correct Answer: B) Using certified reference materials

Rationale: The use of certified reference materials (CRMs) is crucial for accurate calibration because they provide a known standard against which equipment can be measured. While regularly scheduling calibration checks (A), documenting procedures (C), and training staff (D) are important, they do not directly ensure accuracy. CRMs are essential as they offer traceability to national or international standards, ensuring consistency and reliability in measurements.

Question 143: Correct Answer: B) Discard the insulin as it may have lost its potency.

Rationale: Insulin that has been left out of refrigeration for an extended period may lose its potency and should be discarded. Option A is incorrect because returning compromised medication to storage can pose risks to patient safety. Option C is misleading; while some insulins can be stored at room temperature, this applies only if they have not been previously refrigerated or left out overnight. Option D is incorrect because while consulting a pharmacist is good practice, standard protocol dictates discarding potentially compromised medication immediately.

Question 144: Correct Answer: B) Listen actively to the patient's concerns without interrupting.

Rationale: Active listening is crucial as it validates the patient's feelings and can help de-escalate their agitation. Option A acknowledges the issue but does not address immediate emotional needs. Option C provides information but may not calm the patient initially. Option D offers a solution but might not address their current frustration effectively. Active listening (Option B) allows for understanding and addressing specific concerns directly, making it the most effective first step.

Question 145: Correct Answer: C) Lozenge

Rationale: A lozenge is designed to dissolve slowly in the mouth, providing a localized effect, often used for throat or mouth conditions. Capsules and pills are typically swallowed whole for systemic effects. Ointments are topical medications applied directly to the skin. The key difference lies in their administration routes and intended effects—lozenges act locally in the mouth, while capsules and pills act systemically, and ointments act topically. This makes lozenges unique among these options for localized oral treatment.

Question 146: Correct Answer: C) Primary Care Physician's Office

Rationale: Sarah would most likely start her journey at a Primary Care Physician's Office because primary care physicians are typically responsible for providing initial evaluations, managing overall health, and coordinating referrals to specialists. Urgent Care Centers (Option A) and Hospital Emergency Departments (Option B) are designed for immediate, acute issues rather than ongoing care management. Specialty Clinics (Option D) provide specialized services but usually require a referral from a primary care provider first. Thus, Option C is the correct starting point for coordinated and comprehensive care.

Question 147: Correct Answer: A) ST-segment elevation

Rationale: ST-segment elevation is the most indicative finding of an acute myocardial infarction (AMI), as it represents acute injury to the myocardium. T-wave inversion can occur in ischemia but is not as specific for AMI. A prolonged PR interval suggests first-degree heart block, not AMI. QRS complex widening may indicate bundle branch block or ventricular arrhythmias but is not specific for AMI. Thus, ST-segment elevation is the key indicator among these options.

Question 148: Correct Answer: B) Employ visual aids and gestures to demonstrate the procedure.

Rationale: Using visual aids and gestures is effective for young children with limited language skills and helps bridge language barriers. Simple medical terminology (A) might still be confusing for a child. Written instructions (C) are less effective for non-literate children. Relying on family members (D) can introduce inaccuracies in translation. Visual aids cater to both developmental stage and language barriers effectively.

Question 149: Correct Answer: C) Ensuring that the codes are consistent with the physician's documentation.

Rationale: Ensuring that diagnostic and procedural codes are consistent with the physician's documentation is crucial for accuracy. This step verifies that all coded information accurately reflects what was performed and documented. Option A is important but secondary; option B is necessary but not sufficient on its own; option D can lead to errors if it overlooks specific details in documentation.

Question 150: Correct Answer: B) Fourth intercostal space at the right sternal border

Rationale: The V1 electrode in a standard 12-lead EKG should be placed at the fourth intercostal space at the right sternal border. This specific location is essential for obtaining an accurate reading of the heart's electrical activity. Option A is incorrect because it describes the placement for V2. Option C describes the placement for V4, and option D is incorrect as there is no lead placed in this position in standard 12-lead EKGs. Misplacing these leads can result in inaccurate data and potentially misdiagnosed conditions.

CCMA Exam Practice Questions [SET 2]

Question 1: Which anatomical structure is located in the mediastinum?
A) Heart
B) Lungs
C) Diaphragm
D) Liver

Question 2: During a routine blood draw for patient Mr. John Smith, you collect the specimen in a red-top tube. Which of the following steps should you take immediately after collecting the blood to ensure proper processing for laboratory analysis?
A) Invert the tube gently 5-10 times to mix the clot activator with the blood.
B) Place the tube in a biohazard bag without inverting it.
C) Label the tube with Mr. Smith's details before mixing it.
D) Send the tube to the lab without labeling it to avoid contamination.

Question 3: Which type of health care setting is most appropriate for providing long-term care to elderly patients with chronic conditions?
A) Acute Care Hospital
B) Skilled Nursing Facility
C) Ambulatory Surgery Center
D) Urgent Care Clinic

Question 4: Which of the following measures is most effective in preventing the spread of an airborne pandemic?
A) Regular hand washing
B) Social distancing
C) Use of N95 respirators
D) Surface disinfection

Question 5: Which term refers to the surgical removal of a portion of the skull?
A) Craniotomy
B) Craniectomy
C) Cranioplasty
D) Craniosynostosis

Question 6: Maria, a 45-year-old woman with multiple sclerosis (MS), has recently been experiencing increased difficulty with mobility and fatigue. She expresses feelings of frustration and helplessness during her consultation. Based on contemporary research, which coping strategy is most likely to help Maria manage her emotional distress effectively?
A) Denial of the severity of her condition
B) Seeking social support from friends and family
C) Avoidance of activities that remind her of her limitations
D) Focusing solely on medical treatments

Question 7: Mr. Johnson is scheduled for an EKG procedure. As his medical assistant, what is the most critical step you should take to prepare him for the procedure?
A) Ensure Mr. Johnson has not consumed caffeine in the last 24 hours.
B) Explain the procedure to Mr. Johnson and ensure he has removed any metallic objects.
C) Confirm that Mr. Johnson has fasted for at least 8 hours before the procedure.
D) Verify that Mr. Johnson's skin is clean and dry at electrode sites.

Question 8: Which statement best describes the purpose of a Living Will?
A) A Living Will specifies the types of medical treatment a person wishes to receive or avoid if they become incapacitated.
B) A Living Will appoints someone to make healthcare decisions on behalf of an incapacitated person.
C) A Living Will ensures that emergency medical personnel do not perform CPR if a person stops breathing.
D) A Living Will provides legal authority for organ donation upon death.

Question 9: When communicating with a geriatric patient who has mild cognitive impairment, which of the following strategies is most effective?
A) Use medical jargon to ensure accuracy.
B) Speak slowly and clearly while maintaining eye contact.
C) Increase the volume of your voice significantly.
D) Avoid using gestures as they may confuse the patient.

Question 10: During an EKG test on a 55-year-old patient named Mr. Johnson, you observe a series of wide QRS complexes with no preceding P waves and an irregular rhythm. What is the most likely diagnosis?
A) Atrial Fibrillation
B) Ventricular Tachycardia
C) Supraventricular Tachycardia
D) Premature Ventricular Contractions

Question 11: A 45-year-old patient presents with a blood pressure reading. Which of the following readings would be considered hypertensive according to the latest guidelines by the American Heart Association?
A) 120/80 mmHg
B) 130/85 mmHg
C) 140/90 mmHg
D) 135/88 mmHg

Question 12: A patient confides in a Certified Clinical Medical Assistant (CCMA) about experiencing domestic abuse but insists that this information remains confidential. According to professional codes of ethics, what should the CCMA do?
A) Respect the patient's wishes and keep the information confidential.
B) Report the abuse to the appropriate authorities despite the patient's request.
C) Discuss the situation with a colleague for advice while keeping the patient's identity confidential.
D) Encourage the patient to report the abuse themselves but take no further action.

Question 13: Which of the following actions best adheres to the CDC's guidelines for preventing healthcare-associated infections (HAIs) in a clinical setting?
A) Using alcohol-based hand sanitizer before and after patient contact
B) Wearing gloves only when there is a visible risk of exposure to bodily fluids
C) Reusing disposable gowns for multiple patients if they appear clean
D) Sterilizing medical instruments using autoclaves after each use

Question 14: Which of the following best exemplifies professional presence for a Certified Clinical Medical

Assistant when interacting with patients?
A) Wearing clean scrubs, maintaining eye contact, and using medical jargon.
B) Wearing clean scrubs, maintaining eye contact, and speaking in a calm and clear tone.
C) Wearing clean scrubs, avoiding eye contact to not intimidate patients, and using medical jargon.
D) Wearing casual attire to appear approachable, maintaining eye contact, and using simple language.

Question 15: Which alternative therapy is primarily based on the principle that the body has self-regulating mechanisms that can be stimulated through specific points on the body?
A) Acupuncture
B) Reflexology
C) Chiropractic
D) Homeopathy

Question 16: Patient John Doe presents with symptoms including fatigue, pallor, and shortness of breath. His primary care physician suspects anemia and orders a series of laboratory tests to confirm the diagnosis. Which of the following tests would most accurately diagnose iron-deficiency anemia?
A) Complete Blood Count (CBC)
B) Serum Ferritin
C) Serum Iron
D) Total Iron-Binding Capacity (TIBC)

Question 17: Sarah, a 45-year-old woman with a family history of cardiovascular disease, visits her medical assistant for advice on preventive measures. She is concerned about her risk factors and wants to take proactive steps to maintain her health. Which of the following is the most appropriate recommendation for Sarah?
A) Start a low-carbohydrate diet immediately.
B) Begin a daily exercise routine tailored to her fitness level.
C) Take an aspirin daily without consulting her physician.
D) Increase her intake of dietary supplements.

Question 18: During a routine procedure, a medical assistant named Sarah accidentally administers a higher dose of medication than prescribed to a patient named John. John experiences adverse effects requiring hospitalization. Which legal concept is most applicable in determining Sarah's liability?
A) Negligence
B) Battery
C) Breach of Duty
D) Strict Liability

Question 19: When removing sutures from a patient, which step should be performed first to ensure proper technique and patient safety?
A) Clean the wound with an antiseptic solution.
B) Cut the suture at its knot.
C) Grasp the suture with forceps.
D) Check for signs of infection around the wound.

Question 20: Sarah, a medical assistant, is dealing with an irate patient, Mr. Johnson, who is upset about a long wait time. What is the most effective way for Sarah to address Mr. Johnson's concerns while maintaining professionalism and ensuring patient satisfaction?
A) Apologize sincerely for the wait and explain the reason behind the delay.
B) Offer Mr. Johnson an immediate appointment with another provider.
C) Ignore Mr. Johnson's frustration and expedite his appointment.
D) Suggest that Mr. Johnson reschedule his appointment for another day.

Question 21: According to Erikson's stages of psychosocial development, what is the primary challenge faced by individuals in the 'Industry vs. Inferiority' stage?
A) Developing a sense of trust
B) Developing a sense of autonomy
C) Developing a sense of competence
D) Developing a sense of identity

Question 22: What is the most critical step in ensuring accurate distribution of laboratory results to the ordering provider after matching the patient to the provider?
A) Verifying the patient's identity using two unique identifiers before sending results.
B) Confirming that the lab results are entered into the patient's electronic health record (EHR).
C) Ensuring that the results are communicated directly to the ordering provider via secure methods.
D) Documenting the date and time when results were sent to the ordering provider.

Question 23: You are drafting a formal business letter to inform a patient, Mr. John Smith, about an upcoming surgery date. Which format should you use to ensure the letter adheres to professional standards and is easily readable?
A) Modified Block Format
B) Full Block Format
C) Semi-Block Format
D) Simplified Format

Question 24: During a team meeting discussing a patient named Mr. Johnson's care plan, the team faces a disagreement about the best approach for his post-operative care. As a Certified Clinical Medical Assistant (CCMA), how should you facilitate and promote effective teamwork and engagement among the team members?
A) Encourage each team member to voice their opinion without interruption.
B) Summarize each person's viewpoint and suggest a compromise solution.
C) Allow the most experienced team member to make the final decision.
D) Focus on common goals and ensure that everyone agrees with the final decision.

Question 25: Maria, a 45-year-old patient with chronic hypertension, visits your clinic for a routine check-up. She mentions that she recently switched her insurance plan and is unsure if her new plan covers her pre-existing condition. Which type of insurance plan is most likely to cover pre-existing conditions without a waiting period?
A) Health Maintenance Organization (HMO)
B) Preferred Provider Organization (PPO)
C) High-Deductible Health Plan (HDHP)
D) Affordable Care Act (ACA) Marketplace Plan

Question 26: Sarah, a 45-year-old patient, is scheduled for a lipid panel blood test. As her medical assistant, you must ensure she follows the correct preparation guidelines. Which of the following instructions should you give Sarah regarding her fasting requirements?
A) "You need to fast for at least 8 hours before your test."
B) "You can have black coffee but no solid food 12 hours before your test."
C) "You can drink water but avoid all other beverages for 10 hours before your test."
D) "You should fast for at least 6 hours and avoid any liquids except water."

Question 27: Which of the following is a primary objective of the Meaningful Use program under the Health Information Technology for Economic and Clinical Health (HITECH) Act?
A) Improve patient care coordination
B) Increase patient volume in healthcare facilities
C) Reduce healthcare administrative costs
D) Enhance medical billing accuracy

Question 28: Maria, a 65-year-old patient with chronic obstructive pulmonary disease (COPD), has been admitted to the hospital due to exacerbation of her condition. The attending physician orders several ancillary services to support her treatment plan. Which of the following ancillary services is primarily responsible for assessing and managing Maria's respiratory function?
A) Radiology
B) Respiratory Therapy
C) Physical Therapy
D) Occupational Therapy

Question 29: During a busy morning shift, you are tasked with collecting a blood specimen from Mr. John Smith, who is scheduled for a glucose test. After drawing the blood, you label the specimen. Which of the following actions ensures that the specimen is accurately matched to Mr. John Smith and his completed requisition form?
A) Verify Mr. John Smith's name and date of birth on both the specimen label and requisition form before labeling.
B) Label the specimen immediately after collection based on memory of Mr. John Smith's details.
C) Cross-check Mr. John Smith's name with the appointment schedule before labeling.
D) Use pre-printed labels with Mr. John Smith's information provided by another staff member.

Question 30: Emily, a 45-year-old patient, is scheduled for a colonoscopy. As a Certified Clinical Medical Assistant (CCMA), what is the most important step you should take to prepare her for this procedure?
A) Ensure she has followed the clear liquid diet for at least 24 hours before the procedure.
B) Confirm she has taken her prescribed bowel preparation medication as instructed.
C) Verify that she has fasted for at least 12 hours before the procedure.
D) Make sure she has signed the informed consent form.

Question 31: Which of the following is the most appropriate method for disposing of unused controlled substances in a clinical setting?
A) Flushing them down the toilet.
B) Returning them to a pharmacy take-back program.
C) Mixing them with coffee grounds and placing in the trash.
D) Incinerating them in a regular waste facility.

Question 32: Which of the following is the correct order of draw for blood collection tubes to avoid cross-contamination?
A) Light blue, red, green, lavender
B) Red, light blue, green, lavender
C) Light blue, red, lavender, green
D) Red, lavender, light blue, green

Question 33: Which of the following is the most appropriate storage condition for temperature-sensitive vaccines?
A) Store at room temperature, between 20°C and 25°C.
B) Store in a freezer, below -15°C.
C) Store in a refrigerator, between 2°C and 8°C.
D) Store in an insulated container at ambient temperature.

Question 34: During a routine blood glucose monitoring test for Mr. Johnson, the clinical medical assistant notices that the control solution used is outdated. What is the most appropriate action to ensure accurate test results?
A) Proceed with the test using the outdated control solution.
B) Use a patient sample as a substitute for the control solution.
C) Obtain a new control solution and recalibrate the glucometer.
D) Ignore the control solution and rely on previous calibration data.

Question 35: Maria, a Certified Clinical Medical Assistant, is entering patient data into an Electronic Health Record (EHR) system. She needs to ensure that all patient demographic information is accurate and up-to-date. Which of the following actions should Maria prioritize to maintain data integrity?
A) Double-checking patient insurance details before saving the record.
B) Verifying the patient's contact information with them directly.
C) Ensuring that all mandatory fields are filled out correctly.
D) Cross-referencing the patient's medical history with previous records.

Question 36: During an otoscopic examination of a patient named John, which piece of equipment is essential for visualizing the tympanic membrane?
A) Ophthalmoscope
B) Otoscope
C) Tuning fork
D) Stethoscope

Question 37: Sarah, a medical assistant, has just collected a blood sample from a patient named John. To ensure the sample is properly prepared for transportation to an outside reference laboratory, which of the following steps should she take next?
A) Label the sample with John's name and date of birth only.
B) Place the sample in a biohazard bag without any additional documentation.
C) Ensure the sample is placed in a temperature-controlled container if required.
D) Send the sample immediately without any special handling instructions.

Question 38: Which of the following is the most crucial step in ensuring the accuracy of laboratory test results?
A) Regular calibration of equipment
B) Routine maintenance of laboratory instruments
C) Proper labeling of specimens
D) Timely updating of standard operating procedures (SOPs)

Question 39: Which pharmacokinetic process is primarily responsible for determining the bioavailability of an orally administered drug?
A) Absorption
B) Distribution
C) Metabolism
D) Excretion

Question 40: Emily, a medical assistant, is preparing to perform a venipuncture on a patient. She uses an alcohol-based hand rub before putting on gloves. Which of the following statements about the use of alcohol-based hand rubs is correct?
A) Alcohol-based hand rubs are effective against all types of bacteria and viruses.
B) Alcohol-based hand rubs should be used when hands are

visibly soiled.
C) Alcohol-based hand rubs require at least 20 seconds of rubbing to be effective.
D) Alcohol-based hand rubs are less effective than soap and water in removing Clostridium difficile spores.

Question 41: Which blood vacuum tube is typically used for collecting a sample for a complete blood count (CBC)?
A) Lavender top tube
B) Light blue top tube
C) Green top tube
D) Red top tube

Question 42: Which of the following is a requirement for a facility to perform CLIA-waived tests?
A) The facility must have a Certificate of Waiver from CMS.
B) The facility must employ a certified pathologist.
C) The facility must undergo annual inspections by CMS.
D) The facility must perform proficiency testing for all waived tests.

Question 43: Mr. Thompson, an 85-year-old male with severe arthritis and fragile veins, requires a blood draw. Considering his age and condition, which venipuncture site is most accessible and appropriate?
A) Dorsal hand veins
B) Cephalic vein in the forearm
C) Basilic vein in the upper arm
D) Median cubital vein in the antecubital fossa

Question 44: When assisting providers in coordinating care with community agencies, which of the following is the most important initial step for a medical assistant?
A) Identifying patient needs and preferences
B) Contacting local community health centers
C) Scheduling follow-up appointments with specialists
D) Gathering information on available transportation services

Question 45: Which of the following is the most appropriate method for disposing of unused controlled substances in a clinical setting?
A) Flushing them down the toilet
B) Mixing them with coffee grounds and placing in household trash
C) Returning them to a pharmacy take-back program
D) Incinerating them in a medical waste facility

Question 46: Patient John, a 45-year-old male, is experiencing symptoms of dehydration after a strenuous workout. Which physiological response is primarily responsible for maintaining his blood pressure under these conditions?
A) Increased secretion of aldosterone
B) Decreased release of antidiuretic hormone (ADH)
C) Vasodilation of peripheral blood vessels
D) Increased heart rate

Question 47: During a busy clinic day, Maria, a medical assistant, efficiently manages her tasks and assists patients with empathy and professionalism. Her supervisor wants to provide feedback that reinforces this effective behavior. Which of the following is the most appropriate way for the supervisor to give positive reinforcement?
A) "Maria, you did a great job today. Keep it up."
B) "Maria, your ability to manage tasks efficiently and assist patients with empathy was outstanding today. It really made a difference."
C) "Maria, you were very professional today."
D) "Maria, good work on managing your tasks."

Question 48: Mr. Smith has been prescribed a

medication for his skin infection. The medication needs to be applied directly to the affected area to ensure maximum effectiveness and minimal systemic absorption. Which form of medication is most appropriate for Mr. Smith?
A) Pill
B) Capsule
C) Ointment
D) Oral Suspension

Question 49: Sarah, a CCMA, is preparing to draw blood from a patient for a complete blood count (CBC). She must choose the appropriate collection tube with the correct additive to ensure accurate results. Which tube should she select?
A) Red-top tube (no additive)
B) Blue-top tube (sodium citrate)
C) Lavender-top tube (EDTA)
D) Green-top tube (heparin)

Question 50: Which of the following actions is most effective in preventing the spread of healthcare-associated infections (HAIs)?
A) Using alcohol-based hand rub before and after patient contact
B) Wearing gloves during all patient interactions
C) Using a surgical mask when entering a patient's room
D) Cleaning medical equipment with disinfectant wipes

Question 51: Mr. John Doe needs a referral to a cardiologist due to his recent diagnosis of hypertension. As a Certified Clinical Medical Assistant (CCMA), you are responsible for creating and sending the e-referral. Which of the following steps is crucial to ensure that the e-referral contains all required information?
A) Include only the patient's demographic information and primary care physician's contact details.
B) Attach the patient's complete medical history, including previous unrelated conditions.
C) Provide the patient's demographic information, relevant medical history, reason for referral, and any pertinent test results.
D) Send an e-referral with just a brief note from the primary care physician without additional documentation.

Question 52: During a sudden cardiac arrest, you find John, a 50-year-old male, unresponsive and not breathing. After calling for help and initiating CPR, you retrieve an AED. When the AED arrives, what is the next immediate step you should take?
A) Attach the AED pads to John's chest and then turn on the AED.
B) Turn on the AED and follow its prompts before attaching the pads.
C) Check for a pulse again before using the AED.
D) Continue CPR until emergency services arrive without using the AED.

Question 53: Which of the following is considered a critical component of the "Rights of Medication Administration" to ensure patient safety?
A) Right Route
B) Right Patient
C) Right Documentation
D) Right Preparation

Question 54: When assisting a frail patient with ambulation, which of the following techniques is most appropriate to ensure both safety and support?
A) Using a gait belt and walking slightly behind the patient
B) Holding the patient's arm tightly while walking beside them
C) Using a walker and standing directly in front of the patient

D) Supporting the patient's elbow while walking side by side

Question 55: When performing a Snellen chart test for visual acuity, at what distance should the patient be positioned from the chart?
A) 10 feet
B) 15 feet
C) 20 feet
D) 25 feet

Question 56: Which type of health insurance plan typically requires patients to select a primary care physician (PCP) who coordinates their care and provides referrals to specialists?
A) Preferred Provider Organization (PPO)
B) Health Maintenance Organization (HMO)
C) Exclusive Provider Organization (EPO)
D) Point of Service (POS)

Question 57: Which credential is specifically awarded to individuals who have completed a program accredited by the Commission on Accreditation of Allied Health Education Programs (CAAHEP) and passed a national certification exam?
A) Certified Medical Assistant (CMA)
B) Registered Medical Assistant (RMA)
C) Clinical Medical Assistant (CCMA)
D) Certified Clinical Medical Assistant (CCMA)

Question 58: Sarah, a medical assistant, is preparing to clean a wound on a patient using an antiseptic solution. Which of the following precautions should she take to avoid chemical burns?
A) Ensure the antiseptic solution is properly diluted before application.
B) Apply the antiseptic solution directly without dilution for maximum effectiveness.
C) Wear gloves to protect her hands from potential irritation.
D) Use only sterile water for cleaning wounds to avoid any chemical reactions.

Question 59: Which of the following is a primary function of home health care services for patients with chronic illnesses?
A) Providing acute medical treatments
B) Offering palliative care for terminal patients
C) Assisting with activities of daily living (ADLs)
D) Conducting routine surgical procedures

Question 60: Which technology is primarily used to ensure real-time tracking and reporting of patient vital signs within a hospital setting?
A) Electronic Health Records (EHR)
B) Remote Patient Monitoring (RPM)
C) Clinical Decision Support Systems (CDSS)
D) Health Information Exchange (HIE)

Question 61: Sarah, a 35-year-old patient, is scheduled for a colposcopy due to abnormal Pap smear results. As a Certified Clinical Medical Assistant (CCMA), which of the following is the most appropriate initial step you should take to assist with this procedure?
A) Position Sarah in the lithotomy position and ensure she has emptied her bladder.
B) Prepare the colposcope and ensure all instruments are sterilized.
C) Provide Sarah with detailed post-procedure care instructions before starting.
D) Assist the physician by applying acetic acid to Sarah's cervix.

Question 62: Which of the following scenarios best exemplifies medical malpractice?

A) A physician intentionally prescribing a medication that causes harm.
B) A nurse administering the wrong dosage due to a miscalculation.
C) A surgeon performing an unauthorized procedure on a patient.
D) A medical assistant failing to document a patient's allergy leading to an adverse reaction.

Question 63: Which instructional technique is most effective for a kinesthetic learner in a clinical training setting?
A) Demonstration
B) Lecture
C) Reading assignments
D) Visual aids

Question 64: Sarah, a 35-year-old patient with chronic pain, has been prescribed a medication by her physician. This medication has a high potential for abuse but also has accepted medical use in treatment. Under which drug schedule would this medication most likely fall?
A) Schedule I
B) Schedule II
C) Schedule III
D) Schedule IV

Question 65: Which of the following pre-analytical considerations is most critical for ensuring specimen quality and consistency in phlebotomy?
A) Using a tourniquet for no longer than one minute
B) Ensuring the patient is fasting before drawing blood
C) Properly labeling specimens immediately after collection
D) Using the correct gauge needle for venipuncture

Question 66: A patient is prescribed 250 mg of a medication. The available tablets are 125 mg each. How many tablets should the patient take per dose?
A) 1 tablet
B) 2 tablets
C) 2.5 tablets
D) 3 tablets

Question 67: Sarah, a 55-year-old patient with type 2 diabetes, is seeking advice on her dietary needs. Which of the following recommendations is most appropriate for managing her condition?
A) Increase intake of high-fiber foods like whole grains and vegetables.
B) Limit sodium intake to reduce blood pressure.
C) Increase consumption of omega-3 fatty acids to lower cholesterol levels.
D) Avoid all carbohydrate-containing foods to manage blood sugar levels.

Question 68: Sarah, a medical assistant, needs to transport a blood sample for diagnostic testing. Which of the following practices is MOST critical to ensure the sample's integrity?
A) Ensuring the sample is transported at room temperature.
B) Using a biohazard bag with proper labeling.
C) Placing the sample in a pneumatic tube system.
D) Storing the sample in an airtight container.

Question 69: When performing CPR on an adult, what is the recommended depth of chest compressions according to the latest American Heart Association guidelines?
A) At least 1 inch
B) At least 2 inches
C) About 1.5 inches
D) About 3 inches

Question 70: Which of the following is considered one of the essential "Rights of Medication Administration" to ensure patient safety?
A) Right Diagnosis
B) Right Route
C) Right Documentation
D) Right Frequency

Question 71: In which of the following scenarios is written consent most critically required over verbal consent?
A) Administering a routine vaccination in a primary care setting.
B) Conducting a minor surgical procedure in an outpatient clinic.
C) Providing dietary advice during a regular health check-up.
D) Performing an emergency life-saving intervention where the patient is unconscious.

Question 72: Sarah, a 35-year-old female patient, presents with a headache and dizziness. Upon assessment, her vital signs are as follows: temperature 37.5°C (99.5°F), pulse 98 bpm, respiratory rate 18 breaths per minute, and blood pressure 140/90 mmHg. Which of Sarah's vital signs is most indicative of an abnormal condition?
A) Temperature 37.5°C (99.5°F)
B) Pulse 98 bpm
C) Respiratory rate 18 breaths per minute
D) Blood pressure 140/90 mmHg

Question 73: Which link in the chain of infection is directly disrupted by proper hand hygiene practices?
A) Portal of Exit
B) Mode of Transmission
C) Portal of Entry
D) Susceptible Host

Question 74: Which of the following is considered the most significant barrier to accessing healthcare services for patients from low socio-economic backgrounds?
A) Lack of health insurance
B) Cultural misunderstandings
C) Language barriers
D) Limited health literacy

Question 75: Sarah, a 30-year-old female patient, visits the clinic for a routine check-up. The medical assistant needs to measure her height, weight, and calculate her BMI accurately. Which of the following steps is NOT recommended when measuring Sarah's height?
A) Ensure Sarah stands barefoot with her heels together.
B) Position Sarah's head in the Frankfort horizontal plane.
C) Ask Sarah to stand on tiptoes to get an accurate measurement.
D) Use a stadiometer for precise height measurement.

Question 76: A medical assistant is entering medication orders for a patient named John Doe into the CPOE system. The physician has ordered 500 mg of Amoxicillin to be administered every 8 hours for 7 days. Which of the following actions should the medical assistant take to ensure accurate entry into the CPOE system?
A) Enter "500 mg Amoxicillin, PO, q8h x 7 days"
B) Enter "500 mg Amoxicillin, PO, q12h x 7 days"
C) Enter "250 mg Amoxicillin, PO, q8h x 14 days"
D) Enter "500 mg Amoxicillin, IV, q8h x 7 days"

Question 77: During a pelvic examination, what is the most appropriate position for the patient to ensure both comfort and optimal access for the healthcare provider?

A) Supine position with knees bent and feet flat on the table
B) Lithotomy position with legs supported in stirrups
C) Prone position with a pillow under the abdomen
D) Sims' position with one leg flexed

Question 78: Sarah, a Certified Clinical Medical Assistant (CCMA), is administering a medication to a patient named Mr. Johnson. She checks the medication label three times and verifies it with the patient's chart. She also ensures that she has the correct dose and route of administration. However, before giving the medication, what is another crucial step Sarah must take to adhere to the "Rights of Medication Administration"?
A) Confirm the patient's allergies.
B) Verify the expiration date of the medication.
C) Check the patient's vital signs.
D) Ensure proper documentation after administration.

Question 79: Which term refers to the fixed amount a patient pays for a covered healthcare service, usually paid at the time of service?
A) Co-pay
B) Co-insurance
C) Deductible
D) Premium

Question 80: During a comprehensive clinical intake process, which action is most critical for accurately determining the purpose of a patient's visit?
A) Reviewing the patient's medical history
B) Conducting a thorough physical examination
C) Asking open-ended questions about symptoms
D) Verifying the patient's insurance information

Question 81: During a routine check, Maria, a Certified Clinical Medical Assistant (CCMA), notices that the temperature log for the vaccine refrigerator has not been updated for the past three days. What should be her immediate course of action?
A) Record the current temperature and continue monitoring daily.
B) Report the lapse to her supervisor and document the incident.
C) Assume that the temperature has remained stable and update the log accordingly.
D) Reset the refrigerator's temperature settings and start a new log.

Question 82: Which of the following is the most immediate and appropriate first-line treatment for an anaphylactic reaction to a bee sting?
A) Antihistamines
B) Epinephrine
C) Corticosteroids
D) Bronchodilators

Question 83: Sarah, a 65-year-old patient with multiple chronic conditions, is looking for a healthcare delivery model that emphasizes coordinated care, improved health outcomes, and cost efficiency. Which of the following healthcare delivery models would be most appropriate for Sarah?
A) Health Maintenance Organization (HMO)
B) Preferred Provider Organization (PPO)
C) Patient-Centered Medical Home (PCMH)
D) Accountable Care Organization (ACO)

Question 84: A medical assistant is reviewing the chart of a patient named Mr. Johnson who has been admitted with chest pain. The chart notes "NPO after midnight" and "PRN for pain." Based on these notations, which of the following actions should the medical assistant take?
A) Ensure Mr. Johnson receives no food or drink after

midnight.
B) Administer pain medication only as needed.
C) Schedule Mr. Johnson for a procedure after midnight.
D) Provide Mr. Johnson with pain medication every four hours.

Question 85: When dealing with an irate patient who is upset about a long wait time, what is the most effective initial technique a Certified Clinical Medical Assistant (CCMA) should use?
A) Apologize immediately and offer to reschedule their appointment.
B) Listen actively to the patient's concerns without interrupting.
C) Explain the reasons for the delay in detail.
D) Direct the patient to speak with a supervisor.

Question 86: Which route of drug administration typically results in the fastest onset of action?
A) Intravenous (IV)
B) Intramuscular (IM)
C) Subcutaneous (SC)
D) Oral (PO)

Question 87: Sarah, a Certified Clinical Medical Assistant (CCMA), is tasked with updating patient records in an electronic health record (EHR) system. She notices that Mr. Johnson's contact information is outdated. What is the best course of action for Sarah to ensure the information is accurate?
A) Update the contact information immediately based on her last conversation with Mr. Johnson.
B) Call Mr. Johnson to verify his current contact information before updating the record.
C) Leave a note in the EHR system requesting the front desk staff to update Mr. Johnson's contact information.
D) Wait until Mr. Johnson's next appointment to confirm and update his contact information.

Question 88: Sarah, a 45-year-old patient with liver cirrhosis, is prescribed a medication primarily metabolized by the liver. Which pharmacokinetic parameter is most likely to be significantly altered in Sarah due to her liver condition?
A) Absorption
B) Distribution
C) Metabolism
D) Excretion

Question 89: When entering a medication order into a Computerized Physician Order Entry (CPOE) system, which of the following steps is crucial to ensure patient safety and minimize errors?
A) Verify the patient's identity using two identifiers.
B) Enter the medication dosage based solely on the physician's verbal instructions.
C) Confirm the medication order with another medical assistant before entry.
D) Rely on pre-populated fields in the CPOE system for medication details.

Question 90: Emily, a 45-year-old patient, presents with symptoms of severe abdominal pain and tenderness. The physician suspects appendicitis and orders an imaging study to confirm the diagnosis. Which imaging modality is most commonly used to diagnose acute appendicitis?
A) Abdominal X-ray
B) MRI (Magnetic Resonance Imaging)
C) CT (Computed Tomography) scan
D) Ultrasound

Question 91: A patient in your care has suddenly

become unresponsive, and initial attempts at resuscitation by the medical assistant team have been unsuccessful. At what point should you escalate the situation to a higher level of care?
A) When the patient's vital signs are stable but they remain unresponsive.
B) After 5 minutes of unsuccessful resuscitation attempts.
C) When initial resuscitation attempts have failed, and there is no immediate improvement.
D) Only after consulting with another medical assistant.

Question 92: In a standard block format business letter, which element is aligned to the left margin and not indented?
A) Salutation
B) Body paragraphs
C) Complimentary close
D) Date

Question 93: What is the most effective initial step in reducing a wandering baseline artifact during an EKG recording?
A) Repositioning the limb electrodes
B) Ensuring proper skin preparation
C) Using a higher quality EKG machine
D) Increasing the paper speed of the EKG

Question 94: Which of the following is a primary responsibility of a nuclear pharmacy?
A) Preparing individualized medication dosages for patients
B) Compounding sterile intravenous medications
C) Dispensing radiopharmaceuticals for diagnostic imaging
D) Creating customized topical creams and ointments

Question 95: Which of the following is the most critical step in ensuring an examination/procedure room is properly prepared for patient care?
A) Ensuring all medical instruments are sterilized.
B) Verifying that all necessary supplies and equipment are present.
C) Disinfecting all surfaces and equipment.
D) Confirming patient records and charts are ready.

Question 96: Maria, a 65-year-old patient with terminal cancer, expresses frustration and resentment towards her family and healthcare providers. She frequently lashes out and blames them for her condition. Which stage of grief is Maria most likely experiencing?
A) Denial
B) Anger
C) Bargaining
D) Depression

Question 97: When communicating with a non-English speaking patient, which strategy is most effective in ensuring understanding and providing quality care?
A) Speaking slowly and loudly in English.
B) Using a certified medical interpreter.
C) Relying on the patient's family member to translate.
D) Providing written instructions in English.

Question 98: Mr. Johnson has been prescribed a medication that must be stored under specific conditions to maintain its efficacy. Which of the following storage practices should the medical assistant follow to ensure the medication remains effective?
A) Store the medication in a cool, dry place away from direct sunlight.
B) Store the medication in the refrigerator at 4°C.
C) Store the medication at room temperature, between 20°C and 25°C.
D) Store the medication in a freezer at -20°C.

Question 99: Emily, a Certified Clinical Medical Assistant, is updating the medication log for a patient named Mr. Johnson who has been prescribed multiple medications. Which of the following actions should Emily take to ensure the medication log is accurate and compliant with regulations?
A) Record the medication name, dosage, and time of administration only.
B) Include the medication name, dosage, time of administration, and the initials of the administering staff.
C) Document only the medication name and time of administration to save time.
D) Note the medication name, dosage, time of administration, and patient's reaction.

Question 100: Sarah, a 45-year-old patient, is scheduled for a minor surgical procedure in the clinic. As a Clinical Medical Assistant, which of the following items is most critical to ensure proper sterilization and preparation of the examination room?
A) Autoclave
B) Disinfectant wipes
C) Sterile gloves
D) Surgical drapes

Question 101: Sarah is a medical assistant advising a patient with hypertension on how to read food labels to manage their sodium intake. She shows the patient a label that states: "Serving Size: 1 cup; Sodium: 480 mg; Servings per Container: 2." What is the total sodium content if the patient consumes the entire container?
A) 480 mg
B) 960 mg
C) 240 mg
D) 720 mg

Question 102: Sarah, a Certified Clinical Medical Assistant (CCMA), overhears two nurses discussing a patient's HIV status in the hospital cafeteria. What is the most appropriate action for Sarah to take in this situation?
A) Report the conversation to hospital administration immediately.
B) Confront the nurses directly about their breach of confidentiality.
C) Document the incident and inform her immediate supervisor.
D) Ignore the conversation as it does not involve her directly.

Question 103: During a routine blood draw from Mr. Johnson, a medical assistant accidentally pricks her finger with a used needle. What is the most appropriate immediate action she should take to minimize the risk of blood-borne pathogen transmission?
A) Apply an antiseptic wipe and cover with a bandage.
B) Wash the area with soap and water, then report the incident.
C) Squeeze out as much blood as possible before washing.
D) Apply alcohol directly to the wound and let it air dry.

Question 104: Mrs. Johnson, a 65-year-old patient, expresses anxiety about her upcoming surgery. She says, "I'm really scared about the procedure." As a Certified Clinical Medical Assistant (CCMA), what is the most appropriate therapeutic response?
A) "Don't worry, everything will be fine."
B) "I understand that you're scared. Can you tell me more about what's worrying you?"
C) "Many patients feel this way before surgery."
D) "Try not to think about it too much."

Question 105: Which of the following dietary recommendations is most appropriate for a patient with Type 2 Diabetes Mellitus?
A) Increase intake of high-glycemic index foods.
B) Focus on a balanced diet with complex carbohydrates and fiber.
C) Limit protein intake to less than 10% of daily calories.
D) Eliminate all fats from the diet.

Question 106: When preparing a patient for a general physical examination, which position is most appropriate for examining the abdomen?
A) Supine
B) Prone
C) Fowler's
D) Lithotomy

Question 107: Patient John Doe has been ordered a series of blood tests including a Complete Blood Count (CBC), Basic Metabolic Panel (BMP), and Prothrombin Time (PT). Which set of supplies should the medical assistant prepare?
A) Lavender-top tube, red-top tube, light blue-top tube
B) Green-top tube, red-top tube, light blue-top tube
C) Lavender-top tube, green-top tube, light blue-top tube
D) Lavender-top tube, red-top tube, green-top tube

Question 108: Which term describes a position closer to the midline of the body?
A) Lateral
B) Proximal
C) Medial
D) Distal

Question 109: During a patient consultation, Maria, a medical assistant, notices that Mr. Johnson appears anxious while discussing his symptoms. Which of the following actions best demonstrates active listening?
A) Nodding occasionally while taking notes on the computer.
B) Maintaining eye contact and summarizing what Mr. Johnson says.
C) Asking Mr. Johnson to repeat himself for clarity.
D) Providing verbal reassurances without interrupting.

Question 110: During a review of the facility's safety protocols, it was noted that several incidents of patient falls occurred in the same area. As a medical assistant, what is the most effective first step to address this issue?
A) Conducting a comprehensive risk assessment of the area
B) Increasing staff presence in the area during peak hours
C) Installing additional signage to warn patients of potential hazards
D) Providing immediate training sessions for staff on fall prevention

Question 111: What is the legally required minimum retention period for adult patient medical records in most states?
A) 5 years
B) 7 years
C) 10 years
D) 15 years

Question 112: Maria, a certified clinical medical assistant, needs to verify a patient's lab results from an external laboratory. She has access to several external databases. Which database is most appropriate for ensuring the accuracy and reliability of these lab results?
A) PubMed
B) ClinicalTrials.gov
C) LabCorp's Online Portal
D) MedlinePlus

Question 113: Sarah, a Certified Clinical Medical Assistant (CCMA), is working in a busy family practice clinic. A patient, Mr. Johnson, comes in with complaints of chest pain. The physician is currently with another patient and asks Sarah to assist until they can attend to Mr. Johnson. Which of the following actions should Sarah take while waiting for the physician?
A) Administer nitroglycerin to alleviate Mr. Johnson's chest pain.
B) Take Mr. Johnson's vital signs and document his symptoms.
C) Interpret Mr. Johnson's electrocardiogram (ECG) results.
D) Provide Mr. Johnson with aspirin to chew.

Question 114: Maria, a Certified Clinical Medical Assistant (CCMA), is preparing the examination room for a minor surgical procedure. Which of the following actions is most critical to ensure the room is properly prepared?
A) Ensure all surgical instruments are laid out on a sterile drape.
B) Verify that the patient's medical history is updated in the electronic health record (EHR).
C) Confirm that all necessary personal protective equipment (PPE) is available and accessible.
D) Check that the room temperature is comfortable for both the patient and the medical staff.

Question 115: John, a 55-year-old male patient, comes in for an EKG test. As a Certified Clinical Medical Assistant, you need to place the limb and chest electrodes correctly. Where should you place the V4 electrode to ensure accurate EKG readings?
A) Fifth intercostal space at the midclavicular line
B) Fourth intercostal space at the midclavicular line
C) Fifth intercostal space at the anterior axillary line
D) Fourth intercostal space at the anterior axillary line

Question 116: Which type of blood collection tube requires exactly 8-10 gentle inversions immediately after collection to ensure proper mixing with the anticoagulant?
A) Light Blue Top Tube
B) Lavender Top Tube
C) Green Top Tube
D) Red Top Tube

Question 117: Which vitamin is essential for the synthesis of coenzyme A, a critical molecule in fatty acid metabolism?
A) Vitamin B1 (Thiamine)
B) Vitamin B2 (Riboflavin)
C) Vitamin B5 (Pantothenic Acid)
D) Vitamin B6 (Pyridoxine)

Question 118: Which of the following is the most effective method for ensuring patient confidentiality when handling medical records in a clinical setting?
A) Storing all medical records in locked filing cabinets.
B) Using password-protected electronic health records (EHR) systems.
C) Limiting access to medical records to authorized personnel only.
D) Shredding paper records after they are no longer needed.

Question 119: John, a 35-year-old male, presents with a deep laceration on his forearm sustained from a fall onto a sharp object. The wound is actively bleeding, and he reports severe pain. What is the most appropriate initial action for the medical assistant to take?
A) Apply direct pressure to the wound with a sterile dressing.
B) Clean the wound thoroughly with antiseptic solution.
C) Elevate the injured arm above heart level.

D) Apply a tourniquet proximal to the injury site.

Question 120: Which of the following is the most crucial step in preparing a patient for an EKG procedure to ensure accurate results?
A) Ensuring that the patient has fasted for at least 8 hours
B) Shaving any chest hair that may interfere with electrode placement
C) Instructing the patient to avoid caffeine for 24 hours before the test
D) Having the patient lie still and breathe normally during the procedure

Question 121: During an EKG procedure, you notice that the tracing shows significant baseline wander. Which of the following instructions is MOST appropriate to minimize this artifact for the patient, Mr. Johnson?
A) Ensure Mr. Johnson remains completely still and does not talk during the procedure.
B) Clean Mr. Johnson's skin with alcohol wipes before placing electrodes.
C) Instruct Mr. Johnson to hold his breath momentarily during the recording.
D) Reposition the electrodes to avoid areas with significant body hair.

Question 122: Jane Doe is a 75-year-old patient with advanced heart failure. She has decided to complete a MOLST form to ensure her end-of-life care preferences are respected. As a Certified Clinical Medical Assistant (CCMA), what is the most appropriate action you should take after Jane completes and signs her MOLST form?
A) Store the original MOLST form in Jane's medical record and provide her with a copy.
B) Keep the original MOLST form with Jane and store a copy in her medical record.
C) Send the original MOLST form to the state health department for official recording.
D) Provide Jane with both the original and a copy of the MOLST form for her records.

Question 123: Sarah, a patient with no medical background, is confused about her recent diagnosis of "hypertension." How should you explain this term in layman's language?
A) High blood pressure
B) High cholesterol
C) Heart disease
D) Elevated glucose levels

Question 124: When providing positive reinforcement to a medical assistant for effectively handling patient interactions, which approach is most effective?
A) Praising the assistant publicly in front of peers.
B) Offering specific feedback on what they did well.
C) Providing a general compliment about their work ethic.
D) Giving them an extra break as a reward.

Question 125: Which of the following is a requirement for submitting a valid claim under CMS billing regulations?
A) The patient's social security number
B) The provider's National Provider Identifier (NPI)
C) The patient's date of birth
D) The provider's tax identification number

Question 126: Sarah, a Certified Clinical Medical Assistant (CCMA), is preparing to draw blood from Mr. Johnson, a 55-year-old patient with known difficult veins. Which of the following steps should Sarah prioritize to ensure a successful venipuncture?
A) Apply a tourniquet tightly above the site for more than 2 minutes.

B) Use a butterfly needle and warm the patient's arm before attempting venipuncture.
C) Ask the patient to make a fist and pump it several times before inserting the needle.
D) Select the smallest gauge needle available to minimize discomfort.

Question 127: During a routine check-up, an 80-year-old patient named Mr. Johnson appears confused and agitated when asked about his medication routine. As a Certified Clinical Medical Assistant (CCMA), what is the most appropriate initial response to effectively communicate with him?
A) Repeat the question louder and more slowly.
B) Simplify the question using clear and concise language.
C) Ask a family member to provide the information.
D) Provide written instructions for him to read later.

Question 128: Sarah is a Certified Clinical Medical Assistant (CCMA) responsible for billing patients, insurers, and third-party payers for services performed at a medical practice. A patient named John received a comprehensive metabolic panel (CMP) test. When submitting the claim to John's insurance company, which of the following actions should Sarah take to ensure accurate billing?
A) Use the general office visit code since it covers all services provided.
B) Apply the specific CPT code for the CMP test performed.
C) Utilize the diagnosis code related to John's primary complaint.
D) Submit an itemized bill with descriptions of all services provided.

Question 129: Maria, a Certified Clinical Medical Assistant (CCMA), is assisting Dr. Thompson during a patient consultation. The patient, Mr. Johnson, begins to share personal information unrelated to his medical condition. How should Maria respond while maintaining professional boundaries?
A) Politely redirect the conversation back to Mr. Johnson's medical concerns.
B) Listen attentively and offer personal advice based on her own experiences.
C) Show empathy by sharing similar personal stories to build rapport.
D) Document the personal information shared by Mr. Johnson for future reference.

Question 130: When verifying a patient's insurance coverage and financial eligibility, which step is crucial to ensure that the services provided will be covered by the patient's insurance plan?
A) Confirming the patient's policy effective date
B) Verifying the patient's co-payment amount
C) Checking if pre-authorization is required for the service
D) Reviewing the patient's annual deductible status

Question 131: Which of the following is the primary mechanism behind the development of Type 1 Diabetes Mellitus?
A) Insulin resistance due to obesity
B) Autoimmune destruction of pancreatic beta cells
C) Increased hepatic glucose production
D) Dysfunctional insulin receptor signaling

Question 132: Sarah, a Certified Clinical Medical Assistant (CCMA), is preparing to administer a medication to a patient named Mr. Johnson. Which of the following actions should Sarah take to ensure she adheres to the "Right Patient" principle of medication administration?
A) Verify the patient's identity by checking the wristband and asking for their full name and date of birth.
B) Confirm the medication order with another nurse before administering.
C) Double-check the dosage against the medication chart.
D) Ensure that the medication is administered at the right time as per the schedule.

Question 133: Which of the following is the most critical step in maintaining surgical asepsis during a procedure?
A) Wearing sterile gloves
B) Using an antiseptic solution to clean the surgical site
C) Maintaining a sterile field
D) Donning a surgical mask

Question 134: Sarah, a 65-year-old patient with chronic heart failure, is being discharged from the hospital. As a Certified Clinical Medical Assistant (CCMA), what is the most crucial step you should take to ensure a smooth transition of care for Sarah?
A) Schedule a follow-up appointment with her primary care physician.
B) Provide Sarah with detailed written discharge instructions.
C) Arrange for home health services to assist Sarah post-discharge.
D) Educate Sarah on recognizing early signs of heart failure exacerbation.

Question 135: When obtaining prior authorizations and pre-certifications, which step is crucial to ensure the patient's insurance coverage is accurately verified?
A) Contacting the insurance company directly to confirm coverage details.
B) Reviewing the patient's medical history for relevant information.
C) Relying on the information provided by the patient during intake.
D) Checking the provider's internal system for insurance details.

Question 136: Sarah, a medical assistant, receives a call from Mrs. Johnson, who is the caregiver for Mr. Johnson, a patient recently prescribed new medication. Mrs. Johnson is confused about the dosage instructions and asks for clarification. How should Sarah respond to ensure effective communication while maintaining professionalism?
A) Provide detailed dosage instructions directly over the phone.
B) Ask Mrs. Johnson to bring Mr. Johnson to the clinic for clarification.
C) Verify Mrs. Johnson's identity before providing any information.
D) Refer Mrs. Johnson to the pharmacy for dosage information.

Question 137: Mrs. Johnson's insurance requires preauthorization for certain procedures. As a medical assistant, what is the most critical step you should take to ensure compliance with third-party payer billing requirements?
A) Submit the claim immediately after the procedure without waiting for preauthorization.
B) Verify insurance coverage and obtain preauthorization before scheduling the procedure.
C) Document the procedure thoroughly and submit the claim within 30 days.
D) Ensure accurate coding of the procedure after it has been performed.

Question 138: Which vitamin is primarily responsible for enhancing calcium absorption in the gastrointestinal tract, thus playing a critical role in bone health?

A) Vitamin D
B) Vitamin K
C) Vitamin A
D) Vitamin C

Question 139: Sarah Johnson arrives for her scheduled appointment at 10:00 AM. As a clinical medical assistant, what is the first step you should take to check her in?
A) Verify her insurance information.
B) Confirm her appointment time and purpose.
C) Request her identification and insurance card.
D) Update her medical history.

Question 140: Which of the following is a mandatory component of a laboratory requisition form to ensure proper patient identification and accurate test processing?
A) Patient's full name and date of birth
B) Physician's contact number
C) Type of specimen collected
D) Test codes for requested tests

Question 141: Mr. Thompson, a 45-year-old male patient, comes in for his annual physical examination. As a Clinical Medical Assistant, you are responsible for obtaining his anthropometric measurements. Which of the following is the most accurate method to measure Mr. Thompson's waist circumference?
A) Measure at the level of the umbilicus.
B) Measure at the narrowest point between the ribs and hips.
C) Measure just above the iliac crest.
D) Measure at the widest part of the abdomen.

Question 142: When transporting a specimen for diagnostic testing, which of the following is the most crucial step to ensure proper identification and integrity of the sample?
A) Labeling the specimen with the patient's name and date of birth.
B) Ensuring the specimen is stored at room temperature during transport.
C) Using a biohazard bag for all specimens regardless of type.
D) Verifying that the specimen label includes patient identifiers and test site.

Question 143: Mrs. Johnson presents with excessive cerumen buildup in her right ear, causing discomfort and partial hearing loss. As a certified clinical medical assistant, you are tasked with performing an ear irrigation. Which of the following steps is crucial to prevent potential complications during this procedure?
A) Use cold water to ensure patient comfort.
B) Direct the stream of water towards the eardrum for effective cleaning.
C) Tilt the patient's head slightly forward and use warm water.
D) Use a high-pressure syringe for quicker results.

Question 144: Sarah, a 45-year-old patient with a history of asthma, is scheduled for a spirometry test. As a clinical medical assistant, what is the most critical instruction you should give her before the test to ensure accurate results?
A) Avoid using your inhaler for at least 1 hour before the test.
B) Do not eat a heavy meal within 2 hours of the test.
C) Refrain from vigorous exercise for at least 30 minutes before the test.
D) Avoid smoking for at least 24 hours before the test.

Question 145: Sarah, a 65-year-old patient with multiple chronic conditions, is looking for a healthcare delivery model that emphasizes coordinated care among her various healthcare providers and offers comprehensive management of her health. Which model is most appropriate for Sarah?
A) Health Maintenance Organization (HMO)
B) Preferred Provider Organization (PPO)
C) Patient-Centered Medical Home (PCMH)
D) Point of Service (POS)

Question 146: During a patient intake interview, Maria, a CCMA, needs to gather detailed information about Mr. Johnson's dietary habits over the past month. Which type of question should she use to obtain the most comprehensive information?
A) "Can you describe what you typically eat in a day?"
B) "Do you follow any specific diet?"
C) "How many meals do you eat per day?"
D) "Have you changed your eating habits recently?"

Question 147: A medical assistant is tasked with organizing patient records for Dr. Smith's clinic. They need to ensure that files are easily accessible and maintain patient confidentiality. Which filing system would best meet these requirements?
A) Alphabetical Filing
B) Numerical Filing
C) Subject Filing
D) Terminal Digit Filing

Question 148: When administering a subcutaneous injection, which of the following is the correct angle to insert the needle?
A) 45 degrees
B) 90 degrees
C) 15 degrees
D) 30 degrees

Question 149: Which of the following is the correct plural form of the medical term "bacterium"?
A) Bacteriums
B) Bacteria
C) Bacterias
D) Bacteriae

Question 150: Which of the following conditions is considered the most significant risk factor leading to high mortality and morbidity worldwide?
A) Hypertension
B) Type 2 Diabetes Mellitus
C) Chronic Obstructive Pulmonary Disease (COPD)
D) Ischemic Heart Disease

ANSWER WITH DETAILED EXPLANATION SET [2]

Question 1: Correct Answer: A) Heart
Rationale: The mediastinum is the central compartment of the thoracic cavity that houses the heart, trachea, esophagus, and major blood vessels. The lungs (Option B) are located in the pleural cavities on either side of the mediastinum. The diaphragm (Option C) is a muscle that separates the thoracic cavity from the abdominal cavity. The liver (Option D) is located in the abdominal cavity. This makes Option A (Heart) correct as it resides within the mediastinum, unlike the other options which are in different anatomical locations.

Question 2: Correct Answer: A) Invert the tube gently 5-10 times to mix the clot activator with the blood.
Rationale: The correct procedure involves inverting the red-top tube gently 5-10 times immediately after collection to mix the clot activator with the blood, preventing clot formation before analysis. Option B is incorrect because not mixing can lead to inaccurate results. Option C is tricky as labeling is crucial but must occur after mixing. Option D is incorrect since sending an unlabeled specimen risks misidentification and contamination concerns are unfounded.

Question 3: Correct Answer: B) Skilled Nursing Facility
Rationale: A Skilled Nursing Facility (SNF) is designed to provide long-term care for elderly patients with chronic conditions, offering both medical and personal care services. Acute Care Hospitals focus on short-term treatment for severe injuries or illnesses. Ambulatory Surgery Centers are outpatient facilities for surgical procedures not requiring overnight stays. Urgent Care Clinics handle immediate but non-life-threatening issues. SNFs are specialized in managing chronic conditions over extended periods, making them the most suitable setting for long-term elderly care.

Question 4: Correct Answer: C) Use of N95 respirators
Rationale: The use of N95 respirators is most effective in preventing the spread of an airborne pandemic because these masks filter out at least 95% of airborne particles, including viruses. While regular hand washing (Option A) and surface disinfection (Option D) are crucial for preventing contact-based transmission, they are less effective against airborne pathogens. Social distancing (Option B) helps reduce transmission but does not provide direct protection from inhaling airborne particles. Therefore, N95 respirators offer superior protection in airborne pandemics by directly filtering out harmful particles from the air.

Question 5: Correct Answer: B) Craniectomy
Rationale: A craniectomy is the surgical removal of a portion of the skull to relieve pressure on the brain. In contrast, a craniotomy involves temporarily removing a portion of the skull and then replacing it. Cranioplasty refers to the surgical repair of a bone defect in the skull, while craniosynostosis is a condition where one or more of the sutures in an infant's skull close prematurely. Understanding these distinctions is crucial for accurate medical communication and patient care. - A) Craniotomy: Incorrect because it involves temporarily removing and then replacing part of the skull. - B) Craniectomy: Correct because it involves permanently removing part of the skull. - C) Cranioplasty: Incorrect because it refers to repairing a defect in the skull. - D) Craniosynostosis: Incorrect because it is a condition, not a surgical procedure. This question tests deep knowledge of specific medical procedures and conditions, ensuring that only those with thorough understanding can select the correct answer.

Question 6: Correct Answer: B) Seeking social support from friends and family
Rationale: Seeking social support from friends and family is a well-documented effective coping strategy for managing emotional distress in individuals with chronic illnesses like MS. It provides emotional comfort, practical assistance, and a sense of belonging. Denial (Option A) can lead to maladaptive outcomes by preventing necessary adjustments. Avoidance (Option C) may temporarily reduce stress but can lead to isolation and increased distress in the long term. Focusing solely on medical treatments (Option D) neglects the psychosocial aspects critical for holistic well-being.

Question 7: Correct Answer: B) Explain the procedure to Mr. Johnson and ensure he has removed any metallic objects.
Rationale: The most critical step in preparing a patient for an EKG is to explain the procedure and ensure they have removed any metallic objects, which can interfere with the readings. While avoiding caffeine (Option A), fasting (Option C), and ensuring clean skin (Option D) are important considerations, they are not as immediately critical as ensuring patient understanding and removing potential interference sources. Explaining the procedure helps alleviate anxiety and ensures cooperation, while removing metallic objects prevents artifacts in the EKG reading. - Option A is incorrect because while caffeine can affect heart rate, it is not as immediately crucial as removing metallic objects. - Option C is incorrect because fasting is more relevant to other procedures like blood tests or imaging requiring sedation. - Option D is incorrect because although clean skin aids electrode adhesion, it does not address potential electrical interference from metallic objects or patient understanding of the procedure. By focusing on these nuances, we create a challenging question that requires deep knowledge of patient preparation protocols for cardiovascular testing procedures like EKGs.

Question 8: Correct Answer: A) A Living Will specifies the types of medical treatment a person wishes to receive or avoid if they become incapacitated.
Rationale: A Living Will is a document that outlines an individual's preferences regarding medical treatments they wish to receive or avoid if they are unable to communicate their decisions. Option B is incorrect as it describes a Durable Power of Attorney for Healthcare. Option C refers to a Do Not Resuscitate (DNR) order, and Option D pertains to an organ donor card or registry, not a Living Will. The key distinction is that a Living Will directly addresses specific medical treatments rather than appointing decision-makers or addressing organ donation.

Question 9: Correct Answer: B) Speak slowly and clearly while maintaining eye contact.
Rationale: Speaking slowly and clearly while maintaining eye contact helps ensure that the geriatric patient understands the information being conveyed without feeling overwhelmed. This approach respects their cognitive limitations and promotes effective communication. Option A is incorrect because medical jargon can confuse patients with cognitive impairments. Option C is incorrect as increasing volume significantly may be perceived as shouting, which can be distressing. Option D is incorrect because non-verbal cues like gestures can aid in understanding when used appropriately.

Question 10: Correct Answer: B) Ventricular Tachycardia
Rationale: Ventricular tachycardia (VT) is characterized by wide QRS complexes, absence of P waves, and an irregular rhythm. Atrial fibrillation (A) typically presents with narrow QRS complexes and no distinct P waves but is usually irregularly irregular. Supraventricular tachycardia (C) generally has narrow QRS complexes with a regular rhythm. Premature ventricular contractions (D) are isolated wide QRS complexes that occur prematurely but do not form a continuous pattern like VT. The key distinguishing feature for VT is the continuous series of wide QRS complexes without preceding P waves, which differentiates it from other

arrhythmias.

Question 11: Correct Answer: C) 140/90 mmHg

Rationale: According to the latest guidelines by the American Heart Association, a blood pressure reading of 140/90 mmHg is classified as Stage 2 Hypertension. Option A (120/80 mmHg) is considered normal. Option B (130/85 mmHg) falls under Stage 1 Hypertension but is not as severe as Option C. Option D (135/88 mmHg) also indicates elevated blood pressure but does not meet the threshold for Stage 2 Hypertension. Therefore, Option C is correct as it represents an abnormal vital sign indicative of hypertension.

Question 12: Correct Answer: B) Report the abuse to the appropriate authorities despite the patient's request.

Rationale: According to professional codes of ethics, healthcare professionals must prioritize patient safety over confidentiality when there is a risk of harm. Reporting domestic abuse is mandatory in many jurisdictions to protect vulnerable individuals. While respecting patient autonomy is crucial, it does not override legal and ethical obligations to report abuse. Options A, C, and D fail to address immediate safety concerns and legal requirements. Option B correctly identifies the need for mandatory reporting despite patient objections, ensuring adherence to ethical standards and legal mandates.

Question 13: Correct Answer: A) Using alcohol-based hand sanitizer before and after patient contact

Rationale: The CDC emphasizes the importance of hand hygiene as the most effective way to prevent HAIs. Alcohol-based hand sanitizers are recommended for their efficacy in reducing pathogens. Option B is incorrect because gloves should be worn according to standard precautions, not just when there is visible risk. Option C is incorrect as disposable gowns should not be reused. Option D, while important, does not address the broader practice of routine hand hygiene critical in infection prevention.

Question 14: Correct Answer: B) Wearing clean scrubs, maintaining eye contact, and speaking in a calm and clear tone.

Rationale: Option B is correct because it encompasses key elements of professional presence: appropriate attire (clean scrubs), effective non-verbal communication (eye contact), and clear verbal communication (calm tone). Option A is incorrect because using medical jargon can confuse patients. Option C is incorrect as avoiding eye contact can be perceived as unprofessional or disengaged. Option D is incorrect because casual attire may undermine professionalism despite effective communication methods. This question challenges test-takers by presenting nearly correct options that miss one critical aspect of professional presence.

Question 15: Correct Answer: A) Acupuncture

Rationale: Acupuncture is based on Traditional Chinese Medicine principles, which involve stimulating specific points on the body to balance energy flow (Qi). Reflexology involves applying pressure to feet or hands but does not focus on self-regulation through specific points. Chiropractic care emphasizes spinal adjustments to improve health but does not use specific points for stimulation. Homeopathy relies on highly diluted substances to trigger the body's healing process, rather than stimulating points. Therefore, Acupuncture is the correct answer as it directly aligns with the principle of stimulating specific points for self-regulation.

Question 16: Correct Answer: B) Serum Ferritin

Rationale: Serum ferritin is the most accurate test for diagnosing iron-deficiency anemia as it directly measures stored iron levels in the body. While a CBC (Option A) can indicate anemia through low hemoglobin and hematocrit levels, it does not specify iron deficiency. Serum iron (Option C) measures circulating iron but can be affected by various factors such as recent dietary intake. TIBC (Option D) indicates the blood's capacity to bind iron but is less specific than serum ferritin for diagnosing iron deficiency. Thus, serum ferritin is preferred for its specificity in reflecting iron stores.

Question 17: Correct Answer: B) Begin a daily exercise routine tailored to her fitness level.

Rationale: Regular physical activity is one of the most effective preventive measures for reducing cardiovascular risk factors. A tailored exercise routine can improve heart health, lower blood pressure, and aid in weight management. Option A suggests a specific diet without considering individual nutritional needs. Option C could pose risks without medical supervision. Option D overlooks potential interactions and unnecessary supplementation. Thus, B is correct as it aligns with contemporary guidelines on preventive medicine and wellness.

Question 18: Correct Answer: A) Negligence

Rationale: The correct answer is A) Negligence. Negligence occurs when a healthcare provider fails to exercise reasonable care, resulting in harm to the patient. In this scenario, Sarah's mistake in administering the wrong dose constitutes negligence as it deviates from the standard of care expected. B) Battery is incorrect because it involves intentional harm or offensive contact without consent. C) Breach of Duty is part of proving negligence but not the standalone concept applicable here. D) Strict Liability is incorrect as it applies to inherently dangerous activities or defective products, not professional errors.

Question 19: Correct Answer: A) Clean the wound with an antiseptic solution.

Rationale: The first step in removing sutures is to clean the wound with an antiseptic solution to prevent infection. This ensures that any bacteria present on the skin's surface are minimized before manipulating the sutures. Option B (Cutting the suture at its knot) is incorrect because it should be done after cleaning. Option C (Grasping the suture with forceps) is also subsequent to cleaning. Option D (Checking for signs of infection) is important but should occur during initial assessment and not as a first step in removal.

Question 20: Correct Answer: A) Apologize sincerely for the wait and explain the reason behind the delay.

Rationale: Apologizing sincerely and providing an explanation addresses Mr. Johnson's concerns directly and shows empathy, which is crucial in maintaining professionalism and ensuring patient satisfaction. Offering an immediate appointment (Option B) may not be feasible or fair to other patients. Ignoring his frustration (Option C) would likely escalate the situation and damage trust. Suggesting rescheduling (Option D) does not address his immediate concern and could further frustrate him. Thus, Option A is the best approach as it combines empathy with transparency, aligning with effective communication principles in healthcare settings.

Question 21: Correct Answer: C) Developing a sense of competence

Rationale: In Erikson's 'Industry vs. Inferiority' stage, typically occurring between ages 6 and 12, children strive to develop a sense of competence through learning and productivity. Option A refers to 'Trust vs. Mistrust' (infancy), B refers to 'Autonomy vs. Shame and Doubt' (early childhood), and D refers to 'Identity vs. Role Confusion' (adolescence). Thus, C is correct as it precisely aligns with the developmental task for this stage, while the others are relevant but pertain to different stages in Erikson's theory.

Question 22: Correct Answer: C) Ensuring that the results are communicated directly to the ordering provider via secure methods.

Rationale: The most critical step is ensuring that lab results are communicated directly to the ordering provider via secure methods. While verifying patient identity (Option A), entering results into EHR (Option B), and documenting when results were sent (Option D) are important, direct and secure communication ensures immediate and accurate transfer of information, crucial for timely medical decisions. Verifying identity prevents errors but does not guarantee result delivery; EHR entry ensures records but not immediate notification; documentation is essential for tracking but does not facilitate immediate communication.

Question 23: Correct Answer: B) Full Block Format

Rationale: The Full Block Format is widely accepted in professional settings due to its clean and straightforward layout. All text is left-aligned, which enhances readability and maintains a formal tone. - Option A (Modified Block Format) is incorrect because although it is professional, it involves indenting the date and closing lines, which can be less straightforward. - Option C (Semi-Block Format) also includes indentations in paragraphs, making it less uniform. - Option D (Simplified Format) eliminates salutations and closings, which may seem too informal for a medical setting. The Full Block Format ensures clarity and professionalism in communication with patients.

Question 24: Correct Answer: A) Encourage each team member to voice their opinion without interruption.

Rationale: Encouraging each team member to voice their opinion without interruption promotes open communication, mutual respect, and inclusivity, which are essential for effective teamwork. Option B is incorrect because summarizing viewpoints and suggesting compromises may not address underlying issues or ensure full participation. Option C is incorrect as deferring to the most experienced member can undermine team dynamics and collaboration. Option D is incorrect because focusing solely on agreement can suppress diverse perspectives crucial for comprehensive decision-making.

Question 25: Correct Answer: D) Affordable Care Act (ACA) Marketplace Plan

Rationale: The Affordable Care Act (ACA) mandates that all marketplace plans cover pre-existing conditions without a waiting period. HMOs and PPOs may have varying policies on pre-existing conditions, often requiring waiting periods or exclusions. HDHPs typically have higher out-of-pocket costs and may not provide immediate coverage for pre-existing conditions. Therefore, ACA Marketplace Plans are the most reliable option for covering pre-existing conditions without delay. - Option A (HMO): While HMOs offer comprehensive coverage, they often have stricter network rules and may impose waiting periods for pre-existing conditions. - Option B (PPO): PPOs provide more flexibility in choosing healthcare providers but also may have waiting periods or exclusions for pre-existing conditions. - Option C (HDHP): HDHPs generally have higher deductibles and may not cover pre-existing conditions immediately. - Option D (ACA Marketplace Plan): ACA Marketplace Plans are required by law to cover pre-existing conditions without any waiting period, making them the correct answer.

Question 26: Correct Answer: A) "You need to fast for at least 8 hours before your test."

Rationale: For a lipid panel blood test, it is generally recommended that patients fast for at least 8-12 hours to ensure accurate results. Option A is correct because it aligns with this guideline. Option B is incorrect because black coffee can affect certain lipid levels. Option C is close but incorrect due to the specific requirement of fasting duration being less than the typical recommendation. Option D is also incorrect as the fasting period is too short and may not provide accurate results.

Question 27: Correct Answer: A) Improve patient care coordination

Rationale: The primary objective of the Meaningful Use program is to improve patient care coordination by promoting the use of electronic health records (EHRs). This facilitates better communication among healthcare providers, leading to enhanced patient outcomes. Option B is incorrect because increasing patient volume is not a direct goal of Meaningful Use. Option C is misleading as reducing administrative costs is a secondary benefit but not a primary objective. Option D, enhancing medical billing accuracy, while important, is not a core aim of the Meaningful Use initiative.

Question 28: Correct Answer: B) Respiratory Therapy

Rationale: Respiratory therapy is primarily responsible for assessing and managing respiratory function, particularly in patients with conditions like COPD. This service includes treatments such as administering oxygen therapy, performing pulmonary function tests, and providing education on breathing techniques. Radiology (A) involves imaging studies but does not manage respiratory function directly. Physical therapy (C) focuses on improving physical mobility and strength, not specifically respiratory issues. Occupational therapy (D) aims at helping patients perform daily activities but does not specialize in respiratory management.

Question 29: Correct Answer: A) Verify Mr. John Smith's name and date of birth on both the specimen label and requisition form before labeling.

Rationale: The correct answer is A because verifying the patient's name and date of birth on both the specimen label and requisition form ensures accurate matching, reducing errors in patient identification. Option B is incorrect as relying on memory can lead to mistakes. Option C is not sufficient without checking against the requisition form. Option D introduces risk by using pre-printed labels that may not be verified at the time of collection.

Question 30: Correct Answer: B) Confirm she has taken her prescribed bowel preparation medication as instructed.

Rationale: The most critical step in preparing Emily for a colonoscopy is confirming that she has taken her prescribed bowel preparation medication as instructed. This ensures that her colon is adequately cleansed, which is crucial for accurate visualization during the procedure. While A) following a clear liquid diet and C) fasting are important, they are not as critical as B). D) signing the informed consent form is necessary but does not directly impact the procedural readiness.

Question 31: Correct Answer: B) Returning them to a pharmacy take-back program.

Rationale: The correct method for disposing of unused controlled substances is returning them to a pharmacy take-back program (Option B). This ensures they are handled according to regulatory guidelines. Flushing (Option A) can lead to environmental contamination. Mixing with coffee grounds (Option C) is not secure enough for controlled substances. Incineration in a regular waste facility (Option D) does not guarantee safe disposal as it may not meet specific standards for hazardous waste. Each option explained: - Option A: Flushing down the toilet is discouraged due to potential environmental harm. - Option B: Pharmacy take-back programs are designed specifically for safe disposal of controlled substances. - Option C: Mixing with coffee grounds is recommended for non-controlled medications but not secure enough for controlled substances. - Option D: Regular incineration facilities may not have the capability to safely dispose of hazardous materials like controlled substances.

Question 32: Correct Answer: A) Light blue, red, green, lavender

Rationale: The correct order of draw is essential to prevent cross-contamination between additives in different tubes. The standard order is light blue (citrate), red (no additive or clot activator), green (heparin), and lavender (EDTA). Option B incorrectly places the red tube first. Option C correctly starts with light blue and red but incorrectly places lavender before green. Option D starts with the wrong tube and misorders subsequent tubes. Understanding this sequence is critical for accurate lab results and patient safety.

Question 33: Correct Answer: C) Store in a refrigerator, between 2°C and 8°C.

Rationale: Temperature-sensitive vaccines should be stored in a refrigerator at temperatures between 2°C and 8°C to maintain their efficacy. Storing them at room temperature (A) or in a freezer (B) can degrade the vaccines' potency. An insulated container at ambient temperature (D) does not provide the consistent cooling required. Therefore, option C is correct because it ensures the vaccines remain effective for patient use.

Question 34: Correct Answer: C) Obtain a new control solution and recalibrate the glucometer.

Rationale: The correct action is to obtain a new control solution and recalibrate the glucometer (Option C). Using an outdated control solution (Option A) or substituting it with a patient sample (Option B) can lead to inaccurate results. Ignoring the control solution and relying on previous calibration data (Option D) is also inappropriate because calibration needs to be verified regularly with valid controls to ensure accuracy. Regular recalibration with fresh control solutions ensures that equipment provides reliable readings essential for patient care.

Question 35: Correct Answer: C) Ensuring that all mandatory fields are filled out correctly.

Rationale: Ensuring that all mandatory fields are filled out correctly is critical for maintaining data integrity in an EHR system. Mandatory fields often include essential demographic and clinical information necessary for accurate patient care and billing processes. While double-checking insurance details (A), verifying contact information (B), and cross-referencing medical history (D) are important tasks, they do not address the immediate requirement of ensuring comprehensive and accurate data entry in mandatory fields. This step ensures that no crucial information is missing or incorrectly entered, which could lead to significant errors in patient care or administrative processes.

Question 36: Correct Answer: B) Otoscope

Rationale: An otoscope is specifically designed to visualize the ear canal and tympanic membrane, making it essential for an otoscopic examination. An ophthalmoscope (Option A) is used for examining the eyes, not the ears. A tuning fork (Option C) is used for hearing tests, not visualizing internal structures. A stethoscope (Option D) is used for auscultation of heart and lung sounds, not for visual examinations. Thus, while all options are relevant in clinical settings, only the otoscope directly serves the purpose of visualizing the tympanic membrane during an otoscopic examination.

Question 37: Correct Answer: C) Ensure the sample is placed in a temperature-controlled container if required.

Rationale: Proper preparation of samples for transportation includes ensuring they are stored at appropriate temperatures to maintain their integrity. While labeling (A) and using biohazard bags (B) are important, they are incomplete without considering temperature control. Sending samples without special handling instructions (D) can lead to degradation or contamination. Temperature control is crucial for certain tests to ensure accurate results upon analysis at the reference laboratory.

Question 38: Correct Answer: A) Regular calibration of equipment

Rationale: Regular calibration of equipment is essential to ensure that laboratory instruments provide accurate and reliable results. Calibration involves adjusting the instrument to match a known standard, which helps maintain precision over time. While routine maintenance (B), proper labeling (C), and updating SOPs (D) are important, they do not directly impact the accuracy of test results as significantly as calibration does. Maintenance ensures functionality, labeling prevents sample mix-ups, and SOP updates improve overall lab operations, but only calibration directly affects measurement accuracy.

Question 39: Correct Answer: A) Absorption

Rationale: Absorption is the primary pharmacokinetic process that determines the bioavailability of an orally administered drug. Bioavailability refers to the proportion of a drug that enters systemic circulation and is available at the site of action. While distribution (B), metabolism (C), and excretion (D) are crucial for a drug's overall pharmacokinetics, they do not directly determine initial bioavailability. Distribution involves the dispersion of a drug throughout body fluids and tissues, metabolism involves

chemical alterations usually in the liver, and excretion involves removal from the body.

Question 40: Correct Answer: D) Alcohol-based hand rubs are less effective than soap and water in removing Clostridium difficile spores.

Rationale: Option D is correct because alcohol-based hand rubs are indeed less effective against Clostridium difficile spores compared to soap and water. Option A is incorrect as alcohol-based rubs are not effective against all pathogens, particularly certain spores. Option B is misleading because alcohol-based rubs should not be used when hands are visibly soiled; soap and water should be used instead. Option C contains an accurate statement about rubbing duration but does not address the specific limitation regarding Clostridium difficile, making D the most accurate choice.

Question 41: Correct Answer: A) Lavender top tube

Rationale: The lavender top tube contains EDTA (ethylenediaminetetraacetic acid), an anticoagulant that preserves the shape of cells and prevents clotting, making it ideal for hematology tests such as a complete blood count (CBC). The light blue top tube contains sodium citrate, used for coagulation studies. The green top tube contains heparin, suitable for plasma chemistry tests. The red top tube has no anticoagulant or gel and is used for serum chemistry tests. Thus, while other options are valid for specific tests, only the lavender top tube is appropriate for CBC.

Question 42: Correct Answer: A) The facility must have a Certificate of Waiver from CMS.

Rationale: A Certificate of Waiver from the Centers for Medicare & Medicaid Services (CMS) is required for facilities to legally perform CLIA-waived tests. While employing a certified pathologist (Option B), undergoing annual inspections (Option C), and performing proficiency testing (Option D) are important for higher complexity testing, they are not requirements for CLIA-waived tests. This distinction is crucial in understanding the regulatory framework governing different levels of laboratory testing under CLIA regulations.

Question 43: Correct Answer: D) Median cubital vein in the antecubital fossa

Rationale: The median cubital vein in the antecubital fossa is typically the best choice due to its size, stability, and accessibility. The dorsal hand veins (A) are more prone to rolling and may be painful for patients with arthritis. The cephalic vein in the forearm (B) can be harder to locate in elderly patients with fragile skin. The basilic vein (C), while accessible, is near nerves and arteries, increasing complication risk. Thus, D is optimal for minimizing discomfort and complications.

Question 44: Correct Answer: A) Identifying patient needs and preferences

Rationale: The most important initial step in coordinating care is identifying patient needs and preferences, as it ensures that subsequent actions are tailored to the patient's specific circumstances. While contacting local health centers (Option B), scheduling follow-ups (Option C), and gathering transportation information (Option D) are crucial, they come after understanding what the patient actually requires. This foundational step ensures all subsequent coordination efforts are relevant and effective.

Question 45: Correct Answer: C) Returning them to a pharmacy take-back program

Rationale: The most appropriate method for disposing of unused controlled substances is returning them to a pharmacy take-back program. This ensures that they are handled according to regulatory standards and prevents environmental contamination or misuse. Flushing (Option A) can contaminate water supplies, mixing with coffee grounds (Option B) is not secure enough, and incineration (Option D), while effective, is typically reserved for large-scale disposal by professional waste handlers. Pharmacy take-back programs are specifically designed for safe and compliant disposal.

Question 46: Correct Answer: A) Increased secretion of aldosterone

Rationale: Aldosterone plays a crucial role in maintaining blood pressure by promoting sodium and water reabsorption in the kidneys, which increases blood volume. While ADH also helps retain water, its release would increase rather than decrease during dehydration. Vasodilation would lower blood pressure, contrary to the body's need to maintain it. An increased heart rate helps but is not as directly influential as aldosterone in this context.

Question 47: Correct Answer: B) "Maria, your ability to manage tasks efficiently and assist patients with empathy was outstanding today. It really made a difference."

Rationale: Option B is the correct answer because it provides specific feedback on what behaviors were effective (managing tasks efficiently and assisting patients with empathy), making it clear why Maria's actions were commendable. This specificity helps reinforce those exact behaviors in the future. Option A is too generic and lacks specifics about what was done well. Option C mentions professionalism but does not detail what actions demonstrated this trait. Option D focuses only on task management without acknowledging the empathetic patient care.

Question 48: Correct Answer: C) Ointment

Rationale: An ointment is the most appropriate form of medication for Mr. Smith's skin infection because it can be applied directly to the affected area, ensuring localized treatment with minimal systemic absorption. Pills (A) and capsules (B) are oral medications that would not provide targeted treatment for a skin infection. An oral suspension (D) is also an ingested form and would not be suitable for topical application. Ointments allow for direct application, which is crucial for treating localized skin infections effectively.

Question 49: Correct Answer: C) Lavender-top tube (EDTA)

Rationale: The lavender-top tube contains EDTA, which is the appropriate anticoagulant for a CBC as it preserves cell morphology and prevents clotting. The red-top tube lacks additives, making it unsuitable for CBC. The blue-top tube with sodium citrate is used for coagulation studies, not CBC. The green-top tube contains heparin, which can interfere with cell morphology analysis. Thus, only the lavender-top tube ensures accurate CBC results by preserving cellular components.

Question 50: Correct Answer: A) Using alcohol-based hand rub before and after patient contact

Rationale: Hand hygiene, specifically using an alcohol-based hand rub, is the most effective method for preventing HAIs. While wearing gloves (B), using masks (C), and cleaning equipment (D) are important, they do not replace the need for proper hand hygiene. Gloves can become contaminated, masks primarily prevent respiratory droplet spread, and cleaning equipment addresses only one potential source of infection. Alcohol-based hand rubs reduce transient flora more effectively than soap and water, making option A the best choice.

Question 51: Correct Answer: C) Provide the patient's demographic information, relevant medical history, reason for referral, and any pertinent test results.

Rationale: Option C is correct because it ensures that all necessary information is included in the e-referral, facilitating appropriate specialist care for Mr. John Doe. Option A is incorrect as it lacks critical medical history and reason for referral. Option B includes unnecessary unrelated conditions which may overwhelm or confuse the specialist. Option D is too brief and lacks essential details needed by the cardiologist to understand Mr. Doe's condition comprehensively. Properly detailed referrals improve patient outcomes by providing specialists with complete context.

Question 52: Correct Answer: B) Turn on the AED and follow its prompts before attaching the pads.

Rationale: The correct procedure is to turn on the AED first and follow its prompts. This ensures that you are guided through each step correctly. Option A is incorrect because turning on the AED first is crucial for proper guidance. Option C is incorrect because checking for a pulse can delay necessary defibrillation. Option D is incorrect as it omits using the AED, which can significantly improve survival rates in cardiac arrest cases.

Question 53: Correct Answer: B) Right Patient

Rationale: The "Right Patient" is a critical component of the "Rights of Medication Administration" because verifying the patient's identity ensures that the correct individual receives the intended medication. This step prevents potentially harmful errors. - Option A (Right Route) is important but secondary to ensuring the correct patient. - Option C (Right Documentation) is crucial for record-keeping and future reference but does not directly prevent immediate medication errors. - Option D (Right Preparation) involves proper medication handling but is ineffective if administered to the wrong patient. Thus, while all options are essential for safe medication administration, identifying the right patient is paramount.

Question 54: Correct Answer: A) Using a gait belt and walking slightly behind the patient

Rationale: The correct technique involves using a gait belt and walking slightly behind the patient to provide support without obstructing their movement. Option B is incorrect because holding the patient's arm tightly can restrict their mobility and cause discomfort. Option C is not ideal as standing directly in front of the patient can block their view and path, increasing fall risk. Option D, while supportive, does not offer as much control or safety as a gait belt. Understanding these nuances ensures optimal patient care.

Question 55: Correct Answer: C) 20 feet

Rationale: The standard distance for conducting a Snellen chart test is 20 feet. This distance is used to measure visual acuity accurately by determining how well a person can see letters or symbols from a specific distance. Options A (10 feet), B (15 feet), and D (25 feet) are incorrect because they do not adhere to the standardized testing distance, which could result in inaccurate measurements of visual acuity. Using the correct distance ensures consistency and reliability in vision assessment.

Question 56: Correct Answer: B) Health Maintenance Organization (HMO)

Rationale: An HMO requires patients to select a primary care physician (PCP) who manages their overall care and provides referrals to specialists. This coordination is central to the HMO model. In contrast, a PPO offers more flexibility in choosing healthcare providers without needing referrals. An EPO combines elements of HMOs and PPOs but does not require PCP selection or referrals. A POS plan blends features of HMOs and PPOs but also allows out-of-network care at higher costs, often requiring PCP referrals for specialist visits.

Question 57: Correct Answer: A) Certified Medical Assistant (CMA)

Rationale: The Certified Medical Assistant (CMA) credential is awarded to individuals who have completed a program accredited by the CAAHEP and passed the national certification exam administered by the American Association of Medical Assistants (AAMA). While Registered Medical Assistants (RMA) also require certification, their accrediting bodies differ. Both Clinical Medical Assistant (CCMA) and Certified Clinical Medical Assistant (CCMA) are not standard terminologies recognized by CAAHEP, making them incorrect. This highlights the importance of understanding specific accrediting bodies and certification processes in healthcare.

Question 58: Correct Answer: A) Ensure the antiseptic solution is properly diluted before application.

Rationale: Ensuring that the antiseptic solution is properly diluted before application helps prevent chemical burns and irritation. While wearing gloves (Option C) is important for personal protection, it does not address preventing chemical burns on patients. Applying the solution directly (Option B) can increase the risk of burns if not properly diluted. Using only sterile water (Option D) might not provide adequate antisepsis compared to a diluted antiseptic solution. Proper dilution ensures both safety and effectiveness in wound care.

Question 59: Correct Answer: C) Assisting with activities of daily living (ADLs)

Rationale: Home health care services primarily assist patients with activities of daily living (ADLs), such as bathing, dressing, and eating, especially for those with chronic illnesses. While acute medical treatments (Option A) and routine surgical procedures (Option D) are critical, they are typically provided in hospital settings rather than at home. Palliative care (Option B) focuses on comfort for terminal patients but is a specialized service within home health care, not its primary function. Thus, assisting with ADLs is the core function distinguishing it from other healthcare services.

Question 60: Correct Answer: B) Remote Patient Monitoring (RPM)

Rationale: Remote Patient Monitoring (RPM) is specifically designed for real-time tracking and reporting of patient vital signs, providing continuous monitoring and immediate feedback. While Electronic Health Records (EHR) store comprehensive patient data, they are not primarily used for real-time monitoring. Clinical Decision Support Systems (CDSS) assist with decision-making based on data but do not focus on real-time tracking. Health Information Exchange (HIE) facilitates sharing health information across organizations but does not provide real-time monitoring capabilities. RPM's focus on continuous, real-time data makes it the correct choice.

Question 61: Correct Answer: A) Position Sarah in the lithotomy position and ensure she has emptied her bladder.

Rationale: The initial step in assisting with a colposcopy is positioning the patient correctly in the lithotomy position and ensuring she has emptied her bladder to improve comfort and access. Preparing instruments (Option B) is crucial but not the first step. Providing post-procedure care instructions (Option C) occurs after the procedure. Applying acetic acid (Option D) is done during the procedure, not initially.

Question 62: Correct Answer: D) A medical assistant failing to document a patient's allergy leading to an adverse reaction.

Rationale: Medical malpractice involves negligence or failure to provide the standard care resulting in harm. Option D exemplifies this as it shows negligence in documenting critical patient information. Option A describes intentional harm, which is criminal rather than malpractice. Option B involves a calculation error, which could be negligence but lacks the broader context of standard care failure. Option C is unauthorized procedure, more aligned with battery or criminal act than malpractice. Thus, D is most accurate for medical malpractice due to its alignment with negligence and harm from failure in standard care documentation.

Question 63: Correct Answer: A) Demonstration

Rationale: Demonstration is most effective for kinesthetic learners who learn best through hands-on activities and physical engagement. Lectures (B) primarily benefit auditory learners. Reading assignments (C) cater to reading/writing learners. Visual aids (D) are optimal for visual learners. Thus, while all options are valid instructional techniques, demonstration aligns best with the kinesthetic learning style due to its emphasis on active participation and practical application.

Question 64: Correct Answer: B) Schedule II

Rationale: Schedule II drugs have a high potential for abuse but also have accepted medical uses in treatment, requiring strict regulation. Examples include opioids like oxycodone. Schedule I drugs (Option A) have no accepted medical use and are not prescribed. Schedule III drugs (Option C) have less potential for abuse than Schedule II but more than IV,

including certain anabolic steroids. Schedule IV drugs (Option D) have a lower potential for abuse than III and include medications like diazepam. Thus, the correct answer is B) Schedule II.

Question 65: Correct Answer: C) Properly labeling specimens immediately after collection

Rationale: Properly labeling specimens immediately after collection is crucial for ensuring specimen quality and consistency. Mislabeling can lead to incorrect patient identification and erroneous results. While using a tourniquet for no longer than one minute (A), ensuring the patient is fasting (B), and using the correct gauge needle (D) are important, they do not directly address the risk of misidentification as effectively as proper labeling does.

Question 66: Correct Answer: B) 2 tablets

Rationale: The correct answer is B) 2 tablets. To determine the number of tablets needed, divide the prescribed dose by the strength of one tablet: 250 mg / 125 mg/tablet = 2 tablets. Option A (1 tablet) is incorrect because it provides only half the required dose. Option C (2.5 tablets) is incorrect as it exceeds the prescribed dose and typically, partial tablets are not advised unless specified by a healthcare provider. Option D (3 tablets) is incorrect because it also exceeds the required dose, potentially leading to an overdose.

Question 67: Correct Answer: A) Increase intake of high-fiber foods like whole grains and vegetables.

Rationale: Increasing the intake of high-fiber foods helps manage blood sugar levels by slowing glucose absorption. While limiting sodium (Option B) is crucial for hypertension, it does not directly address diabetes management. Increasing omega-3 fatty acids (Option C) benefits heart health but is not specific to blood sugar control. Avoiding all carbohydrates (Option D) is impractical and can lead to nutrient deficiencies; instead, managing carbohydrate quality and quantity is recommended. Thus, Option A is the most appropriate recommendation for Sarah's condition.

Question 68: Correct Answer: B) Using a biohazard bag with proper labeling.

Rationale: The most critical practice is using a biohazard bag with proper labeling (B). This ensures safety and compliance with regulations, preventing contamination and ensuring accurate identification. While transporting at room temperature (A) might be necessary for some samples, it is not universally critical. Using a pneumatic tube system (C) can be helpful but isn't always available or appropriate. An airtight container (D) may be useful for certain samples but doesn't address labeling and biohazard safety comprehensively. Proper labeling and use of biohazard bags are essential for maintaining sample integrity during transportation.

Question 69: Correct Answer: B) At least 2 inches

Rationale: The American Heart Association recommends that chest compressions for adults should be at least 2 inches deep to ensure adequate perfusion during CPR. Option A is incorrect as it is too shallow to be effective. Option C is also incorrect as it does not meet the minimum depth requirement. Option D is incorrect because compressions deeper than 2.4 inches could cause injury. Therefore, option B is correct as it aligns with current AHA guidelines.

Question 70: Correct Answer: B) Right Route

Rationale: The "Right Route" is a fundamental aspect of the "Rights of Medication Administration," ensuring that medications are given via the correct method (e.g., oral, intravenous). While "Right Diagnosis," "Right Documentation," and "Right Frequency" are important in clinical practice, they do not specifically belong to the core rights aimed at medication administration safety. The other options can lead to errors if misunderstood but are not part of the standard five rights that directly prevent medication errors.

Question 71: Correct Answer: B) Conducting a minor

surgical procedure in an outpatient clinic.

Rationale: Written consent is most critically required for conducting a minor surgical procedure in an outpatient clinic because it involves more significant risks and potential complications compared to other scenarios. Routine vaccinations (A) typically require verbal consent, dietary advice (C) does not usually necessitate formal consent, and emergency interventions (D) often operate under implied consent due to the urgency and patient's incapacity to provide consent. Written consent ensures that patients are fully informed about the risks, benefits, and alternatives of surgical procedures, safeguarding their autonomy and legal rights.

Question 72: Correct Answer: D) Blood pressure 140/90 mmHg

Rationale: Blood pressure of 140/90 mmHg is indicative of hypertension according to current guidelines. While the other vital signs (temperature, pulse, and respiratory rate) fall within normal or slightly elevated ranges for an adult female, they do not indicate a significant abnormality. Hypertension requires clinical attention due to its potential risks for cardiovascular events. - Option A (Temperature 37.5°C): This is slightly elevated but still within the normal range. - Option B (Pulse 98 bpm): This is on the higher end but can be considered normal under certain conditions. - Option C (Respiratory rate 18 breaths per minute): This is within the normal range for adults. - Option D (Blood pressure 140/90 mmHg): This indicates Stage 1 hypertension requiring further evaluation and management. Each option was crafted based on contemporary research and recognized theories regarding normal and abnormal vital signs in clinical practice.

Question 73: Correct Answer: B) Mode of Transmission

Rationale: Proper hand hygiene practices primarily disrupt the 'Mode of Transmission' by removing or killing pathogens that could be transferred from one person or surface to another. While options A (Portal of Exit) and C (Portal of Entry) are related to how pathogens leave and enter hosts, respectively, they do not directly address the interruption caused by hand hygiene. Option D (Susceptible Host) pertains to the vulnerability of the host rather than breaking the transmission chain. Thus, 'Mode of Transmission' is the most accurate answer.

Question 74: Correct Answer: A) Lack of health insurance

Rationale: Lack of health insurance is widely recognized as the most significant barrier to accessing healthcare services for patients from low socio-economic backgrounds. Without insurance, individuals are less likely to seek medical care due to high out-of-pocket costs. While cultural misunderstandings (B), language barriers (C), and limited health literacy (D) are also important barriers, they do not have as direct an impact on access as the financial barrier posed by lack of insurance. Cultural and language issues can often be mitigated through interpreter services and culturally competent care, while health literacy can be improved through patient education programs.

Question 75: Correct Answer: C) Ask Sarah to stand on tiptoes to get an accurate measurement.

Rationale: Asking Sarah to stand on tiptoes would result in an inaccurate height measurement. The correct procedure involves ensuring she stands barefoot with heels together (Option A), positioning her head in the Frankfort horizontal plane (Option B), and using a stadiometer for precision (Option D). Standing on tiptoes skews the true height, leading to erroneous BMI calculations.

Question 76: Correct Answer: A) Enter "500 mg Amoxicillin, PO, q8h x 7 days"

Rationale: The correct answer is A because it accurately reflects the physician's order of administering 500 mg of Amoxicillin orally every 8 hours for 7 days. Option B is incorrect because it changes the frequency to every 12 hours instead of every 8 hours. Option C is incorrect as it changes both the dosage and duration to an incorrect regimen. Option D is incorrect because it changes the route of administration from oral (PO) to intravenous (IV), which could lead to significant clinical implications. Properly entering orders into CPOE ensures accurate medication administration and patient safety.

Question 77: Correct Answer: B) Lithotomy position with legs supported in stirrups

Rationale: The lithotomy position with legs supported in stirrups is the most appropriate for a pelvic examination as it provides optimal access to the pelvic area while ensuring patient comfort. Option A (supine position) does not provide adequate access. Option C (prone position) is inappropriate for pelvic exams as it positions the patient face down. Option D (Sims' position) is typically used for rectal exams and does not offer sufficient access for a pelvic examination.

Question 78: Correct Answer: A) Confirm the patient's allergies.

Rationale: The correct answer is A) Confirm the patient's allergies. This step is essential to prevent adverse drug reactions and is part of ensuring patient safety under the "Rights of Medication Administration." While verifying expiration dates (Option B), checking vital signs (Option C), and documenting administration (Option D) are important, they do not directly address preventing allergic reactions, which is critical for safe medication administration.

Question 79: Correct Answer: A) Co-pay

Rationale: A co-pay is a fixed amount paid by a patient for a covered healthcare service at the time of service. Co-insurance (Option B) is the percentage of costs a patient pays after meeting their deductible. A deductible (Option C) is the amount a patient must pay before insurance starts covering services. A premium (Option D) is the regular payment made to maintain an insurance policy. The key difference lies in when and how these payments are made, making co-pay the correct answer as it specifically refers to a fixed payment made at the time of service.

Question 80: Correct Answer: C) Asking open-ended questions about symptoms

Rationale: Asking open-ended questions about symptoms is essential because it allows patients to describe their concerns in detail, providing crucial information about the purpose of their visit. While reviewing medical history (Option A) and conducting a physical examination (Option B) are important, they come after understanding the patient's current issues. Verifying insurance information (Option D), although necessary for administrative purposes, does not directly determine the visit's purpose.

Question 81: Correct Answer: B) Report the lapse to her supervisor and document the incident.

Rationale: The correct action is to report the lapse to her supervisor and document it. This ensures accountability and addresses any potential issues with vaccine efficacy due to improper storage conditions. Option A is incorrect because it ignores the missed days. Option C is incorrect as it assumes stability without evidence, risking patient safety. Option D is incorrect because resetting settings without addressing the lapse could mask underlying problems.

Question 82: Correct Answer: B) Epinephrine

Rationale: The first-line treatment for an anaphylactic reaction is epinephrine, which rapidly reverses severe allergic symptoms. Antihistamines (A) are used for milder allergic reactions but do not act quickly enough in anaphylaxis. Corticosteroids (C) are useful for preventing delayed reactions but are not immediate treatments. Bronchodilators (D) help with respiratory symptoms but do not address the systemic nature of anaphylaxis. Therefore, epinephrine is the most immediate and effective treatment.

Question 83: Correct Answer: D) Accountable Care Organization (ACO)

Rationale: An Accountable Care Organization (ACO) is designed to improve care coordination, enhance health outcomes, and reduce costs for patients with chronic conditions like Sarah. ACOs achieve this by promoting collaboration among healthcare providers. While HMOs and

PPOs provide network-based care and cost management, they do not emphasize the same level of coordinated care as ACOs. The PCMH model also focuses on coordinated care but primarily within primary care settings, whereas ACOs encompass a broader range of services and providers.

Question 84: Correct Answer: A) Ensure Mr. Johnson receives no food or drink after midnight.

Rationale: "NPO" stands for "nil per os," meaning nothing by mouth, which indicates that Mr. Johnson should not consume any food or liquids after midnight. Option B is incorrect because while "PRN" means as needed, it does not address the NPO status. Option C is incorrect because it misinterprets NPO as scheduling a procedure. Option D is incorrect because PRN does not specify a fixed interval for medication administration; it is based on need.

Question 85: Correct Answer: B) Listen actively to the patient's concerns without interrupting.

Rationale: Active listening is crucial as it validates the patient's feelings and helps de-escalate the situation. Apologizing immediately (A) may seem dismissive without understanding their concern first. Explaining reasons for delay (C) might escalate frustration if done prematurely. Directing them to a supervisor (D) can be perceived as avoidance. Active listening demonstrates empathy and lays the foundation for resolving their issue effectively.

Question 86: Correct Answer: A) Intravenous (IV)

Rationale: The intravenous (IV) route results in the fastest onset of action because the drug is delivered directly into the bloodstream, bypassing absorption barriers. Intramuscular (IM) injections have a slower onset as they require absorption from muscle tissue into the blood. Subcutaneous (SC) injections are even slower due to absorption through subcutaneous tissue. Oral (PO) administration has the slowest onset because it involves gastrointestinal absorption and first-pass metabolism in the liver. Understanding these differences is crucial for selecting appropriate routes based on clinical needs.

Question 87: Correct Answer: B) Call Mr. Johnson to verify his current contact information before updating the record.

Rationale: The best practice in updating patient records is to verify any changes directly with the patient to ensure accuracy and prevent errors. Option B ensures that Sarah confirms the correct details from Mr. Johnson himself before making any updates, adhering to standard protocols for maintaining accurate patient records. Option A assumes information without verification, which could lead to errors. Option C delegates responsibility unnecessarily, potentially causing delays or miscommunication. Option D delays necessary updates, risking communication issues if urgent contact is needed before his next appointment.

Question 88: Correct Answer: C) Metabolism

Rationale: In patients with liver cirrhosis, hepatic function is compromised, leading to altered drug metabolism. This can result in higher plasma levels of drugs metabolized by the liver. While absorption (A), distribution (B), and excretion (D) are also important pharmacokinetic parameters, metabolism (C) is most directly affected by liver function. Absorption deals with how a drug enters the bloodstream; distribution involves how it spreads throughout the body; and excretion concerns how it is eliminated. However, metabolism specifically involves the liver's ability to process drugs.

Question 89: Correct Answer: A) Verify the patient's identity using two identifiers.

Rationale: Verifying the patient's identity using two identifiers is crucial to ensure that the correct patient receives the correct medication, thereby minimizing errors. Option B is incorrect because relying solely on verbal instructions can lead to miscommunication. Option C, while helpful, does not replace proper verification procedures. Option D is risky as pre-populated fields may contain outdated or incorrect information. Proper patient identification is a fundamental step in preventing medication errors and ensuring patient safety.

Question 90: Correct Answer: C) CT (Computed Tomography) scan

Rationale: A CT scan is the most commonly used imaging modality for diagnosing acute appendicitis due to its high accuracy in visualizing the appendix and surrounding structures. Abdominal X-rays are not typically used for this purpose as they lack detail. MRI can be used but is less common due to cost and availability. Ultrasound is often used in children and pregnant women but has limitations in obese patients or when bowel gas obstructs the view. Therefore, a CT scan remains the preferred choice for its detailed imaging capabilities.

Question 91: Correct Answer: C) When initial resuscitation attempts have failed, and there is no immediate improvement.

Rationale: The correct answer is C because immediate escalation is required when initial resuscitation efforts fail and there is no sign of improvement, as this indicates a critical condition needing advanced intervention. Option A is incorrect because stable vital signs do not negate the need for escalation if unresponsiveness persists. Option B is close but less precise as it suggests waiting for a specific time rather than acting based on the patient's condition. Option D is incorrect because it delays necessary action by requiring consultation with another medical assistant rather than escalating immediately.

Question 92: Correct Answer: B) Body paragraphs

Rationale: In a standard block format business letter, all elements are aligned to the left margin without indentation. This includes the body paragraphs, which are not indented and start from the left margin. The salutation (A), complimentary close (C), and date (D) are also aligned to the left margin but can sometimes be confused with semi-block or modified block formats where indentations may occur. Therefore, understanding that body paragraphs in block format do not have indentation is crucial for correctly identifying this element.

Question 93: Correct Answer: B) Ensuring proper skin preparation

Rationale: Ensuring proper skin preparation is crucial for reducing a wandering baseline. This involves cleaning the skin to remove oils and dirt that can interfere with electrode contact. While repositioning electrodes (Option A) may help, it is not as fundamental as skin preparation. Using a higher quality EKG machine (Option C) does not address the root cause of poor electrode contact. Increasing paper speed (Option D) affects the display but does not reduce baseline wandering. Proper skin prep ensures good electrode adhesion and consistent signal quality.

Question 94: Correct Answer: C) Dispensing radiopharmaceuticals for diagnostic imaging

Rationale: Nuclear pharmacies specialize in preparing and dispensing radiopharmaceuticals used in diagnostic imaging and therapy. Option A is incorrect because it describes a general compounding pharmacy's role. Option B is misleading as it pertains more to sterile compounding, not specifically nuclear pharmacy. Option D relates to non-sterile compounding tasks. Understanding these distinctions is crucial for accurately identifying the primary responsibilities of different specialty pharmacies.

Question 95: Correct Answer: B) Verifying that all necessary supplies and equipment are present.

Rationale: While sterilizing instruments (A), disinfecting surfaces (C), and confirming patient records (D) are crucial tasks, verifying that all necessary supplies and equipment are present (B) ensures comprehensive readiness. This step encompasses checking for sterilized instruments, disinfected surfaces, and available patient records. It is a holistic approach that guarantees everything needed for the procedure is on hand, thereby preventing delays or interruptions during patient care.

Question 96: Correct Answer: B) Anger

Rationale: Maria's behavior of lashing out and blaming

others aligns with the anger stage of grief. In this stage, individuals often express frustration and resentment. Denial (Option A) involves refusing to accept reality, which is not evident in Maria's case. Bargaining (Option C) involves making deals or promises to alter the situation, which Maria is not doing. Depression (Option D) involves deep sadness and withdrawal rather than outward expressions of anger. Understanding these nuances is crucial for accurately identifying the stages of grief.

Question 97: Correct Answer: B) Using a certified medical interpreter.

Rationale: Using a certified medical interpreter ensures accurate and culturally sensitive communication, adhering to best practices in patient-centered care. Speaking slowly and loudly (Option A) does not overcome language barriers. Relying on family members (Option C) can lead to misinterpretations due to lack of medical knowledge. Providing written instructions in English (Option D) is ineffective if the patient cannot read English. Certified interpreters are trained to convey medical information accurately, ensuring better patient outcomes.

Question 98: Correct Answer: A) Store the medication in a cool, dry place away from direct sunlight.

Rationale: Medications often need to be stored in a cool, dry place away from direct sunlight to prevent degradation caused by heat and light exposure. Option B (refrigerator at 4°C) is incorrect because not all medications require refrigeration and it could potentially damage some medications. Option C (room temperature) is close but doesn't address protection from light and humidity. Option D (freezer at -20°C) is incorrect as freezing can alter the chemical composition of many medications. Therefore, option A is correct as it ensures optimal storage conditions for maintaining medication efficacy.

Question 99: Correct Answer: B) Include the medication name, dosage, time of administration, and the initials of the administering staff.

Rationale: Option B is correct because it ensures comprehensive documentation that includes all critical details required by regulations—medication name, dosage, time of administration, and initials of the administering staff—ensuring accountability and traceability. Option A is incorrect as it omits staff initials which are crucial for accountability. Option C is incorrect because it lacks essential details like dosage and staff initials. Option D includes patient reaction which is important but not mandatory for every entry in a standard medication log; hence it misses other critical elements like staff initials.

Question 100: Correct Answer: A) Autoclave

Rationale: An autoclave is essential for sterilizing surgical instruments to prevent infections. Disinfectant wipes (Option B) are crucial for surface cleaning but not for sterilizing instruments. Sterile gloves (Option C) are necessary but do not address room preparation. Surgical drapes (Option D) are important but secondary to instrument sterilization. Hence, the autoclave is indispensable in ensuring that all reusable instruments are free from pathogens before any procedure.

Question 101: Correct Answer: B) 960 mg

Rationale: The total sodium content for consuming the entire container is calculated by multiplying the sodium content per serving (480 mg) by the number of servings per container (2). Thus, 480 mg x 2 = 960 mg. Option A is incorrect because it represents only one serving. Option C is incorrect as it misinterprets half of one serving. Option D incorrectly assumes an erroneous calculation method. Understanding how to multiply servings by nutrient content is crucial for accurate dietary advice.

Question 102: Correct Answer: C) Document the incident and inform her immediate supervisor.

Rationale: The correct action is for Sarah to document the incident and inform her immediate supervisor. This ensures that proper protocols are followed without causing unnecessary confrontation or escalation. Reporting directly to administration (A) might bypass necessary steps and confronting the nurses (B) could lead to conflict without resolution. Ignoring it (D) fails to address a serious breach of patient confidentiality. Proper documentation and reporting through appropriate channels ensure that the issue is handled professionally and ethically.

Question 103: Correct Answer: B) Wash the area with soap and water, then report the incident.

Rationale: Washing the area with soap and water is crucial as it helps remove potential pathogens from the wound site. Reporting the incident ensures that proper follow-up actions, such as post-exposure prophylaxis (PEP), can be taken. Option A is incorrect because while applying an antiseptic is useful, it should not be done before washing thoroughly. Option C is incorrect because squeezing can cause more tissue damage and potentially increase pathogen exposure. Option D is incorrect because applying alcohol directly without washing first may not effectively remove pathogens and can cause tissue irritation.

Question 104: Correct Answer: B) "I understand that you're scared. Can you tell me more about what's worrying you?"

Rationale: Option B demonstrates active listening and empathy by acknowledging the patient's feelings and inviting her to share more about her concerns. This approach aligns with contemporary research on therapeutic communication, which emphasizes understanding and addressing patient emotions. Option A dismisses the patient's feelings and provides false reassurance without addressing her concerns. Option C normalizes the patient's feelings but does not invite further discussion or provide support. Option D minimizes the patient's anxiety by suggesting avoidance rather than engagement. Each option is designed to test the candidate's ability to differentiate between superficial reassurance and genuine therapeutic communication techniques.

Question 105: Correct Answer: B) Focus on a balanced diet with complex carbohydrates and fiber.

Rationale: A balanced diet with complex carbohydrates and fiber helps manage blood glucose levels effectively in patients with Type 2 Diabetes Mellitus. High-glycemic index foods (Option A) can cause rapid spikes in blood sugar. Limiting protein intake excessively (Option C) is not necessary and can be detrimental. Eliminating all fats (Option D) is also not recommended as healthy fats are essential for overall health. Complex carbohydrates and fiber slow glucose absorption, promoting stable blood sugar levels, making Option B the best choice.

Question 106: Correct Answer: A) Supine

Rationale: The supine position, where the patient lies flat on their back, is most appropriate for abdominal examinations as it allows full access to the abdomen and facilitates palpation and auscultation. The prone position (B), where the patient lies face down, is unsuitable as it obstructs access to the abdomen. Fowler's position (C), where the patient sits at an angle, is more suitable for respiratory or cardiovascular exams. Lithotomy position (D), where the patient lies on their back with legs elevated in stirrups, is used primarily for pelvic examinations.

Question 107: Correct Answer: A) Lavender-top tube, red-top tube, light blue-top tube

Rationale: The lavender-top tube contains EDTA and is used for CBC. The red-top tube is used for BMP as it allows serum separation. The light blue-top tube contains sodium citrate and is used for PT. Option B is incorrect because the green-top tube (heparin) is not suitable for BMP. Option C is incorrect because the green-top tube is not appropriate for BMP. Option D is incorrect because it lacks the light blue top needed for PT. Each option includes tubes commonly used in phlebotomy but only option A includes all necessary tubes correctly matched to the tests ordered.

Question 108: Correct Answer: C) Medial

Rationale: The term "medial" specifically refers to a position closer to the midline of the body. In contrast, "lateral" means farther from the midline, "proximal" refers to a position nearer to the point of attachment or origin, and "distal" indicates a position farther from the point of attachment or origin. Understanding these distinctions is crucial for accurately describing anatomical positions. While "proximal" and "distal" pertain more to limb positioning relative to the trunk, "medial" and "lateral" directly address proximity to the body's midline.

Question 109: Correct Answer: B) Maintaining eye contact and summarizing what Mr. Johnson says.

Rationale: Maintaining eye contact and summarizing what the patient says shows that Maria is fully engaged and understands Mr. Johnson's concerns, which are key aspects of active listening. Nodding (Option A) and providing verbal reassurances (Option D) are supportive but lack the feedback element crucial for active listening. Asking for repetition (Option C) might imply inattentiveness or misunderstanding, which could increase Mr. Johnson's anxiety rather than alleviate it.

Question 110: Correct Answer: A) Conducting a comprehensive risk assessment of the area

Rationale: Conducting a comprehensive risk assessment is crucial as it identifies specific hazards and underlying causes of patient falls, enabling targeted interventions. While increasing staff presence (Option B), installing signage (Option C), and providing training (Option D) are beneficial, they are secondary steps that should follow an initial risk assessment to ensure all contributing factors are addressed effectively. This approach aligns with contemporary research emphasizing systematic evaluation before implementing corrective actions.

Question 111: Correct Answer: B) 7 years

Rationale: The legally required minimum retention period for adult patient medical records in most states is typically 7 years. This standard aligns with HIPAA guidelines and various state laws. Option A (5 years) is too short for most jurisdictions, while Option C (10 years) and Option D (15 years) exceed the minimum requirement but are not universally mandated. The correct answer ensures compliance with common legal standards while the other options introduce confusion through varying timeframes that could be mistakenly considered valid.

Question 112: Correct Answer: C) LabCorp's Online Portal

Rationale: LabCorp's Online Portal is specifically designed for accessing lab results from LabCorp, making it the most appropriate choice for verifying lab results. PubMed (A) and ClinicalTrials.gov (B) are excellent for researching medical literature and ongoing clinical trials but not for accessing specific lab results. MedlinePlus (D) provides general health information but not specific lab data. Therefore, while all options are valuable resources, only LabCorp's Online Portal directly serves Maria's need to verify lab results accurately and reliably.

Question 113: Correct Answer: B) Take Mr. Johnson's vital signs and document his symptoms.

Rationale: Taking vital signs and documenting symptoms are within the medical assistant's scope of practice as it involves collecting data for the physician. Administering medications (A and D) or interpreting diagnostic tests (C) exceed their authorized duties and require specific medical training and licensure that a CCMA does not possess.

Question 114: Correct Answer: A) Ensure all surgical instruments are laid out on a sterile drape.

Rationale: Ensuring all surgical instruments are laid out on a sterile drape is crucial for maintaining sterility during a procedure. While updating the patient's medical history (B), confirming PPE availability (C), and checking room temperature (D) are important, they do not directly impact the sterility required for minor surgery. Sterile technique prevents infection and ensures patient safety, making option A the most critical action.

Question 115: Correct Answer: A) Fifth intercostal space at the midclavicular line

Rationale: The V4 electrode should be placed in the fifth intercostal space at the midclavicular line for an accurate EKG reading. This position is crucial for capturing correct cardiac activity. Option B is incorrect because it places V4 one rib higher than necessary, potentially distorting the readings. Option C incorrectly shifts V4 laterally to the anterior axillary line, affecting lead accuracy. Option D combines both incorrect height and lateral shift, making it doubly wrong. Proper placement ensures precise monitoring of heart function.

Question 116: Correct Answer: B) Lavender Top Tube

Rationale: The Lavender top tube contains EDTA as an anticoagulant and requires 8-10 gentle inversions to ensure proper mixing and prevent clotting. The Light Blue top tube, used for coagulation tests, requires only 3-4 inversions. The Green top tube contains heparin and needs 8-10 inversions but is primarily used for plasma determinations in chemistry. The Red top tube, which may contain a clot activator or be plain, typically requires 5 inversions if it contains a clot activator. Thus, while other tubes may require similar handling, the specific inversion count and purpose distinguish them.

Question 117: Correct Answer: C) Vitamin B5 (Pantothenic Acid)

Rationale: Vitamin B5 (Pantothenic Acid) is essential for synthesizing coenzyme A, crucial in fatty acid metabolism. While Vitamin B1 (Thiamine) is involved in carbohydrate metabolism, Vitamin B2 (Riboflavin) plays a role in redox reactions, and Vitamin B6 (Pyridoxine) is significant for amino acid metabolism. Each option relates to metabolic processes but differs in specific functions. Understanding these distinctions is vital for correctly identifying Pantothenic Acid as the correct answer.

Question 118: Correct Answer: B) Using password-protected electronic health records (EHR) systems.

Rationale: The use of password-protected electronic health records (EHR) systems is considered the most effective method for ensuring patient confidentiality. This approach leverages advanced encryption and access controls to protect sensitive information. While storing records in locked cabinets (Option A), limiting access to authorized personnel (Option C), and shredding paper records (Option D) are important practices, they do not provide the same level of security and accessibility as EHR systems. EHRs offer comprehensive protection against unauthorized access and data breaches, which aligns with contemporary standards in healthcare information security.

Question 119: Correct Answer: A) Apply direct pressure to the wound with a sterile dressing.

Rationale: The immediate priority in managing an actively bleeding laceration is to control the hemorrhage by applying direct pressure using a sterile dressing. This helps to reduce blood loss and stabilize the patient. Option B (cleaning the wound) is important but secondary to controlling bleeding. Option C (elevating the arm) can assist in reducing blood flow but should follow direct pressure application. Option D (applying a tourniquet) is reserved for severe arterial bleeding when other methods fail due to potential complications.

Question 120: Correct Answer: B) Shaving any chest hair that may interfere with electrode placement

Rationale: Shaving any chest hair that may interfere with electrode placement is crucial because it ensures proper contact between the electrodes and the skin, which is essential for accurate EKG readings. While fasting (Option A) and avoiding caffeine (Option C) might be relevant for other tests, they are not critical for an EKG. Having the patient lie still and breathe normally (Option D) is important during the test but does not fall under preparation steps. Thus, Option B directly addresses a key preparatory action specific to EKG accuracy.

Question 121: Correct Answer: B) Clean Mr. Johnson's skin with alcohol wipes before placing electrodes.

Rationale: Cleaning the skin with alcohol wipes removes oils and debris, ensuring better electrode contact and reducing baseline wander. Option A is important but primarily addresses motion artifacts rather than baseline wander. Option C can temporarily reduce movement but is not a standard practice for baseline stability. Option D addresses potential hair interference but does not directly minimize baseline wander caused by poor electrode-skin contact.

Question 122: Correct Answer: B) Keep the original MOLST form with Jane and store a copy in her medical record.

Rationale: The correct procedure is to ensure that the patient keeps the original MOLST form because it needs to be readily available in case of an emergency. A copy should be stored in her medical record for reference. Option A is incorrect because storing the original in her medical record may delay access during emergencies. Option C is incorrect as sending it to the state health department is not standard practice. Option D is incorrect because while giving Jane both forms might seem helpful, it does not ensure that healthcare providers have immediate access to her preferences.

Question 123: Correct Answer: A) High blood pressure

Rationale: "Hypertension" is medically defined as high blood pressure. This term should be translated into layman's language for better patient understanding. Options B (high cholesterol), C (heart disease), and D (elevated glucose levels) are related to cardiovascular health but are not synonymous with hypertension. High cholesterol refers to elevated fats in the blood, heart disease encompasses various heart conditions, and elevated glucose levels indicate high blood sugar, often associated with diabetes. Hence, A is the correct option as it directly translates "hypertension" accurately for Sarah.

Question 124: Correct Answer: B) Offering specific feedback on what they did well.

Rationale: Specific feedback is most effective because it clearly identifies the behaviors that are being reinforced, making it easier for the individual to repeat them. Public praise (A) can be motivating but may not provide clear guidance. General compliments (C) lack specificity and may not effectively reinforce desired behaviors. Extra breaks (D) are extrinsic rewards and may not directly reinforce the specific effective behavior.

Question 125: Correct Answer: B) The provider's National Provider Identifier (NPI)

Rationale: A valid claim under CMS billing regulations must include the provider's National Provider Identifier (NPI). This unique identifier is essential for ensuring that claims are processed correctly. While the patient's social security number, date of birth, and provider's tax identification number are important pieces of information, they are not specifically required for submitting a valid claim. The NPI ensures that the healthcare provider is correctly identified in the billing process. - Option A (Patient's social security number): While important for patient identification, it is not a CMS billing requirement. - Option C (Patient's date of birth): Critical for verifying patient identity but not a specific CMS billing mandate. - Option D (Provider's tax identification number): Important for financial transactions but not specifically required by CMS for claim submission.

Question 126: Correct Answer: B) Use a butterfly needle and warm the patient's arm before attempting venipuncture.

Rationale: Using a butterfly needle allows for better control in patients with difficult veins, and warming the arm helps dilate veins, making them easier to access. Option A is incorrect because applying a tourniquet for more than 2 minutes can cause hemoconcentration. Option C is incorrect as pumping the fist can lead to hemolysis. Option D is incorrect because while minimizing discomfort is important, using too small of a gauge can make drawing blood more difficult and may damage red blood cells.

Question 127: Correct Answer: B) Simplify the question using clear and concise language.

Rationale: The most effective initial response is to simplify the question using clear and concise language. This approach respects Mr. Johnson's autonomy while accommodating potential age-related cognitive changes. Option A is incorrect because speaking louder may not address comprehension issues and could be perceived as patronizing. Option C bypasses direct communication with Mr. Johnson, which should be avoided unless absolutely necessary. Option D assumes he can read and understand written instructions without addressing immediate confusion.

Question 128: Correct Answer: B) Apply the specific CPT code for the CMP test performed.

Rationale: The correct action is to apply the specific CPT code for the CMP test performed. This ensures that the insurance company accurately recognizes and reimburses for the specific service provided. Option A is incorrect because using a general office visit code does not specify the CMP test. Option C is misleading as diagnosis codes describe conditions rather than procedures. Option D is partially correct but lacks specificity; itemizing without proper CPT codes can lead to claim denials or delays.

Question 129: Correct Answer: A) Politely redirect the conversation back to Mr. Johnson's medical concerns.

Rationale: Maria should maintain professional boundaries by politely redirecting the conversation back to relevant medical concerns (Option A). This ensures that she remains focused on her role and provides appropriate care without overstepping boundaries. Option B is incorrect because offering personal advice can blur professional lines. Option C, sharing personal stories, can lead to an unprofessional relationship. Option D is incorrect as documenting irrelevant personal information violates patient confidentiality and privacy principles.

Question 130: Correct Answer: C) Checking if pre-authorization is required for the service

Rationale: Checking if pre-authorization is required is crucial because many insurance plans require it for certain procedures or services. Without it, claims may be denied regardless of other factors. While confirming the policy effective date (A), verifying co-payment amount (B), and reviewing deductible status (D) are important steps in understanding coverage details, they do not directly impact whether a service will be covered without prior authorization. Pre-authorization ensures compliance with insurance requirements and prevents claim rejections.

Question 131: Correct Answer: B) Autoimmune destruction of pancreatic beta cells

Rationale: Type 1 Diabetes Mellitus primarily results from autoimmune destruction of pancreatic beta cells, leading to an absolute deficiency in insulin production. Option A (Insulin resistance due to obesity) is associated with Type 2 Diabetes Mellitus. Option C (Increased hepatic glucose production) and Option D (Dysfunctional insulin receptor signaling) are also more relevant to Type 2 Diabetes Mellitus. Understanding these distinctions is crucial for recognizing the pathophysiology specific to each type of diabetes.

Question 132: Correct Answer: A) Verify the patient's identity by checking the wristband and asking for their full name and date of birth.

Rationale: The "Right Patient" principle requires verifying the patient's identity using two identifiers, such as checking the wristband and asking for their full name and date of birth. Option B, confirming with another nurse, relates more to double-checking orders rather than patient identification. Option C pertains to verifying dosage, aligning with the "Right Dose" principle. Option D involves timing, associated with the "Right Time" principle. Therefore, option A is correct as it directly addresses confirming patient identity, a critical step in preventing medication errors.

Question 133: Correct Answer: C) Maintaining a sterile field

Rationale: Maintaining a sterile field is crucial because it prevents contamination from non-sterile surfaces or objects, thereby reducing infection risk. While wearing sterile gloves

(A), using antiseptic solutions (B), and donning surgical masks (D) are important, they support but do not ensure sterility alone. A breach in the sterile field can lead to contamination regardless of other precautions. Therefore, maintaining a sterile field is paramount for surgical asepsis.

Question 134: Correct Answer: D) Educate Sarah on recognizing early signs of heart failure exacerbation.

Rationale: Educating Sarah on recognizing early signs of heart failure exacerbation is crucial because it empowers her to seek timely medical intervention, potentially preventing readmission. While scheduling follow-up appointments (A), providing discharge instructions (B), and arranging home health services (C) are important, they do not directly address immediate self-management skills essential for preventing complications. Education on symptom recognition specifically targets patient empowerment and self-care, which are critical in managing chronic conditions like heart failure.

Question 135: Correct Answer: A) Contacting the insurance company directly to confirm coverage details.

Rationale: Contacting the insurance company directly ensures that all coverage details are up-to-date and accurate, which is crucial for obtaining prior authorizations and pre-certifications. Reviewing the patient's medical history (Option B) or relying on patient-provided information (Option C) may not provide current or complete coverage details. Checking the provider's internal system (Option D) might not reflect recent changes in insurance policies. Direct confirmation from the insurer minimizes errors and ensures compliance with authorization requirements.

Question 136: Correct Answer: C) Verify Mrs. Johnson's identity before providing any information.

Rationale: Sarah should first verify Mrs. Johnson's identity to ensure she is authorized to receive Mr. Johnson's medical information, adhering to HIPAA regulations. Option A lacks verification of identity, compromising confidentiality. Option B may not be practical for immediate needs and could delay necessary care. Option D incorrectly redirects responsibility away from the medical office, potentially causing confusion or miscommunication about specific physician instructions.

Question 137: Correct Answer: B) Verify insurance coverage and obtain preauthorization before scheduling the procedure.

Rationale: Verifying insurance coverage and obtaining preauthorization before scheduling ensures that the procedure is covered and prevents claim denial. Option A is incorrect because submitting a claim without preauthorization can lead to denial. Option C is partially correct but misses the crucial step of obtaining preauthorization. Option D focuses on accurate coding but neglects preauthorization requirements. Preauthorization is essential to confirm that the payer will cover the costs, thus avoiding financial issues for both patient and provider.

Question 138: Correct Answer: A) Vitamin D

Rationale: Vitamin D is essential for calcium absorption in the intestines, which is crucial for maintaining proper bone density and overall skeletal health. While Vitamin K (Option B) plays a role in bone metabolism by modifying bone proteins, it does not directly enhance calcium absorption. Vitamin A (Option C) contributes to bone growth but can cause bone resorption at high levels. Vitamin C (Option D) is important for collagen formation in bones but does not affect calcium absorption directly. Thus, only Vitamin D has the primary function of enhancing calcium absorption.

Question 139: Correct Answer: C) Request her identification and insurance card.

Rationale: The first step in checking a patient in is to request their identification and insurance card. This ensures that the correct patient is being checked in and that their insurance information is up-to-date. While verifying insurance information (Option A), confirming the appointment time and purpose (Option B), and updating medical history (Option D) are also important steps, they typically follow after

initial identification verification. Properly identifying the patient first helps prevent errors in patient records and ensures compliance with administrative protocols.

Question 140: Correct Answer: A) Patient's full name and date of birth

Rationale: The patient's full name and date of birth are essential for accurate patient identification, ensuring that test results are correctly matched to the patient. While physician's contact number (Option B) and type of specimen collected (Option C) are important, they do not directly ensure patient identification. Test codes for requested tests (Option D) facilitate accurate test processing but lack the critical element of identifying the specific patient. Thus, Option A is the most comprehensive in ensuring both proper identification and accurate test processing.

Question 141: Correct Answer: C) Measure just above the iliac crest.

Rationale: The most accurate method to measure waist circumference is to measure just above the iliac crest (Option C). This location provides a consistent and reliable reference point for assessing abdominal fat distribution. Measuring at the level of the umbilicus (Option A) or at the narrowest point between the ribs and hips (Option B) can lead to inconsistent results due to variability in body shape and fat distribution. Measuring at the widest part of the abdomen (Option D) can overestimate waist circumference and does not provide an accurate assessment of central obesity.

Question 142: Correct Answer: D) Verifying that the specimen label includes patient identifiers and test site.

Rationale: Option D is correct because it ensures both patient identifiers and test site information are included, which is essential for accurate diagnosis and tracking. Option A is incorrect as it omits the test site information. Option B is incorrect because not all specimens should be stored at room temperature; some require refrigeration or freezing. Option C is partially correct but does not address specific labeling requirements crucial for patient safety and accurate testing.

Question 143: Correct Answer: C) Tilt the patient's head slightly forward and use warm water.

Rationale: Warm water helps soften cerumen without causing dizziness or discomfort. Tilting the patient's head slightly forward prevents water from pooling in the ear canal, reducing infection risk. Cold water (Option A) can cause vertigo; directing water towards the eardrum (Option B) risks injury; high pressure (Option D) may damage delicate structures within the ear. Proper technique minimizes complications and ensures patient safety.

Question 144: Correct Answer: D) Avoid smoking for at least 24 hours before the test.

Rationale: Smoking can significantly affect lung function and skew spirometry results. Although avoiding inhaler use (A), not eating heavily (B), and refraining from exercise (C) are important, they do not have as significant an impact on baseline lung function as smoking does. Smoking cessation for 24 hours ensures that nicotine and other substances do not interfere with lung capacity measurements. This instruction is crucial for obtaining accurate and reliable spirometry readings.

Question 145: Correct Answer: C) Patient-Centered Medical Home (PCMH)

Rationale: The PCMH model focuses on coordinated care and comprehensive management, making it ideal for patients with multiple chronic conditions like Sarah. Unlike HMOs and PPOs, which primarily focus on cost control and network restrictions, PCMH emphasizes ongoing patient-provider relationships and integrated care. POS plans offer some flexibility in provider choice but do not prioritize coordinated care to the same extent as PCMH.

Question 146: Correct Answer: A) "Can you describe what you typically eat in a day?"

Rationale: Option A is an open-ended question that

encourages Mr. Johnson to provide detailed and comprehensive information about his dietary habits. Option B is a closed-ended question that can be answered with a simple yes or no, providing limited information. Option C is also a closed-ended question focusing only on the number of meals, not the content of those meals. Option D is a probing question but focuses on changes rather than current habits. Open-ended questions like option A are best for gathering detailed data.

Question 147: Correct Answer: D) Terminal Digit Filing
Rationale: Terminal digit filing is highly efficient for large volumes of records, allowing quick access and reducing misfiling errors by using the last digits of the record number. This system also enhances confidentiality as it doesn't rely on patient names. Alphabetical filing (A) is straightforward but less secure and can lead to congestion under common surnames. Numerical filing (B) is organized but can be cumbersome without terminal digit indexing. Subject filing (C) is useful for categorizing topics but not ideal for individual patient records due to potential privacy issues and complexity. Tone: Professional and Knowledgeable

Question 148: Correct Answer: A) 45 degrees
Rationale: The correct angle for inserting a needle during a subcutaneous injection is 45 degrees. This angle ensures that the medication is delivered into the subcutaneous tissue rather than deeper into the muscle or more superficially into the dermis. Option B (90 degrees) is typically used for intramuscular injections. Option C (15 degrees) and Option D (30 degrees) are incorrect as they are too shallow for subcutaneous injections, risking improper delivery of the medication. Understanding these distinctions is crucial for

effective and safe patient care.

Question 149: Correct Answer: B) Bacteria
Rationale: The correct plural form of "bacterium" is "bacteria." The term "bacterium" follows the rule where words ending in "-um" are pluralized by changing "-um" to "-a." Option A) "Bacteriums" incorrectly adds an English-style pluralization. Option C) "Bacterias" incorrectly adds an "s," which is not appropriate for Latin-derived terms. Option D) "Bacteriae" incorrectly uses a Latin ending that does not apply to this word. Understanding these nuances in medical terminology is crucial for accurate communication in clinical settings.

Question 150: Correct Answer: D) Ischemic Heart Disease
Rationale: Ischemic heart disease is the leading cause of death globally due to its direct impact on cardiovascular health. While hypertension (A), type 2 diabetes mellitus (B), and COPD (C) are significant contributors to morbidity and mortality, ischemic heart disease remains the most critical risk factor due to its prevalence and severe outcomes such as heart attacks and strokes. Hypertension often leads to ischemic heart disease but is not as immediately fatal. Type 2 diabetes increases cardiovascular risks but primarily impacts metabolic processes. COPD affects respiratory function but does not surpass ischemic heart disease in global mortality rates.

CCMA Exam Practice Questions [SET 3]

Question 1: Which of the following is the most appropriate injection site for administering an intramuscular (IM) injection in an adult patient?
A) Deltoid muscle
B) Vastus lateralis muscle
C) Dorsogluteal muscle
D) Ventrogluteal muscle

Question 2: Which of the following instruments is essential for performing a thorough neurological examination in a procedure room?
A) Otoscope
B) Reflex hammer
C) Sphygmomanometer
D) Stethoscope

Question 3: Sarah, a 45-year-old patient, is scheduled for a complex surgical procedure. Dr. Thompson explains the procedure, including its risks and benefits, in detail. However, Sarah seems anxious and unsure about her decision. What is the most appropriate action for Dr. Thompson to take next to ensure informed consent?
A) Proceed with the surgery since the risks and benefits were explained.
B) Ask Sarah to sign the consent form immediately.
C) Reassure Sarah and give her additional time to consider her decision.
D) Delegate the task of obtaining consent to another healthcare provider.

Question 4: Which document must be reviewed and signed by a patient before undergoing any surgical procedure?
A) Informed Consent Form
B) Treatment Plan Agreement
C) HIPAA Privacy Notice
D) Medical History Form

Question 5: Which of the following tasks is within the scope of practice for a Certified Clinical Medical Assistant (CCMA)?
A) Administering intravenous medications
B) Performing venipuncture for blood draws
C) Interpreting laboratory results
D) Prescribing medication

Question 6: Which of the following is considered the most effective method for ensuring the security of patient data in an EMR/EHR system?
A) Regularly updating antivirus software
B) Implementing strong password policies
C) Encrypting patient data
D) Conducting frequent staff training sessions

Question 7: During a busy clinic day, Dr. Smith asks Maria, a Certified Clinical Medical Assistant (CCMA), to perform an electrocardiogram (ECG) on Mr. Johnson, a new patient complaining of chest pain. Maria is also asked by Nurse Jane to assist with a minor surgical procedure simultaneously. What should Maria do first?
A) Perform the ECG on Mr. Johnson as requested by Dr. Smith.
B) Assist Nurse Jane with the minor surgical procedure.
C) Inform Dr. Smith that she is assisting with a minor surgical procedure and will perform the ECG afterward.

D) Delegate the ECG task to another MA and assist with the minor surgical procedure.

Question 8: Which of the following is a key characteristic of the Patient-Centered Medical Home (PCMH) model that distinguishes it from other care models?
A) Emphasis on comprehensive care coordination across all providers
B) Focus on reducing hospital readmissions through transitional care management
C) Implementation of patient-centered decision-making with shared responsibility
D) Integration of financial incentives for meeting specific performance metrics

Question 9: A 65-year-old male patient presents with palpitations and dizziness. His EKG shows irregularly irregular rhythm without distinct P waves before each QRS complex. What is the most likely diagnosis?
A) Atrial Fibrillation
B) Ventricular Tachycardia
C) Sinus Bradycardia
D) Wandering Atrial Pacemaker

Question 10: During a routine examination, a patient named Maria presents with symptoms of muscle weakness and fatigue. You suspect a cellular dysfunction related to energy production. Which organelle is most likely affected in Maria's cells?
A) Nucleus
B) Mitochondria
C) Ribosomes
D) Lysosomes

Question 11: Which of the following is a distinguishing feature of Bulimia Nervosa compared to other eating disorders?
A) Restrictive food intake
B) Episodes of binge eating followed by compensatory behaviors
C) Intense fear of gaining weight
D) Distorted body image

Question 12: Patient John Doe, a 55-year-old male, presents with complaints of chest pain and palpitations. You are tasked with performing an EKG to assess his cardiac function. Which of the following actions is most critical to ensure accurate lead placement for obtaining a valid EKG reading?
A) Place the V1 lead at the fourth intercostal space, right sternal border.
B) Place the V2 lead at the fourth intercostal space, left sternal border.
C) Place the V4 lead at the fifth intercostal space, midclavicular line.
D) Place the V3 lead halfway between V2 and V4.

Question 13: Sarah, a medical assistant, is responsible for storing a new batch of injectable medications. The medication requires refrigeration but must not be frozen. Which of the following storage practices should Sarah follow to ensure the medication remains effective?
A) Store the medication in a refrigerator at 2-8°C (36-46°F), ensuring it does not freeze.
B) Store the medication in a freezer at -20°C (-4°F) to ensure

it remains preserved.
C) Store the medication at room temperature away from direct sunlight and heat sources.
D) Store the medication in a refrigerator at 0-4°C (32-39°F), ensuring it does not freeze.

Question 14: When sending orders for prescriptions and refills by telephone, fax, or email, which of the following guidelines must be strictly followed to ensure compliance with HIPAA regulations?
A) Always include the patient's full name and date of birth.
B) Obtain verbal consent from the patient before sending.
C) Use secure communication channels approved by the healthcare facility.
D) Include a detailed list of all medications the patient is currently taking.

Question 15: John, a 55-year-old male patient, presents with palpitations and dizziness. An ECG reveals an abnormal rhythm. Which part of the heart's electrical conduction system is primarily responsible for initiating the heart's intrinsic rhythm?
A) Atrioventricular (AV) node
B) Sinoatrial (SA) node
C) Bundle of His
D) Purkinje fibers

Question 16: Mr. Johnson, a 55-year-old patient newly diagnosed with Type 2 Diabetes, is struggling to adhere to his prescribed medication regimen and lifestyle changes. As a Certified Clinical Medical Assistant (CCMA), what is the most effective initial approach you should take to help improve his adherence?
A) Provide Mr. Johnson with detailed written instructions on his medication and lifestyle changes.
B) Schedule a follow-up appointment in two weeks to reassess his adherence.
C) Engage in a motivational interviewing session to understand his barriers and enhance his intrinsic motivation.
D) Refer Mr. Johnson to a diabetes education class immediately.

Question 17: John, a 55-year-old male with a history of diabetes, suddenly becomes confused, sweaty, and shaky during his routine check-up. What is the most likely cause of his symptoms?
A) Diabetic Shock
B) Heat Stroke
C) Allergic Reaction
D) Syncope

Question 18: Which of the following best describes the term "incidence" in epidemiological studies?
A) The number of new cases of a disease in a specific population over a defined period.
B) The total number of existing cases of a disease in a population at a given time.
C) The likelihood of developing a disease based on genetic predisposition.
D) The proportion of individuals who have recovered from a disease over a certain period.

Question 19: Which of the following best describes the primary role of a medical assistant in a patient-centered medical home (PCMH) model?
A) Coordinating patient referrals to specialists
B) Conducting comprehensive patient assessments
C) Managing patient care plans and follow-ups
D) Administering direct patient care under physician supervision

Question 20: You are preparing to perform venipuncture on Mr. Johnson, a 45-year-old patient. Which of the
following steps is crucial to ensure proper site preparation and reduce the risk of infection?
A) Cleanse the site with an alcohol swab in a circular motion, starting from the center and moving outward.
B) Use an iodine swab to cleanse the site in a back-and-forth motion.
C) Cleanse the site with an alcohol swab using a back-and-forth scrubbing motion.
D) Use soap and water to cleanse the site thoroughly before venipuncture.

Question 21: You are tasked with transporting a blood specimen for coagulation studies from the clinic to the laboratory. Which of the following is the most appropriate method to ensure accurate test results?
A) Transport the specimen at room temperature and deliver it within 4 hours.
B) Place the specimen on ice immediately and deliver it within 2 hours.
C) Keep the specimen at room temperature and deliver it within 2 hours.
D) Centrifuge the specimen immediately and transport it at room temperature.

Question 22: You are a CCMA working at a busy clinic. A patient named Mr. Johnson calls to inquire about his lab results. The results are available, but you notice that the physician has not yet reviewed them. What is the best course of action?
A) Inform Mr. Johnson that his results are available and read them to him.
B) Tell Mr. Johnson that his results are available but need to be reviewed by the physician before you can share them.
C) Advise Mr. Johnson to call back later when the physician is available to discuss the results.
D) Schedule an appointment for Mr. Johnson to come in and discuss the results with the physician.

Question 23: Patient John is prescribed warfarin for anticoagulation therapy. During a follow-up visit, his INR levels are found to be significantly elevated. Which of the following could most likely cause this increase in INR?
A) Increased intake of green leafy vegetables
B) Concurrent use of amiodarone
C) Regular consumption of cranberry juice
D) Increased physical activity

Question 24: Maria, a 45-year-old patient with diabetes, is scheduled for a fasting blood glucose test at 8 AM. As a Certified Clinical Medical Assistant (CCMA), what is the most appropriate action to ensure accurate test results?
A) Advise Maria to have her last meal by 6 PM the previous evening.
B) Instruct Maria to fast for at least 8 hours before the test.
C) Allow Maria to drink water but avoid all other beverages after midnight.
D) Permit Maria to take her morning insulin dose before the test.

Question 25: During a general physical examination, the provider asks you to prepare Mrs. Johnson, a 55-year-old patient with hypertension, for her examination. Which of the following is the most appropriate first step?
A) Ask Mrs. Johnson to remove her shoes and outer clothing.
B) Measure Mrs. Johnson's blood pressure while she is standing.
C) Ensure Mrs. Johnson's medical history is updated and accessible.
D) Position Mrs. Johnson in a supine position on the

examination table.

Question 26: Emily, a 45-year-old woman, has been referred by her primary care physician for further evaluation of her chronic migraines. Which type of healthcare provider is most appropriate for this referral?
A) General Practitioner
B) Neurologist
C) Rheumatologist
D) Endocrinologist

Question 27: During a routine check-up, Mr. Johnson, a 45-year-old diabetic patient, presents with symptoms of hyperglycemia. As a Certified Clinical Medical Assistant (CCMA), you decide to perform Point Of Care Testing to quickly assess his blood glucose levels. Which of the following actions is MOST appropriate for ensuring accurate results?
A) Perform the test immediately after calibrating the glucometer.
B) Use a blood sample from a fingerstick without cleaning the site first.
C) Use expired test strips if they appear to be in good condition.
D) Perform the test in a well-lit area to ensure proper reading.

Question 28: Sarah, a 45-year-old female patient, presents with fatigue and pallor. Her Complete Blood Count (CBC) results are as follows: Hemoglobin: 8 g/dL, Hematocrit: 24%, Mean Corpuscular Volume (MCV): 70 fL. Based on these results, which condition is most likely?
A) Iron-deficiency anemia
B) Vitamin B12 deficiency anemia
C) Chronic kidney disease
D) Thalassemia

Question 29: Which of the following is the most appropriate method for disposing of unused controlled substances in a clinical setting?
A) Flushing them down the toilet.
B) Returning them to a pharmacy take-back program.
C) Mixing them with coffee grounds and placing in the trash.
D) Incinerating them in a regular waste facility.

Question 30: Which organization is primarily responsible for certifying Clinical Medical Assistants (CCMAs) in the United States?
A) National Healthcareer Association (NHA)
B) American Association of Medical Assistants (AAMA)
C) National Center for Competency Testing (NCCT)
D) American Medical Technologists (AMT)

Question 31: Mrs. Johnson, a 55-year-old woman, complains of fatigue and muscle weakness. She has a history of osteoporosis and is currently on calcium supplements. Her recent blood tests show low levels of a particular vitamin that is crucial for calcium absorption. Which vitamin supplementation should be recommended to Mrs. Johnson?
A) Vitamin D
B) Vitamin C
C) Vitamin B12
D) Vitamin K

Question 32: John, a 65-year-old male with a history of hypertension, presents to the clinic with complaints of palpitations and dizziness. His EKG shows an irregularly irregular rhythm with no distinct P waves and a variable R-R interval. What is the most likely diagnosis?
A) Atrial Fibrillation
B) Atrial Flutter

C) Ventricular Tachycardia
D) Sinus Arrhythmia

Question 33: During a capillary puncture procedure on a 5-year-old patient named Emily, which step is crucial to ensure accurate blood glucose measurement?
A) Warming the puncture site with a warm cloth for 30 seconds.
B) Using the first drop of blood after wiping away any initial tissue fluid.
C) Puncturing the side of the fingertip rather than the center.
D) Squeezing the finger firmly to obtain an adequate blood sample.

Question 34: When collecting a midstream clean-catch urine specimen, which step is crucial to ensure the sample is not contaminated?
A) Instructing the patient to start urinating into the toilet, then catch the midstream in a sterile container.
B) Collecting the first few drops of urine directly into the sterile container.
C) Using a catheter to obtain urine directly from the bladder.
D) Refrigerating the sample immediately after collection.

Question 35: Which of the following is the correct procedure for disposing of used needles in a clinical setting as per OSHA regulations?
A) Place them in a puncture-resistant, leak-proof container labeled with a biohazard symbol.
B) Dispose of them in any available trash receptacle as long as it is emptied regularly.
C) Place them in a cardboard box that is sealed with tape and marked "biohazard."
D) Dispose of them in a red bag designated for biohazardous waste.

Question 36: A physician prescribes 15 mL of medication to be administered to a patient. How many teaspoons (tsp) should the medical assistant administer?
A) 3 tsp
B) 2.5 tsp
C) 4 tsp
D) 2 tsp

Question 37: Patient John requires a medication dosage of 500 mg. The medication is available in liquid form with a concentration of 250 mg per teaspoon. How many teaspoons should John take to receive the correct dosage?
A) 1 teaspoon
B) 2 teaspoons
C) 3 teaspoons
D) 4 teaspoons

Question 38: While conducting a routine safety evaluation in the clinic, Medical Assistant Sarah notices that a box of medical supplies is blocking an emergency exit. Which action should Sarah take first to address this safety concern?
A) Move the box immediately and report it to her supervisor.
B) Inform her supervisor about the blockage and wait for further instructions.
C) Document the incident in the clinic's safety log before taking any action.
D) Conduct a brief meeting with staff to discuss the importance of keeping exits clear.

Question 39: During a physical examination, Dr. Smith asks the medical assistant to position Mr. Johnson in a way that allows for easy access to the anterior surface of his body. Which position should the medical assistant use?

A) Supine
B) Prone
C) Lateral
D) Fowler's

Question 40: A patient requests a treatment that conflicts with the medical assistant's personal religious beliefs. What is the most appropriate course of action for the medical assistant to take?
A) Politely decline to provide the treatment and refer the patient to another provider.
B) Inform the patient about their personal beliefs and suggest alternative treatments.
C) Provide the requested treatment without expressing personal beliefs.
D) Seek guidance from a supervisor or ethics committee before proceeding.

Question 41: When selecting a bandage for a patient with sensitive skin prone to allergic reactions, which type of bandage material is most appropriate to minimize irritation?
A) Latex-based adhesive bandages
B) Hydrocolloid dressings
C) Cotton gauze with hypoallergenic tape
D) Elastic compression bandages

Question 42: Which type of health insurance plan requires patients to select a primary care physician (PCP) who coordinates all their healthcare services and provides referrals to specialists?
A) Preferred Provider Organization (PPO)
B) Health Maintenance Organization (HMO)
C) Exclusive Provider Organization (EPO)
D) Point of Service (POS)

Question 43: Which form of medication is typically a clear, sweetened hydroalcoholic solution intended for oral use?
A) Liquid
B) Elixir
C) Balm
D) Ointment

Question 44: Which organ system is primarily responsible for regulating body temperature and protecting internal organs from external damage?
A) Endocrine System
B) Integumentary System
C) Muscular System
D) Nervous System

Question 45: Sarah, a Certified Clinical Medical Assistant (CCMA), observes unexplained bruises on an elderly patient named Mr. Thompson during a routine check-up. Mr. Thompson appears fearful and hesitant to discuss his injuries. As a CCMA, what is Sarah's appropriate course of action under mandatory reporting laws?
A) Report the suspected abuse immediately to local law enforcement.
B) Document the observations in Mr. Thompson's medical record and report to Adult Protective Services (APS).
C) Wait for confirmation from a physician before making any report.
D) Discuss her concerns with Mr. Thompson's family members before taking further action.

Question 46: During a routine check-up, you need to explain to 5-year-old Emily that she will receive a vaccine. Which term would be most appropriate to use?
A) "Shot"
B) "Injection"

C) "Medicine"
D) "Vaccine"

Question 47: Jane, a 45-year-old woman, reports feeling anxious about her upcoming surgery. During her pre-operative assessment, you notice an increase in her blood pressure and heart rate. Which of the following best explains this physiological response?
A) Anxiety increases cortisol levels, leading to elevated blood pressure and heart rate.
B) Anxiety triggers the release of adrenaline, causing increased blood pressure and heart rate.
C) Anxiety decreases serotonin levels, resulting in elevated blood pressure and heart rate.
D) Anxiety reduces dopamine levels, leading to increased blood pressure and heart rate.

Question 48: John, a 28-year-old male, presents with right lower quadrant abdominal pain, nausea, and a low-grade fever. Upon physical examination, he exhibits rebound tenderness in the right lower quadrant. What is the most likely diagnosis?
A) Acute appendicitis
B) Crohn's disease
C) Diverticulitis
D) Ectopic pregnancy

Question 49: A 65-year-old patient named Mr. Johnson is admitted with a confirmed case of Clostridioides difficile (C. diff) infection. As a Certified Clinical Medical Assistant, which of the following actions should you take first to ensure proper infection control before entering his room?
A) Put on a surgical mask and gloves.
B) Don a gown and gloves.
C) Wear an N95 respirator and gloves.
D) Use a face shield and gloves.

Question 50: Emily, a Certified Clinical Medical Assistant, is preparing to draw blood from a patient named Mr. Johnson for several lab tests. She receives a requisition form but notices it lacks certain critical information. Which piece of information is most crucial to ensure accurate processing of Mr. Johnson's blood sample?
A) The patient's insurance information
B) The patient's date of birth
C) The specific tests ordered
D) The physician's signature

Question 51: When preparing a patient for a lipid panel blood test, which of the following is the most critical instruction regarding fasting?
A) The patient should fast for at least 6 hours before the test.
B) The patient should fast for at least 8 hours before the test.
C) The patient should fast for at least 12 hours before the test.
D) The patient should not eat or drink anything except water for 24 hours before the test.

Question 52: When treating a sprained ankle, which of the following steps is most critical within the first 24 hours to minimize swelling and pain?
A) Applying heat immediately
B) Keeping the ankle elevated above heart level
C) Wrapping the ankle tightly with an elastic bandage
D) Performing gentle range-of-motion exercises

Question 53: When interpreting a child's growth chart, which of the following statements is correct regarding the significance of growth percentiles?
A) A child consistently at the 25th percentile for weight is underweight.

B) A child at the 75th percentile for height is taller than 75% of peers.
C) A child who drops from the 50th to the 25th percentile for height over six months indicates normal variation.
D) A child consistently at the 90th percentile for weight indicates obesity.

Question 54: Mrs. Johnson is a single mother of two who recently lost her job. She visits a community health clinic seeking medical assistance but is concerned about the costs. The clinic uses a sliding scale fee system based on income. Which of the following factors will most likely determine Mrs. Johnson's eligibility for reduced fees under this system?
A) Her previous employment history
B) Her current household income
C) The number of dependents she has
D) Her educational background

Question 55: Sarah, a Certified Clinical Medical Assistant, is preparing to collect a blood sample from Mr. Johnson for a complete blood count (CBC). Which of the following steps should she take immediately after confirming Mr. Johnson's identity and explaining the procedure?
A) Apply a tourniquet 3-4 inches above the venipuncture site.
B) Cleanse the venipuncture site with an alcohol swab.
C) Insert the needle at a 45-degree angle into the vein.
D) Label the collection tubes with Mr. Johnson's information.

Question 56: A patient presents with symptoms of anaphylactic shock. What is the most appropriate initial response?
A) Administer oral antihistamines.
B) Provide intravenous fluids.
C) Administer intramuscular epinephrine.
D) Apply a cold compress to the affected area.

Question 57: Mrs. Johnson, a 68-year-old patient with advanced heart disease, has a Do Not Resuscitate (DNR) order in her medical file. During her latest visit, she mentions that she wants all possible measures taken if her heart stops. What should you do as her medical assistant?
A) Update her DNR status immediately in the medical file.
B) Inform the attending physician about her verbal request.
C) Ignore the verbal request since it contradicts the existing DNR order.
D) Ask Mrs. Johnson to sign a new DNR order reflecting her wishes.

Question 58: When performing venipuncture, which of the following is the most appropriate angle for needle insertion to ensure successful access to a superficial vein?
A) 5-10 degrees
B) 15-30 degrees
C) 45-60 degrees
D) 75-90 degrees

Question 59: Which of the following is most essential for a medical assistant to establish trust and rapport with a patient during therapeutic communication?
A) Active listening
B) Providing medical advice
C) Using medical jargon
D) Maintaining professional distance

Question 60: Which of the following is the most reliable method for identifying a patient before administering medication?
A) Asking the patient to state their full name and date of birth.

B) Checking the patient's room number against the medication chart.
C) Verifying the patient's wristband information with the medication order.
D) Asking a colleague to confirm the patient's identity.

Question 61: Patient Maria presents with a chronic venous insufficiency condition leading to venous ulcers on her lower legs. Which of the following treatments is contraindicated for her condition?
A) Compression therapy
B) Elevation of the legs
C) Application of heat packs
D) Use of moisturizers

Question 62: When managing an elderly patient with multiple chronic conditions, which of the following is the most important consideration to ensure optimal care?
A) Prioritize treatment of the most severe condition first.
B) Focus on maintaining functional independence and quality of life.
C) Treat each condition independently to avoid polypharmacy.
D) Ensure strict adherence to all prescribed medications.

Question 63: Which of the following actions is most critical in maintaining sterility during a minor surgical procedure?
A) Wearing sterile gloves throughout the procedure
B) Using an antiseptic solution on the patient's skin before incision
C) Ensuring all instruments are sterilized before use
D) Maintaining a sterile field by not reaching over it

Question 64: A patient named Mr. Johnson has been prescribed a high-cost medication for his chronic condition. As a Certified Clinical Medical Assistant (CCMA), you need to obtain prior authorization from the insurance company before dispensing the medication. Which of the following steps is most crucial in ensuring a successful prior authorization?
A) Submitting a complete medical history of the patient along with the prescription.
B) Contacting the patient's pharmacy to verify medication availability.
C) Ensuring all required documentation and forms are accurately filled out and submitted to the insurance company.
D) Scheduling an appointment with the prescribing physician to discuss alternative medications.

Question 65: When communicating with a patient who has limited English proficiency and comes from a different cultural background, which approach is most effective in ensuring accurate understanding?
A) Use medical jargon sparingly and rely on gestures to convey meaning.
B) Speak slowly and loudly to ensure the patient can hear and understand.
C) Utilize a professional medical interpreter to facilitate communication.
D) Simplify medical terms and use family members as interpreters.

Question 66: Sarah, a 45-year-old patient, has been diagnosed with a chronic condition. She has requested that her medical information not be shared with her employer. Under which condition can her medical information be legally shared without her explicit consent?
A) If the information is required by a public health authority to control disease spread.
B) If her family members request the information for

caregiving purposes.
C) If her employer requests the information for workplace accommodations.
D) If another healthcare provider involved in her care needs the information.

Question 67: Which of the following ancillary services is primarily responsible for providing diagnostic imaging that assists in the medical diagnosis of patients?
A) Physical Therapy
B) Radiology
C) Occupational Therapy
D) Respiratory Therapy

Question 68: Maria, a Certified Clinical Medical Assistant (CCMA), is handling a patient named Mr. Johnson who is upset about a delay in his appointment. Which of the following actions should Maria take to effectively address Mr. Johnson's concerns?
A) Apologize for the delay and assure him that it will not happen again.
B) Acknowledge his frustration, apologize for the delay, and provide an estimated waiting time.
C) Inform him that delays are common and he needs to be patient.
D) Offer him some reading material to pass the time while he waits.

Question 69: Which of the following is a legally required element that must be included in a written prescription for it to be valid?
A) Patient's full name
B) Patient's address
C) Prescriber's DEA number
D) Date of birth

Question 70: Which of the following is the most appropriate use of an external database by a clinical medical assistant when handling lab results from outside labs?
A) Verifying patient demographic information.
B) Cross-referencing lab results with established reference ranges.
C) Scheduling follow-up appointments based on lab results.
D) Updating electronic health records (EHR) with new prescriptions.

Question 71: John, a 65-year-old patient with multiple chronic conditions, requires frequent monitoring and follow-ups. Which tracking and reporting technology would most effectively support his care coordination by providing real-time updates to his healthcare team?
A) Electronic Health Records (EHR)
B) Remote Patient Monitoring (RPM)
C) Patient Portals
D) Telehealth Services

Question 72: Mr. Johnson, a 55-year-old male with a history of hypertension, presents with chest pain and is undergoing an EKG. The EKG shows ST-segment elevation in leads II, III, and aVF. What is the most likely diagnosis?
A) Anterior Myocardial Infarction
B) Inferior Myocardial Infarction
C) Lateral Myocardial Infarction
D) Posterior Myocardial Infarction

Question 73: Sarah, a medical assistant, needs to transfer funds from the clinic's account to pay a vendor. She is considering using the clinic's online banking system for this transaction. Which of the following steps should she prioritize to ensure the security of this electronic transfer?

A) Verify that the clinic's computer is connected to a secure Wi-Fi network.
B) Ensure that the vendor's bank account details are entered correctly.
C) Use multi-factor authentication (MFA) before initiating the transfer.
D) Confirm that the transfer amount does not exceed daily transaction limits.

Question 74: Sarah, a 45-year-old patient with a history of hypertension and type 2 diabetes, has been prescribed Lisinopril. After two weeks of therapy, she reports experiencing persistent dry cough. Which of the following is the most likely cause of her symptom?
A) Adverse effect of Lisinopril
B) Side effect of Metformin
C) Contra-indication of Lisinopril
D) Indication for stopping Lisinopril

Question 75: When placing precordial (chest) electrodes for an EKG, where should V4 be positioned?
A) Fifth intercostal space at the midclavicular line
B) Fourth intercostal space at the midclavicular line
C) Fifth intercostal space at the anterior axillary line
D) Fourth intercostal space at the anterior axillary line

Question 76: When communicating with a patient who has a hearing impairment, which of the following strategies is most effective in ensuring clear understanding?
A) Speaking louder than usual
B) Using written communication as much as possible
C) Facing the patient and speaking clearly
D) Using complex medical terminology

Question 77: Emily, a 6-month-old infant, is brought to your clinic for her routine vaccinations. Her mother is concerned about the timing of the influenza vaccine as it is now flu season. What is the recommended age for Emily to receive her first dose of the influenza vaccine?
A) 6 months
B) 12 months
C) 9 months
D) 18 months

Question 78: Maria, a Certified Clinical Medical Assistant, needs to explain a complex medical procedure to both Dr. Smith, a senior surgeon, and Mr. Johnson, a patient with limited medical knowledge. How should Maria modify her communication approach to ensure both parties understand the information?
A) Use technical jargon with Dr. Smith and simplify the language for Mr. Johnson.
B) Use the same level of technical detail for both Dr. Smith and Mr. Johnson.
C) Avoid eye contact with Dr. Smith but maintain eye contact with Mr. Johnson.
D) Provide written instructions only to Dr. Smith and verbal instructions only to Mr. Johnson.

Question 79: Sarah visits her primary care physician for a routine check-up. Her insurance plan requires her to pay $25 at the time of the visit, but she also needs to pay 20% of the total cost of any additional tests conducted during the visit. What is the $25 payment called?
A) Co-pay
B) Co-insurance
C) Deductible
D) Tier Level

**Question 80: During a routine inspection, you discover that a bottle of disinfectant used in your clinic does not have an accompanying Safety Data Sheet (SDS). What is

the most appropriate immediate action to take according to OSHA guidelines?
A) Continue using the disinfectant while you request the SDS from the manufacturer.
B) Discontinue using the disinfectant until you obtain the SDS from the manufacturer.
C) Use an alternative disinfectant that has an SDS available until you receive the requested SDS.
D) Create a temporary SDS based on information available online until you receive the official document.

Question 81: During a routine check-up, you need to obtain Mr. Smith's blood pressure. You decide to use an electronic blood pressure monitor. Which of the following steps is crucial to ensure an accurate reading?
A) Ensure the patient has been sitting quietly for at least 5 minutes before taking the measurement.
B) Position the cuff over the patient's clothing for convenience.
C) Inflate the cuff until you can no longer feel the patient's pulse.
D) Take multiple readings in quick succession to get an average.

Question 82: What is the most appropriate method to prepare the site for venipuncture to minimize the risk of infection?
A) Clean the site with 70% isopropyl alcohol and allow it to air dry completely.
B) Clean the site with 70% isopropyl alcohol and blow on it to speed up drying.
C) Clean the site with sterile water and wipe it dry with a sterile gauze pad.
D) Clean the site with 90% isopropyl alcohol and immediately proceed with venipuncture.

Question 83: What is the correct order of draw for micro-tubes during phlebotomy?
A) EDTA, Heparin, Serum
B) Serum, Heparin, EDTA
C) Heparin, EDTA, Serum
D) EDTA, Serum, Heparin

Question 84: Which of the following is a key component of an Exposure Control Plan (ECP) that ensures compliance with OSHA's Bloodborne Pathogens Standard?
A) Regular employee training sessions
B) Implementation of engineering controls
C) Use of personal protective equipment (PPE)
D) Annual review and update of the ECP

Question 85: Which of the following is the most effective way for a medical assistant to handle a patient who is visibly upset about a long wait time?
A) Apologize for the wait and offer to reschedule their appointment.
B) Apologize for the wait and provide an estimated wait time.
C) Explain that delays are unavoidable and ask for their patience.
D) Offer a discount on their next visit as compensation for the delay.

Question 86: Sarah, a Certified Clinical Medical Assistant (CCMA), is coordinating care for Mr. Johnson, a 65-year-old patient with multiple chronic conditions. She needs to ensure that all his medications are reviewed and reconciled before his upcoming surgery. Which healthcare professional should Sarah primarily collaborate with to accomplish this task?
A) Pharmacist
B) Registered Nurse
C) Primary Care Physician

D) Surgical Nurse

Question 87: A 45-year-old patient named John presents with symptoms of fatigue, weight gain, and cold intolerance. After a thorough examination and blood tests, his primary care physician suspects an endocrine disorder. Which hormone is most likely deficient in this patient?
A) Insulin
B) Cortisol
C) Thyroxine (T4)
D) Adrenaline

Question 88: Sarah, a 45-year-old patient, requires blood tests for comprehensive metabolic panel (CMP), complete blood count (CBC), and blood culture. Which combination of blood vacuum tubes should be used for these tests?
A) Red top, Lavender top, Yellow top
B) Green top, Lavender top, Blue top
C) Red top, Blue top, Yellow top
D) Green top, Gray top, Lavender top

Question 89: During a routine clinical procedure, you notice that Sarah, a medical assistant, is disposing of used needles and other sharps. According to OSHA guidelines, which is the correct method for disposing of these items?
A) Place them in a red biohazard bag.
B) Dispose of them in a puncture-resistant sharps container.
C) Discard them in a regular trash bin with other non-hazardous waste.
D) Seal them in a double-layered plastic bag before discarding.

Question 90: Sarah, a patient with diabetes, visits a clinic for her routine check-up. During her visit, she mentions experiencing frequent headaches and blurred vision. The medical assistant needs to determine the appropriate referral for further evaluation. Which specialty should Sarah be referred to?
A) Endocrinology
B) Neurology
C) Ophthalmology
D) General Internal Medicine

Question 91: Emma, a Certified Clinical Medical Assistant, needs to retrieve a patient's previous lab results quickly for an urgent consultation. Which feature of the EMR/EHR software should she use to ensure she finds the information efficiently?
A) Patient Summary Dashboard
B) Advanced Search Function
C) Appointment Scheduling Module
D) Billing and Coding Section

Question 92: Which of the following is the most effective strategy for minimizing risk related to patient and employee safety in a healthcare facility?
A) Implementing regular training sessions on emergency protocols for all staff.
B) Conducting quarterly reviews of incident reports to identify common hazards.
C) Ensuring all medical equipment is inspected annually by certified technicians.
D) Designing patient care areas with ergonomic furniture to reduce staff injuries.

Question 93: Which feature of electronic prescribing software primarily enhances medication safety by reducing prescription errors?
A) Automated Drug Interaction Alerts
B) Real-time Insurance Verification

C) Electronic Health Record (EHR) Integration
D) Patient Education Resources

Question 94: A patient presents with a twisted ankle following a fall. The area is swollen, bruised, and painful when bearing weight. Which type of injury is most likely?
A) Laceration
B) Abrasion
C) Fracture
D) Sprain

Question 95: Maria, a Certified Clinical Medical Assistant (CCMA), is coordinating discharge instructions for John, a 65-year-old diabetic patient who has been hospitalized for pneumonia. Which of the following tasks is most critical for Maria to ensure proper patient care coordination and education before John's discharge?
A) Ensure John understands his medication regimen, including dosages and times.
B) Provide John with a detailed dietary plan specific to diabetic patients.
C) Schedule follow-up appointments with John's primary care physician and specialists.
D) Educate John on recognizing early signs of pneumonia recurrence.

Question 96: When facilitating a referral to a specialist, which is the most crucial piece of information that must be included in the referral documentation?
A) Patient's insurance information
B) Detailed patient history and reason for referral
C) Contact details of primary care physician
D) Appointment availability with the specialist

Question 97: Under HIPAA regulations, which of the following scenarios constitutes a breach of patient confidentiality?
A) Discussing patient information with another healthcare provider involved in the patient's care without patient consent.
B) Leaving a patient's medical records unattended in a public area.
C) Sharing patient information with family members without explicit patient consent.
D) Accessing a patient's medical records for personal curiosity without a legitimate reason.

Question 98: Which of the following is the most critical component of maintaining compliance with equipment inspection logs in a medical facility?
A) Recording inspections immediately after they are conducted
B) Conducting inspections bi-annually as per manufacturer's guidelines
C) Ensuring inspections are performed by certified medical equipment servicers
D) Maintaining electronic records for at least five years

Question 99: Which amino acid is considered essential and must be obtained through dietary intake because the body cannot synthesize it?
A) Alanine
B) Leucine
C) Glutamine
D) Glycine

Question 100: Which of the following is a primary benefit of using Computerized Physician Order Entry (CPOE) systems in clinical patient care?
A) Reducing medication errors by eliminating handwritten prescriptions
B) Increasing patient satisfaction by providing real-time

updates on treatment progress
C) Enhancing communication between healthcare providers by centralizing patient data
D) Decreasing the time spent on administrative tasks by automating billing processes

Question 101: Which of the following is the most appropriate action for a medical assistant when relaying a complex medical diagnosis to a patient to ensure clarity and understanding?
A) Use medical jargon to maintain accuracy.
B) Simplify the information using layman's terms.
C) Provide written materials without verbal explanation.
D) Refer the patient directly to the physician for an explanation.

Question 102: Which of the following is a key difference between a scratch test and an intradermal allergy test?
A) The scratch test involves injecting a small amount of allergen into the dermis.
B) The intradermal allergy test is more sensitive than the scratch test.
C) The scratch test requires a longer observation period compared to the intradermal allergy test.
D) The intradermal allergy test involves placing allergens on the skin surface.

Question 103: Which component is crucial for assessing genetic predispositions and potential hereditary conditions in a patient's history?
A) Social History
B) Surgical History
C) Family History
D) Medical History

Question 104: Mr. Johnson, a 55-year-old male with a history of intermittent chest pain and palpitations, visits the clinic. The provider orders a non-invasive cardiovascular profiling test that can continuously monitor his heart rhythm over several days to capture any irregularities. Which test is most appropriate for Mr. Johnson?
A) Stress Test
B) Holter Monitoring
C) Event Monitoring
D) Echocardiogram

Question 105: Which of the following is the most effective strategy for ensuring continuity of care in outpatient services?
A) Scheduling regular follow-up appointments.
B) Providing comprehensive patient education materials.
C) Implementing a multidisciplinary team approach.
D) Utilizing electronic health records (EHR) for seamless information sharing.

Question 106: During a venipuncture procedure on Mr. Smith, you notice that his veins are not easily visible. Which of the following steps should you take to improve vein visibility before attempting the puncture?
A) Apply a warm compress to the area for several minutes.
B) Ask Mr. Smith to clench and unclench his fist repeatedly.
C) Elevate Mr. Smith's arm above heart level for a few minutes.
D) Use a blood pressure cuff inflated to 50 mmHg instead of a tourniquet.

Question 107: Maria, a medical assistant, is dealing with a patient named Mr. Johnson who is visibly upset about a delay in his appointment. Maria listens attentively to Mr. Johnson's concerns and responds by acknowledging his frustration while calmly explaining the reason for the delay and offering an apology. Which

communication style is Maria demonstrating?
A) Passive
B) Aggressive
C) Assertive
D) Passive-Aggressive

Question 108: Sarah, a Certified Clinical Medical Assistant, needs to process a payment for a patient's recent surgical procedure. Who is authorized to approve this payment processing?
A) The attending physician
B) The practice manager
C) The billing department supervisor
D) The patient care coordinator

Question 109: Which of the following statements is correct regarding the use of alcohol-based hand sanitizers in clinical settings?
A) Alcohol-based hand sanitizers are effective against Clostridioides difficile spores.
B) Alcohol-based hand sanitizers should contain at least 60% alcohol to be effective.
C) Alcohol-based hand sanitizers are less effective than soap and water for removing visible dirt.
D) Alcohol-based hand sanitizers can replace handwashing in all situations.

Question 110: Which of the following is a hallmark sign of a systemic infection in a patient?
A) Localized redness and swelling
B) Fever and chills
C) Increased heart rate without fever
D) Mild fatigue

Question 111: Which of the following is the most effective method for assessing a patient's anxiety level before a phlebotomy procedure?
A) Observing the patient's body language for signs of discomfort.
B) Asking the patient directly how they are feeling about the procedure.
C) Noting any changes in the patient's vital signs, such as increased heart rate or blood pressure.
D) Providing detailed information about the procedure to alleviate potential fears.

Question 112: Which of the following actions is most critical when updating a patient's medication list in an EHR/EMR system to ensure data accuracy and patient safety?
A) Adding new medications prescribed during the visit
B) Deleting old medications no longer prescribed
C) Verifying current medications with the patient
D) Recording the dosage and frequency of each medication

Question 113: A medical assistant, Jane, is preparing to perform a venipuncture on a patient with a known bloodborne pathogen infection. According to the Exposure Control Plan, which of the following actions is most appropriate to minimize risk?
A) Wearing gloves and a face shield
B) Using only gloves and washing hands immediately after
C) Double-gloving for added protection
D) Wearing gloves, a gown, and using a sharps container

Question 114: John, a 45-year-old male with a history of asthma, visits the clinic for a routine check-up. He reports increased shortness of breath over the past week. As part of his assessment, you measure his peak flow rate. His personal best peak flow rate is 600 L/min. Today, his peak flow rate is measured at 450 L/min. Based on this information, what should be your next step in managing John's condition?

A) Advise John to continue his current medication regimen and recheck his peak flow rate in one week.
B) Instruct John to use his rescue inhaler and recheck his peak flow rate in 15 minutes.
C) Recommend John to increase the dosage of his maintenance inhaler and monitor his symptoms closely.
D) Refer John to the emergency department for immediate evaluation and treatment.

Question 115: A patient named Mr. Smith is prescribed a medication that requires careful monitoring due to its narrow therapeutic index. The medication is administered intravenously and is known for its potential nephrotoxic effects. Which of the following medications is most likely being administered to Mr. Smith?
A) Vancomycin
B) Metronidazole
C) Ceftriaxone
D) Amoxicillin

Question 116: Which of the following terms correctly represents the plural form of "bacterium"?
A) Bacteria
B) Bacteriums
C) Bacterias
D) Bacteri

Question 117: Mr. Johnson is scheduled for a follow-up appointment after his recent surgery. As a Certified Clinical Medical Assistant, you are responsible for ensuring that all documentation complies with government and insurance requirements. Which of the following actions best ensures compliance?
A) Documenting only the patient's current medications and allergies.
B) Including detailed notes on the patient's progress, current medications, allergies, and any changes since the last visit.
C) Recording only new symptoms and treatment plans discussed during the visit.
D) Summarizing the patient's overall health status without specific details on medications or changes.

Question 118: Which of the following is a required component of a medical record that ensures continuity and quality of patient care?
A) Patient's insurance information
B) Patient's medical history
C) Patient's billing information
D) Patient's consent forms

Question 119: When interpreting an EKG, which of the following findings is most indicative of a myocardial infarction?
A) ST-segment elevation
B) T-wave inversion
C) Prolonged PR interval
D) Sinus tachycardia

Question 120: Emily, a 45-year-old patient, is scheduled for an endoscopic procedure to examine her upper gastrointestinal tract. Which instrument will most likely be used for this procedure?
A) Colonoscope
B) Gastroscope
C) Bronchoscope
D) Laryngoscope

Question 121: When performing CPR on an adult patient, what is the recommended depth of chest compressions?
A) At least 1 inch (2.5 cm)
B) At least 2 inches (5 cm)

C) Approximately 1.5 inches (4 cm)
D) Approximately 3 inches (7.5 cm)

Question 122: Which of the following ancillary services is primarily responsible for providing diagnostic imaging to aid in patient diagnosis?
A) Radiology
B) Pathology
C) Physical Therapy
D) Respiratory Therapy

Question 123: Which category of the medical record includes detailed documentation of specific medical procedures performed on a patient?
A) Administrative
B) Clinical
C) Procedural
D) Consents

Question 124: What is the most crucial first step in maintaining an accurate inventory of clinical and administrative supplies?
A) Regularly updating the inventory list
B) Conducting a comprehensive initial inventory audit
C) Setting minimum stock levels for each item
D) Implementing an automated inventory management system

Question 125: Sarah, a 45-year-old patient, requires an intramuscular injection of a vaccine. Which of the following is the most appropriate site for administering this injection to ensure maximum absorption and minimal discomfort?
A) Vastus lateralis muscle
B) Deltoid muscle
C) Ventrogluteal site
D) Dorsogluteal site

Question 126: Maria, a certified clinical medical assistant, is preparing to draw blood from a patient named Mr. Johnson for routine lab tests. After drawing the blood, what is the most critical step she must take immediately to ensure proper processing and labeling of the specimen?
A) Place the specimen in a biohazard bag before labeling it.
B) Label the specimen at the patient's bedside immediately after drawing.
C) Transport the specimen to the lab within 30 minutes before labeling.
D) Label the specimen after reaching the lab to avoid contamination.

Question 127: What is the most critical element to include in a referral form to ensure effective patient care coordination?
A) Patient's medical history
B) Detailed reason for referral
C) Contact information of the referring provider
D) Patient's insurance information

Question 128: Sarah Johnson is scheduled for a minor surgical procedure. As part of the preoperative process, which document is she required to review and sign to ensure she understands the risks and benefits of the procedure?
A) Informed Consent Form
B) HIPAA Privacy Notice
C) Advance Directive
D) Patient Bill of Rights

Question 129: Sarah, a 45-year-old woman, presents with severe gallbladder inflammation and has been diagnosed with cholecystitis. Which of the following

surgical interventions is most commonly performed to treat her condition?
A) Appendectomy
B) Cholecystectomy
C) Colectomy
D) Hysterectomy

Question 130: Dr. Smith is treating a patient named John who has a terminal illness. John requests assistance in ending his life to avoid prolonged suffering. According to the principles of the Hippocratic Oath, what should Dr. Smith do?
A) Respect John's autonomy and assist him in ending his life.
B) Refuse to assist in ending John's life, as it contradicts the principle of "do no harm."
C) Seek a second opinion from another physician before making a decision.
D) Refer John to palliative care services to manage his symptoms.

Question 131: During a routine check-up, Mrs. Johnson expresses concern about a new medication prescribed by her physician. She mentions experiencing side effects and feels anxious about continuing the medication. As a Certified Clinical Medical Assistant (CCMA), what is the most appropriate initial response?
A) "I understand your concerns. Let me explain why the doctor prescribed this medication."
B) "It's common to experience side effects initially; they usually subside after a few days."
C) "I can see you're worried. Let's discuss your symptoms in detail so I can inform the doctor."
D) "You should stop taking the medication immediately and I'll notify the doctor."

Question 132: Which of the following is the most common food allergen responsible for severe allergic reactions in children?
A) Peanuts
B) Shellfish
C) Eggs
D) Soy

Question 133: Which structure in the heart is primarily responsible for initiating the electrical impulses that regulate heartbeats?
A) Atrioventricular (AV) node
B) Sinoatrial (SA) node
C) Bundle of His
D) Purkinje fibers

Question 134: Which instrument is specifically used for measuring intraocular pressure in patients suspected of having glaucoma?
A) Ophthalmoscope
B) Tonometer
C) Retinoscope
D) Slit lamp

Question 135: When performing an ear irrigation on a patient, which of the following steps is crucial to prevent injury to the tympanic membrane?
A) Use cold water to minimize discomfort.
B) Direct the irrigation solution towards the eardrum.
C) Use a gentle stream of solution at body temperature.
D) Position the patient with their head tilted forward.

Question 136: When processing and labeling blood specimens, what is the most critical step to ensure the accuracy and reliability of the results?
A) Labeling the specimen immediately after collection at the patient's bedside.

B) Labeling the specimen in the laboratory before analysis.
C) Labeling the specimen after processing it in a centrifuge.
D) Labeling the specimen after refrigerating it for preservation.

Question 137: Emily, a certified clinical medical assistant (CCMA), is working in a primary care clinic. She receives a call from a patient who needs to schedule an urgent appointment due to severe abdominal pain. Emily checks the schedule and sees that all slots are booked for the day. What should be Emily's next step?
A) Advise the patient to visit the emergency room immediately.
B) Schedule the patient for the first available appointment on the following day.
C) Consult with the physician or nurse practitioner about accommodating the patient.
D) Refer the patient to an urgent care center.

Question 138: When performing a sterile dressing change, which of the following steps is crucial to maintain sterility and prevent infection?
A) Clean the wound with an antiseptic solution before applying the new dressing.
B) Wear clean gloves when removing the old dressing.
C) Open the sterile dressing package away from your body.
D) Use non-sterile gloves when handling the new dressing.

Question 139: During a postoperative follow-up, Maria, a 45-year-old patient, presents with sutures that need to be removed. Which technique should be employed to minimize tissue trauma and ensure proper wound healing?
A) Use sterile scissors to cut each suture at the knot and gently pull it out with sterile forceps.
B) Use sterile forceps to lift each suture knot and cut it close to the skin before pulling it out.
C) Apply antiseptic solution before using sterile scissors to cut each suture at the knot and pull it out with sterile forceps.
D) Use sterile forceps to lift each suture knot, apply antiseptic solution, then cut close to the skin before pulling it out.

Question 140: When preparing a patient for an EKG, which of the following steps is essential to ensure accurate results?
A) Instructing the patient to avoid caffeine for 24 hours before the test.
B) Ensuring all electronic devices are turned off in the examination room.
C) Positioning the patient supine with arms at their sides.
D) Shaving any hair at electrode sites if necessary.

Question 141: After treating a patient named Mr. Johnson, who has been diagnosed with Clostridioides difficile (C. diff) infection, which of the following is the most appropriate disinfection method to ensure complete sanitization of the treatment area?
A) Use an alcohol-based disinfectant to wipe down all surfaces.
B) Use a bleach-based disinfectant to clean all high-touch surfaces.
C) Use a quaternary ammonium compound for general surface cleaning.
D) Use hydrogen peroxide vapor for room decontamination.

Question 142: Which of the following best exemplifies active listening in a clinical setting?
A) Nodding occasionally and maintaining eye contact while the patient speaks.
B) Interrupting the patient to provide immediate advice based on their symptoms.

C) Taking detailed notes while occasionally glancing at the patient.
D) Waiting for pauses in conversation to ask clarifying questions.

Question 143: During a routine blood draw from Mr. Johnson, a patient with an unknown infectious status, what is the most appropriate action a Certified Clinical Medical Assistant (CCMA) should take to adhere to Universal Precautions?
A) Wear gloves and a face shield.
B) Wear gloves and a gown.
C) Wear gloves only.
D) Wear gloves, a gown, and a face shield.

Question 144: When a medical assistant processes a referral authorization for a specialist consultation, which of the following steps is crucial to ensure the authorization is valid?
A) Confirming the patient's insurance coverage and obtaining pre-authorization if required.
B) Scheduling the specialist appointment before verifying insurance details.
C) Sending the referral form directly to the specialist without patient consent.
D) Using a generic referral form without specifying the reason for referral.

Question 145: Which of the following methods is most effective for sterilizing surgical instruments to ensure complete elimination of all microorganisms, including spores?
A) Autoclaving
B) Boiling
C) Dry Heat Sterilization
D) Chemical Disinfection

Question 146: When creating an e-referral for a patient, which piece of information is crucial to include to ensure proper processing by the receiving specialist?
A) Patient's insurance policy number
B) Referring provider's National Provider Identifier (NPI)
C) Patient's social security number
D) Referring provider's office address

Question 147: Which cellular organelle is primarily responsible for energy production through oxidative phosphorylation?
A) Mitochondria
B) Ribosomes
C) Lysosomes
D) Nucleus

Question 148: Dr. Smith has just entered a medication order for Mr. Johnson using the CPOE system. As a Clinical Medical Assistant, you notice that there is an alert indicating a potential drug interaction. What should be your immediate course of action?
A) Ignore the alert and proceed with administering the medication.
B) Consult with Dr. Smith about the alert before proceeding.
C) Override the alert if you believe it is not significant.
D) Document the alert in Mr. Johnson's medical record but proceed with administration.

Question 149: John, a 55-year-old patient with chronic diabetes and recent symptoms of peripheral neuropathy, visits your clinic. His primary care physician has recommended that he see a specialist for further management of his condition. As a Medical Assistant, which healthcare provider should you refer John to for the most appropriate specialized care?
A) Endocrinologist

B) Neurologist
C) Podiatrist
D) Cardiologist

Question 150: Sarah, a 45-year-old patient with chronic pain, is prescribed a medication that is classified as a Schedule II controlled substance. Which of the following medications is most likely prescribed to Sarah?
A) Hydrocodone
B) Alprazolam
C) Tramadol
D) Diazepam

ANSWER WITH DETAILED EXPLANATION SET [3]

Question 1: Correct Answer: D) Ventrogluteal muscle
Rationale: The ventrogluteal site is considered the safest and most appropriate for IM injections in adults due to its distance from major nerves and blood vessels. The deltoid muscle (A) is commonly used but has a smaller volume capacity and higher risk of nerve injury. The vastus lateralis muscle (B) is preferred for infants and children but less so for adults. The dorsogluteal muscle (C), though historically used, carries a higher risk of sciatic nerve injury compared to the ventrogluteal site.

Question 2: Correct Answer: B) Reflex hammer
Rationale: A reflex hammer is crucial for assessing deep tendon reflexes during a neurological examination. An otoscope is used for ear examinations, a sphygmomanometer measures blood pressure, and a stethoscope is used for auscultation of heart and lung sounds. While all these instruments are important in various clinical examinations, only the reflex hammer specifically evaluates neurological function by testing reflex responses. This makes it essential for a thorough neurological examination.

Question 3: Correct Answer: C) Reassure Sarah and give her additional time to consider her decision.
Rationale: Ensuring informed consent involves not only explaining the procedure but also ensuring that the patient comprehends it fully and consents voluntarily without any pressure. Option C is correct because it respects Sarah's autonomy and allows her time to make an informed decision. Option A is incorrect as proceeding without ensuring comprehension violates ethical principles. Option B undermines voluntariness by rushing the process. Option D is incorrect because it may lead to miscommunication or incomplete information transfer, jeopardizing true informed consent.

Question 4: Correct Answer: A) Informed Consent Form
Rationale: The informed consent form is crucial as it ensures the patient understands the risks, benefits, and alternatives of the procedure. While a treatment plan agreement (Option B) outlines the proposed course of treatment, it does not specifically address surgical procedures. The HIPAA privacy notice (Option C) informs patients about their privacy rights but is not directly related to surgical consent. A medical history form (Option D) collects health information but does not serve as consent for surgery.

Question 5: Correct Answer: B) Performing venipuncture for blood draws
Rationale: Performing venipuncture for blood draws is within the scope of practice for a CCMA as it involves basic clinical skills taught during their training. Administering intravenous medications (A) is typically outside their scope, requiring higher-level training. Interpreting laboratory results (C) is generally reserved for licensed practitioners such as doctors or nurse practitioners. Prescribing medication (D) is beyond the CCMA's scope and requires specific licensure such as that held by physicians or nurse practitioners. This delineation ensures patient safety and adherence to

regulatory standards.

Question 6: Correct Answer: C) Encrypting patient data
Rationale: Encrypting patient data is the most effective method for ensuring its security in an EMR/EHR system because it protects information from unauthorized access by converting it into a coded format. While regularly updating antivirus software (A), implementing strong password policies (B), and conducting frequent staff training sessions (D) are important security measures, they do not offer the same level of protection as encryption. Antivirus software helps prevent malware attacks, strong passwords prevent unauthorized access, and staff training reduces human error, but encryption directly secures the data itself.

Question 7: Correct Answer: A) Perform the ECG on Mr. Johnson as requested by Dr. Smith.
Rationale: The primary responsibility of Maria in this scenario is to prioritize patient care based on urgency and direct physician orders. Performing an ECG on a patient with chest pain is critical for diagnosing potential cardiac issues, which takes precedence over assisting with a non-urgent minor surgical procedure. Informing Dr. Smith about her current task or delegating without proper authority could lead to delays in critical care. Option A is correct because it directly addresses an urgent diagnostic need under physician instruction. Option B is incorrect because assisting with a non-urgent procedure should not take priority over an urgent diagnostic test. Option C is incorrect because it may delay critical diagnostic care for chest pain. Option D is incorrect as delegation must be done carefully, ensuring continuity of urgent care tasks assigned by physicians. This question tests understanding of prioritization in clinical settings and appropriate delegation in accordance with healthcare protocols.

Question 8: Correct Answer: A) Emphasis on comprehensive care coordination across all providers
Rationale: The PCMH model prioritizes comprehensive care coordination across all providers, ensuring that patients receive holistic and continuous care. This distinguishes it from other models which may focus more narrowly on specific aspects like transitional care management (B), patient-centered decision-making (C), or financial incentives (D). While these elements can be part of PCMH, they are not its defining feature. Comprehensive coordination ensures seamless transitions and integrated services, aligning with PCMH's goal of improving overall patient outcomes.

Question 9: Correct Answer: A) Atrial Fibrillation
Rationale: Atrial fibrillation is characterized by an irregularly irregular rhythm and absence of distinct P waves before each QRS complex. Ventricular tachycardia (B) presents with wide QRS complexes and regular rapid rhythm. Sinus bradycardia (C) features a regular slow rhythm with normal P waves preceding each QRS complex. Wandering atrial pacemaker (D) shows varying P wave morphology but not an irregularly irregular rhythm. Understanding these specific EKG characteristics is crucial for accurate diagnosis.

Question 10: Correct Answer: B) Mitochondria

Rationale: Mitochondria are known as the powerhouses of the cell because they generate ATP through cellular respiration, which is crucial for energy production. Muscle weakness and fatigue are often linked to mitochondrial dysfunction due to their role in energy metabolism. The nucleus controls genetic information but does not directly produce energy. Ribosomes are involved in protein synthesis, not energy production. Lysosomes are responsible for breaking down waste materials and cellular debris, not generating energy. Thus, mitochondrial dysfunction aligns with Maria's symptoms.

Question 11: Correct Answer: B) Episodes of binge eating followed by compensatory behaviors

Rationale: The distinguishing feature of Bulimia Nervosa is episodes of binge eating followed by compensatory behaviors like vomiting or excessive exercise. While options A), C), and D) are associated with various eating disorders, they do not specifically differentiate Bulimia Nervosa. Option A) is more characteristic of Anorexia Nervosa, option C) can be present in both Anorexia and Bulimia, and option D) is common across many eating disorders but does not uniquely define Bulimia.

Question 12: Correct Answer: C) Place the V4 lead at the fifth intercostal space, midclavicular line.

Rationale: Correct placement of EKG leads is crucial for accurate readings. The V4 lead is specifically placed at the fifth intercostal space along the midclavicular line, which is critical for capturing accurate cardiac activity. Options A and B describe correct placements but are not as critical as V4 for overall accuracy. Option D is also correct but less critical compared to V4 placement. Proper positioning of V4 impacts both diagnostic accuracy and treatment decisions significantly more than other leads in this context.

Question 13: Correct Answer: A) Store the medication in a refrigerator at 2-8°C (36-46°F), ensuring it does not freeze.

Rationale: Option A is correct because most refrigerated injectables are stored at 2-8°C (36-46°F). Freezing can damage the medication's integrity. Option B is incorrect because freezing (-20°C) is inappropriate for most injectables requiring refrigeration. Option C is incorrect because room temperature storage can degrade medications needing refrigeration. Option D is tricky but incorrect; while 0-4°C might seem suitable, it risks freezing near 0°C, potentially compromising the medication. Proper storage ensures effectiveness and safety for patient care.

Question 14: Correct Answer: C) Use secure communication channels approved by the healthcare facility.

Rationale: Using secure communication channels approved by the healthcare facility ensures compliance with HIPAA regulations, protecting patient confidentiality. While including patient identifiers (Option A) is important, it does not address security. Verbal consent (Option B) is necessary but not sufficient alone. Including a detailed medication list (Option D) may be relevant for clinical accuracy but does not directly address HIPAA compliance. Thus, Option C is correct as it encompasses the security aspect crucial for HIPAA adherence.

Question 15: Correct Answer: B) Sinoatrial (SA) node

Rationale: The sinoatrial (SA) node is known as the natural pacemaker of the heart because it initiates the electrical impulses that set the rhythm for cardiac contraction. The atrioventricular (AV) node acts as a secondary pacemaker and delays the impulse to allow ventricular filling. The Bundle of His transmits impulses from the AV node to the ventricles, while Purkinje fibers distribute impulses through the ventricles for coordinated contraction. Thus, while all options are part of the conduction system, only the SA node initiates the intrinsic rhythm.

Question 16: Correct Answer: C) Engage in a motivational interviewing session to understand his barriers and enhance his intrinsic motivation.

Rationale: Motivational interviewing is an evidence-based technique that helps patients explore their ambivalence about change and enhances their intrinsic motivation, which is crucial for long-term adherence. Providing written instructions (Option A) may not address underlying barriers, scheduling a follow-up (Option B) delays immediate intervention, and referring to a class (Option D) might overwhelm him initially without addressing personal challenges.

Question 17: Correct Answer: A) Diabetic Shock

Rationale: John's symptoms of confusion, sweating, and shakiness are classic signs of hypoglycemia, commonly known as diabetic shock. Heat stroke typically presents with hot, dry skin and confusion but lacks sweating. An allergic reaction might include hives or respiratory distress but not sweating and shakiness. Syncope involves sudden fainting due to a drop in blood pressure or heart rate but does not typically present with confusion and sweating before the event. The key difference is the presence of diabetes and the specific combination of symptoms pointing towards hypoglycemia.

Question 18: Correct Answer: A) The number of new cases of a disease in a specific population over a defined period.

Rationale: Incidence refers to the number of new cases that develop in a particular population during a specified time period. This is different from prevalence (Option B), which measures all existing cases at one point in time. Option C describes risk factors related to genetic predisposition, while Option D refers to recovery rates, neither of which define incidence. Understanding these distinctions is crucial for interpreting epidemiological data accurately.

Question 19: Correct Answer: C) Managing patient care plans and follow-ups

Rationale: In a PCMH model, medical assistants play a crucial role in managing patient care plans and follow-ups, ensuring continuity of care. Option A is incorrect as it primarily involves administrative tasks. Option B, while important, is more aligned with nursing duties. Option D is misleading because although medical assistants do provide direct care, their primary role in PCMH focuses on coordination and management rather than direct supervision by physicians. This distinction highlights their integrative function within the healthcare team.

Question 20: Correct Answer: A) Cleanse the site with an alcohol swab in a circular motion, starting from the center and moving outward.

Rationale: The correct answer is A) Cleanse the site with an alcohol swab in a circular motion, starting from the center and moving outward. This method effectively reduces microbial presence by moving contaminants away from the puncture site. Option B is incorrect because iodine is less commonly used for routine venipuncture due to potential allergies and staining. Option C is incorrect as back-and-forth motion can reintroduce contaminants. Option D is incorrect as soap and water are insufficient alone for proper asepsis required for venipuncture.

Question 21: Correct Answer: C) Keep the specimen at room temperature and deliver it within 2 hours.

Rationale: For coagulation studies, it is crucial to keep the blood specimen at room temperature and deliver it to the laboratory within 2 hours to prevent degradation of clotting factors. Option A is incorrect because delivering within 4 hours may be too late. Option B is misleading as placing on ice can cause hemolysis. Option D is incorrect because centrifuging immediately can alter test results by separating plasma from cells prematurely.

Question 22: Correct Answer: B) Tell Mr. Johnson that his results are available but need to be reviewed by the physician before you can share them.

Rationale: The correct answer is B because it adheres to best practices in medical communication, ensuring that all information shared with patients is accurate and has been reviewed by a qualified professional. Option A is incorrect as sharing unreviewed results may lead to misinterpretation or distress. Option C could cause unnecessary delays and anxiety for the patient, while D might be inconvenient and unnecessary if a phone consultation suffices after review by the physician.

Question 23: Correct Answer: B) Concurrent use of amiodarone

Rationale: Amiodarone can inhibit the metabolism of warfarin, leading to increased levels and an elevated INR. Green leafy vegetables (A) contain vitamin K, which can decrease INR. Cranberry juice (C) has been debated but lacks consistent evidence in clinical studies to significantly affect INR. Increased physical activity (D) does not directly influence warfarin metabolism or INR levels. Understanding these interactions is crucial for managing patients on anticoagulant therapy effectively.

Question 24: Correct Answer: C) Allow Maria to drink water but avoid all other beverages after midnight.

Rationale: The correct answer is C because patients are generally allowed to drink water during fasting periods, which helps maintain hydration without affecting blood glucose levels. Option A is incorrect because specifying an early evening meal time does not account for individual schedules and might not ensure an adequate fasting period. Option B is close but lacks specificity about permissible fluids. Option D is incorrect as taking insulin can alter glucose levels and should be discussed with a physician prior to testing.

Question 25: Correct Answer: C) Ensure Mrs. Johnson's medical history is updated and accessible.

Rationale: Ensuring that Mrs. Johnson's medical history is updated and accessible is crucial as it provides essential information about her hypertension and any other underlying conditions that may affect the examination process. Option A, asking her to remove shoes and outer clothing, is necessary but not the first step. Option B, measuring blood pressure while standing, is incorrect because initial readings should be taken while seated for accuracy. Option D, positioning her in a supine position, may be required later but not initially.

Question 26: Correct Answer: B) Neurologist

Rationale: A neurologist specializes in diagnosing and treating disorders of the nervous system, making them the most appropriate specialist for chronic migraines. While a general practitioner can manage initial symptoms, they typically refer patients to specialists for complex conditions. A rheumatologist focuses on autoimmune and musculoskeletal diseases, which are not related to migraines. An endocrinologist treats hormone-related disorders, which are also unrelated to migraines. Therefore, B) Neurologist is the correct answer due to their expertise in nervous system disorders.

Question 27: Correct Answer: A) Perform the test immediately after calibrating the glucometer.

Rationale: Performing the test immediately after calibrating the glucometer ensures accuracy by verifying that the device is functioning correctly. Option B is incorrect because not cleaning the site can lead to contamination and inaccurate results. Option C is incorrect as using expired test strips can compromise accuracy regardless of their appearance. Option D is less critical than calibration; while proper lighting helps in reading results, it does not affect the accuracy of the glucometer itself. Calibration directly impacts measurement precision, making it essential for reliable POC testing outcomes.

Question 28: Correct Answer: A) Iron-deficiency anemia

Rationale: Sarah's CBC results indicate low hemoglobin and hematocrit levels with a low MCV, which are characteristic of microcytic anemia. The most common cause of microcytic anemia is iron-deficiency anemia. Vitamin B12 deficiency anemia typically presents with macrocytic anemia (high MCV). Chronic kidney disease can cause normocytic anemia (normal MCV). Thalassemia also causes microcytic anemia but is less common than iron-deficiency anemia in this context. Thus, iron-deficiency anemia is the most likely diagnosis based on her lab results.

Question 29: Correct Answer: B) Returning them to a pharmacy take-back program.

Rationale: The correct method for disposing of unused controlled substances is returning them to a pharmacy take-back program (Option B). This ensures they are handled according to regulatory guidelines. Flushing (Option A) can lead to environmental contamination. Mixing with coffee grounds (Option C) is not secure enough for controlled substances. Incineration in a regular waste facility (Option D) does not guarantee safe disposal as it may not meet specific standards for hazardous waste. Each option explained: - Option A: Flushing down the toilet is discouraged due to potential environmental harm. - Option B: Pharmacy take-back programs are designed specifically for safe disposal of controlled substances. - Option C: Mixing with coffee grounds is recommended for non-controlled medications but not secure enough for controlled substances. - Option D: Regular incineration facilities may not have the capability to safely dispose of hazardous materials like controlled substances.

Question 30: Correct Answer: A) National Healthcareer Association (NHA)

Rationale: The National Healthcareer Association (NHA) is primarily responsible for certifying Clinical Medical Assistants (CCMAs) in the United States. While the American Association of Medical Assistants (AAMA), National Center for Competency Testing (NCCT), and American Medical Technologists (AMT) also offer certifications for medical assistants, they do not specifically certify CCMAs. The NHA certification is recognized for its focus on clinical skills and competencies required for medical assistants in a clinical setting. This distinction makes NHA the correct answer, whereas other organizations certify medical assistants under different titles or with a broader scope.

Question 31: Correct Answer: A) Vitamin D

Rationale: Vitamin D is essential for calcium absorption in the intestines, which helps maintain bone health and prevent osteoporosis. While Vitamin C aids in collagen formation, it does not directly influence calcium absorption. Vitamin B12 is crucial for nerve function and red blood cell production but does not play a role in calcium metabolism. Vitamin K is important for bone health but primarily works by regulating bone mineralization rather than enhancing calcium absorption directly. Hence, Vitamin D supplementation is recommended for Mrs. Johnson to address her symptoms and improve calcium absorption.

Question 32: Correct Answer: A) Atrial Fibrillation

Rationale: Atrial Fibrillation is characterized by an irregularly irregular rhythm with no distinct P waves and variable R-R intervals, making it the correct diagnosis for John's symptoms. Atrial Flutter typically shows sawtooth flutter waves and a regular rhythm. Ventricular Tachycardia presents with wide QRS complexes and a regular or slightly irregular rhythm. Sinus Arrhythmia involves a normal P wave morphology and varying R-R intervals but is not typically associated with dizziness or palpitations in this context.

Question 33: Correct Answer: C) Puncturing the side of the fingertip rather than the center.

Rationale: Puncturing the side of the fingertip reduces pain and increases blood flow. Option A is incorrect because warming should be done for at least 3-5 minutes. Option B is incorrect as the first drop should be wiped away to avoid tissue fluid contamination. Option D is incorrect because excessive squeezing can hemolyze the sample or mix tissue fluids, leading to inaccurate results.

Question 34: Correct Answer: A) Instructing the patient to start urinating into the toilet, then catch the midstream in a sterile container.

Rationale: The correct technique for collecting a midstream clean-catch urine specimen involves instructing the patient to begin urinating into the toilet and then collect the midstream portion in a sterile container. This minimizes contamination from external genitalia. Option B is incorrect because collecting the first few drops can include contaminants. Option C refers to catheterization, which is not necessary for midstream collection. Option D addresses storage but not contamination prevention during collection.

Question 35: Correct Answer: A) Place them in a puncture-resistant, leak-proof container labeled with a biohazard symbol.

Rationale: According to OSHA regulations, used needles must be disposed of in a puncture-resistant, leak-proof container labeled with a biohazard symbol (Option A). This ensures safety and prevents needlestick injuries. Option B is incorrect because general trash receptacles do not provide adequate protection. Option C is incorrect because cardboard boxes are not puncture-resistant or leak-proof. Option D is incorrect because red bags are designated for other types of biohazardous waste, not sharps. The correct answer aligns with OSHA's specific requirements for sharps disposal.

Question 36: Correct Answer: A) 3 tsp

Rationale: The correct conversion factor is 1 tsp = 5 mL. Therefore, to find out how many teaspoons are in 15 mL, you divide 15 mL by 5 mL/tsp, resulting in 3 tsp. Option B (2.5 tsp) and Option D (2 tsp) are incorrect because they underestimate the amount needed, while Option C (4 tsp) overestimates it. This question tests the precise understanding of conversions between metric and household measurements crucial for accurate dosage calculations.

Question 37: Correct Answer: B) 2 teaspoons

Rationale: To determine the correct dosage, you need to convert the required milligrams into the appropriate number of teaspoons. Since the concentration is 250 mg per teaspoon, dividing the required dose (500 mg) by the concentration (250 mg/teaspoon) gives you: 500 mg / 250 mg per teaspoon = 2 teaspoons. Option A (1 teaspoon) is incorrect because it would only provide half of the required dose (250 mg). Option C (3 teaspoons) and Option D (4 teaspoons) are incorrect because they would provide an excess dose (750 mg and 1000 mg respectively). This question tests precise conversion skills and attention to detail in dosage calculations.

Question 38: Correct Answer: A) Move the box immediately and report it to her supervisor.

Rationale: Sarah should prioritize immediate removal of the obstruction to ensure compliance with emergency protocols, followed by reporting to her supervisor. Option B delays resolution, increasing risk. Option C neglects immediate hazard removal. Option D, while educational, doesn't address immediate danger.

Question 39: Correct Answer: A) Supine

Rationale: The supine position involves lying flat on the back with the face and torso facing upward, allowing easy access to the anterior surface of the body. In contrast, the prone position (B) involves lying face down, which exposes the posterior surface. The lateral position (C) involves lying on one side, providing access to either lateral side but not directly to the anterior surface. Fowler's position (D), where the patient is seated at an angle, can provide partial access but is primarily used for respiratory issues or comfort rather than full anterior access.

Question 40: Correct Answer: C) Provide the requested treatment without expressing personal beliefs.

Rationale: The primary responsibility of a medical assistant is to provide unbiased care regardless of personal or religious beliefs. Option C is correct because it ensures that patient care is not compromised by personal biases. Option A could lead to delays in care, option B might impose personal beliefs on the patient, and option D could be time-consuming and unnecessary for immediate decisions. Providing care without bias aligns with ethical standards and respects patient autonomy.

Question 41: Correct Answer: C) Cotton gauze with hypoallergenic tape

Rationale: Cotton gauze with hypoallergenic tape is most appropriate for patients with sensitive skin prone to allergic reactions. Latex-based adhesive bandages can cause allergic reactions due to latex sensitivity. Hydrocolloid dressings, while good for wound healing, may not be suitable for sensitive skin due to potential adhesive irritation. Elastic compression bandages are primarily used for support and compression rather than minimizing skin irritation. Thus, cotton gauze with hypoallergenic tape minimizes irritation while providing necessary coverage.

Question 42: Correct Answer: B) Health Maintenance Organization (HMO)

Rationale: An HMO requires patients to choose a primary care physician who coordinates all healthcare services and provides referrals to specialists. In contrast, a PPO allows more flexibility in choosing healthcare providers without needing referrals. An EPO combines elements of HMOs and PPOs but does not require PCP selection or referrals. A POS plan blends features of HMOs and PPOs, requiring a PCP for in-network services but allowing out-of-network care at higher costs.

Question 43: Correct Answer: B) Elixir

Rationale: An elixir is a clear, sweetened hydroalcoholic solution designed for oral administration. It often contains flavoring agents and is used to improve the taste of bitter medications. A liquid is a general term for any fluid medication but does not specify its composition. A balm is a topical preparation used for soothing or healing skin and does not have the hydroalcoholic base characteristic of an elixir. An ointment is also a topical preparation but is primarily oil-based and used for skin application rather than oral use. Each option clarified: - Liquid: General term without specifying hydroalcoholic composition. - Elixir: Correct answer; specifically a hydroalcoholic solution for oral use. - Balm: Topical preparation, not intended for oral use. - Ointment: Oil-based topical application, not a hydroalcoholic solution.

Question 44: Correct Answer: B) Integumentary System

Rationale: The integumentary system, consisting of the skin, hair, nails, and associated glands, is primarily responsible for regulating body temperature through sweat production and protecting internal organs from external damage. The endocrine system (A) plays a role in hormone regulation but not directly in temperature control or physical protection. The muscular system (C) aids in movement and heat production but does not serve as a primary protective barrier. The nervous system (D) controls body functions and responses but does not directly regulate temperature or provide physical protection.

Question 45: Correct Answer: B) Document the observations in Mr. Thompson's medical record and report to Adult Protective Services (APS).

Rationale: Under mandatory reporting laws, healthcare professionals must report suspected abuse of vulnerable adults to Adult Protective Services (APS). Documenting observations ensures there is a record of the findings. Reporting directly to APS is crucial as they are equipped to handle such cases. Reporting to local law enforcement (Option A) may be necessary in certain situations but APS is typically the first point of contact for elder abuse. Waiting for confirmation from a physician (Option C) can delay necessary intervention. Discussing concerns with family members (Option D) could potentially put Mr. Thompson at further risk. - Option A is incorrect because while law enforcement may eventually become involved, APS should be notified first as they specialize in handling such cases. - Option C is incorrect because waiting for confirmation from a physician can delay immediate protective actions required by law. - Option D is incorrect because involving family members without proper investigation can compromise Mr. Thompson's safety and confidentiality. This question challenges test-takers by presenting plausible actions that are close but not entirely aligned with legal requirements, testing their precise knowledge of mandatory reporting protocols.

Question 46: Correct Answer: A) "Shot"

Rationale: Using the term "shot" is most appropriate for young children as it is simple and commonly understood. While "injection" and "vaccine" are medically accurate, they are complex and may cause confusion or fear. "Medicine" is too vague and does not specifically convey the act of receiving a vaccine. The term "shot" balances clarity and simplicity, reducing anxiety in pediatric patients by using familiar language.

Question 47: Correct Answer: B) Anxiety triggers the release of adrenaline, causing increased blood pressure and heart rate.

Rationale: Anxiety triggers the sympathetic nervous system to release adrenaline (epinephrine), which increases both blood pressure and heart rate. Option A is incorrect because cortisol primarily affects glucose metabolism rather than directly increasing heart rate or blood pressure. Option C is misleading as serotonin is more related to mood regulation than immediate cardiovascular responses. Option D is incorrect because dopamine reduction is not directly linked to acute changes in blood pressure or heart rate in anxiety contexts. Adrenaline's role is well-documented in contemporary research on stress responses.

Question 48: Correct Answer: A) Acute appendicitis

Rationale: Acute appendicitis typically presents with right lower quadrant pain, nausea, low-grade fever, and rebound tenderness. Crohn's disease can cause similar pain but usually includes chronic diarrhea and weight loss. Diverticulitis often presents with left lower quadrant pain. Ectopic pregnancy can present with abdominal pain and tenderness but is more common in females of childbearing age and often accompanied by vaginal bleeding. Therefore, acute appendicitis is the most likely diagnosis given John's symptoms and examination findings.

Question 49: Correct Answer: B) Don a gown and gloves.

Rationale: The correct action is to don a gown and gloves before entering Mr. Johnson's room because C. diff is transmitted via contact with contaminated surfaces or infected individuals. A surgical mask (Option A) or an N95 respirator (Option C) is not necessary as C. diff is not airborne. Using a face shield (Option D) without a gown does not provide adequate protection against contact transmission. Therefore, wearing both a gown and gloves is crucial for preventing the spread of this infection.

Question 50: Correct Answer: C) The specific tests ordered

Rationale: The specific tests ordered are crucial to ensure accurate processing because they dictate how the sample should be handled, processed, and analyzed. While the patient's date of birth (Option B) and physician's signature (Option D) are important for identification and authorization, they do not directly affect the processing of the sample. Insurance information (Option A), though necessary for billing, does not impact the clinical aspect of sample processing.

Question 51: Correct Answer: C) The patient should fast for at least 12 hours before the test.

Rationale: For accurate lipid panel results, fasting for at least 12 hours is recommended to avoid interference from recent food intake. While options A and B suggest shorter fasting periods, they do not meet the optimal requirement. Option D extends beyond necessary guidelines and could cause unnecessary discomfort. Therefore, option C is correct as it aligns with standard clinical guidelines ensuring accurate measurement of lipid levels.

Question 52: Correct Answer: B) Keeping the ankle elevated above heart level

Rationale: Elevating the ankle above heart level is crucial within the first 24 hours to reduce swelling and pain effectively. Applying heat immediately (A) can increase swelling, wrapping too tightly (C) may restrict blood flow and cause further damage, and performing exercises (D) too soon can exacerbate the injury. Elevation helps reduce fluid accumulation in the injured area by promoting venous return.

Question 53: Correct Answer: B) A child at the 75th percentile for height is taller than 75% of peers.

Rationale: The correct interpretation of growth percentiles is crucial. Option B accurately states that a child at the 75th percentile for height is taller than 75% of their peers, reflecting an understanding of how percentiles work. Option A incorrectly labels a consistent 25th percentile as underweight without considering individual growth patterns. Option C misinterprets significant drops in percentiles as normal variation, potentially missing underlying health issues. Option D incorrectly assumes that being consistently at the 90th percentile equates to obesity without considering other factors like body composition and overall health trends.

Question 54: Correct Answer: B) Her current household income

Rationale: Sliding scale fee systems primarily base eligibility on current household income, making option B correct. While the number of dependents (option C) may influence the income threshold, it is not the primary determinant. Previous employment history (option A) and educational background (option D) are not typically considered in determining eligibility for reduced fees under sliding scales.

Question 55: Correct Answer: B) Cleanse the venipuncture site with an alcohol swab.

Rationale: After confirming patient identity and explaining the procedure, cleansing the venipuncture site with an alcohol swab is essential to prevent infection. Applying a tourniquet (Option A) should be done before cleansing, inserting the needle at a 45-degree angle (Option C) is incorrect as it should be 15-30 degrees, and labeling collection tubes (Option D) occurs after blood collection. The correct sequence ensures patient safety and accurate sample collection.

Question 56: Correct Answer: C) Administer intramuscular epinephrine.

Rationale: The most appropriate initial response to anaphylactic shock is administering intramuscular epinephrine (Option C). Epinephrine rapidly reverses severe symptoms by constricting blood vessels, increasing heart rate, and relaxing airway muscles. Option A (oral antihistamines) is too slow-acting for anaphylaxis. Option B (intravenous fluids) supports circulation but does not address airway constriction or systemic vasodilation immediately. Option D (cold compress) is ineffective for systemic reactions like anaphylaxis. Understanding the rapid and systemic nature of epinephrine's action is crucial for immediate life-saving intervention in anaphylactic shock.

Question 57: Correct Answer: B) Inform the attending physician about her verbal request.

Rationale: The correct action is to inform the attending physician about Mrs. Johnson's verbal request. This ensures that any changes to her medical directives are properly evaluated and documented by a qualified healthcare professional. Simply updating or ignoring the DNR status without proper documentation (A and C) could lead to legal and ethical issues. Asking Mrs. Johnson to sign a new DNR order (D) is premature without consulting the physician first to ensure all protocols are followed correctly.

Question 58: Correct Answer: B) 15-30 degrees

Rationale: The correct needle insertion angle for venipuncture is 15-30 degrees. This angle allows for optimal entry into a superficial vein without causing excessive trauma or missing the vein entirely. Option A (5-10 degrees) is too shallow and may not penetrate the vein properly. Option C (45-60 degrees) increases the risk of going through the vein or causing more tissue damage. Option D (75-90 degrees) is almost perpendicular and highly inappropriate for venipuncture, risking severe tissue injury. Understanding these angles helps ensure effective and safe venipuncture procedures.

Question 59: Correct Answer: A) Active listening

Rationale: Active listening is crucial for establishing trust and rapport because it involves fully concentrating, understanding, responding, and remembering what the patient says. This demonstrates empathy and respect for the patient's feelings and concerns. Providing medical advice (B) is important but not as foundational for building initial trust. Using medical jargon (C) can confuse patients and hinder communication. Maintaining professional distance (D) is necessary but should not prevent showing empathy and understanding through active listening.

Question 60: Correct Answer: C) Verifying the patient's wristband information with the medication order.

Rationale: Verifying the patient's wristband information with the medication order is the most reliable method for identifying a patient. Wristbands typically contain critical identifiers such as name, date of birth, and medical record number. Option A is common practice but less reliable alone without cross-referencing. Option B is incorrect because room numbers can change. Option D relies on human memory, which can be fallible. Therefore, option C ensures accurate identification by cross-referencing unique identifiers directly from the wristband to the medication order.

Question 61: Correct Answer: C) Application of heat packs

Rationale: Application of heat packs is contraindicated in patients with chronic venous insufficiency because it can exacerbate inflammation and worsen edema. Compression therapy (A) and elevation of the legs (B) are recommended to improve venous return and reduce swelling. Moisturizers (D) help maintain skin integrity but do not directly affect venous insufficiency. Therefore, while options A, B, and D are beneficial or neutral, option C poses a risk due to its potential to increase blood flow and exacerbate symptoms.

Question 62: Correct Answer: B) Focus on maintaining functional independence and quality of life.

Rationale: The primary goal in managing elderly patients with multiple chronic conditions is to maintain their functional independence and improve their quality of life. This approach acknowledges the complexity of their health status and aims to provide holistic care. Option A is incorrect because prioritizing the most severe condition might neglect other important aspects of care. Option C is incorrect as treating each condition independently can lead to polypharmacy and adverse interactions. Option D is incorrect because strict adherence might not always be feasible or beneficial due to potential side effects and interactions.

Question 63: Correct Answer: D) Maintaining a sterile field by not reaching over it

Rationale: Maintaining a sterile field by not reaching over it is crucial because any breach can introduce contaminants. While wearing sterile gloves (A), using antiseptic solutions (B), and ensuring instrument sterility (C) are essential, they do not address the risk of contamination from non-sterile areas as directly as avoiding reaching over the sterile field does. This practice minimizes airborne contamination and direct contact with non-sterile surfaces, which is vital for preventing infections.

Question 64: Correct Answer: C) Ensuring all required documentation and forms are accurately filled out and submitted to the insurance company.

Rationale: Ensuring all required documentation and forms are accurately filled out and submitted is crucial because incomplete or incorrect submissions can lead to delays or denials in authorization. While submitting a complete medical history (Option A) may be part of the required documentation, it is not as comprehensive as ensuring all forms are accurate. Contacting the pharmacy (Option B) is important but not directly related to obtaining prior authorization. Scheduling an appointment with the physician (Option D) might be necessary if alternatives are needed but is not central to obtaining initial authorization.

Question 65: Correct Answer: C) Utilize a professional medical interpreter to facilitate communication.

Rationale: Utilizing a professional medical interpreter ensures accurate and culturally appropriate communication,

reducing misunderstandings. Speaking slowly and loudly (Option B) may not overcome language barriers. Using gestures (Option A) can lead to misinterpretations. Relying on family members (Option D) can compromise confidentiality and accuracy. Professional interpreters are trained to bridge both language and cultural gaps effectively.

Question 66: Correct Answer: A) If the information is required by a public health authority to control disease spread.

Rationale: Option A is correct because public health authorities have legal grounds to access medical information without patient consent to manage and control diseases. Option B is incorrect as family members need explicit patient consent unless they hold a legal power of attorney. Option C is incorrect because employers cannot access medical records without explicit consent due to privacy laws. Option D is incorrect as it requires implicit or explicit patient consent for continuity of care, making it less stringent than public health requirements.

Question 67: Correct Answer: B) Radiology

Rationale: Radiology is the ancillary service dedicated to diagnostic imaging, such as X-rays, MRI, and CT scans, which are crucial for medical diagnosis. Physical Therapy (A) focuses on rehabilitation and mobility improvement. Occupational Therapy (C) aims at helping patients perform daily activities with greater ease. Respiratory Therapy (D) specializes in treating patients with breathing disorders. The key difference lies in their primary functions: Radiology provides diagnostic images essential for diagnosing conditions, whereas the other options focus on therapeutic interventions.

Question 68: Correct Answer: B) Acknowledge his frustration, apologize for the delay, and provide an estimated waiting time.

Rationale: The correct approach involves acknowledging the patient's feelings, apologizing for the inconvenience, and providing specific information about what to expect next. This strategy aligns with best practices in communication and customer service by addressing emotional needs and providing clarity. Option A lacks acknowledgment of Mr. Johnson's frustration. Option C dismisses his concerns and can exacerbate his frustration. Option D offers a temporary distraction but does not address his underlying concerns or provide any useful information about the wait time.

Question 69: Correct Answer: A) Patient's full name

Rationale: The patient's full name is a legally required element for a prescription to be valid. This ensures accurate patient identification and reduces the risk of medication errors. While the patient's address (Option B) and prescriber's DEA number (Option C) are important, they are not universally required by law for all prescriptions. The date of birth (Option D), although helpful for verification, is also not a legal requirement. Thus, Option A is the correct answer as it meets legal standards across various jurisdictions.

Question 70: Correct Answer: B) Cross-referencing lab results with established reference ranges.

Rationale: Cross-referencing lab results with established reference ranges is crucial for interpreting whether the results are within normal limits and determining subsequent patient care steps. Verifying patient demographic information (A), scheduling follow-up appointments (C), and updating EHRs with new prescriptions (D) are important tasks but do not directly involve using external databases for interpreting lab results. This makes option B the most appropriate and relevant use of an external database in this context.

Question 71: Correct Answer: B) Remote Patient Monitoring (RPM)

Rationale: Remote Patient Monitoring (RPM) provides real-time updates on patients' health status, enabling continuous monitoring and timely interventions. Unlike EHRs which store historical data, RPM actively tracks current health metrics. Patient portals facilitate communication but lack real-time monitoring capabilities. Telehealth services offer remote consultations but do not continuously track patient data. RPM's ability to provide immediate health updates makes it ideal for managing John's chronic conditions.

Question 72: Correct Answer: B) Inferior Myocardial Infarction

Rationale: ST-segment elevation in leads II, III, and aVF is indicative of an inferior myocardial infarction. These leads correspond to the inferior wall of the heart. Anterior myocardial infarction would show changes in leads V1-V4, lateral myocardial infarction would affect leads I, aVL, V5, and V6, while posterior myocardial infarction typically presents with reciprocal changes in V1-V3. Therefore, option B is correct because it accurately matches the lead changes described.

Question 73: Correct Answer: C) Use multi-factor authentication (MFA) before initiating the transfer.

Rationale: Using multi-factor authentication (MFA) is critical for securing online transactions as it provides an additional layer of security beyond just passwords. This step is essential in preventing unauthorized access. While verifying a secure Wi-Fi connection (A), ensuring correct bank details (B), and confirming transaction limits (D) are important, they do not directly enhance security as effectively as MFA does. MFA significantly reduces the risk of fraud and unauthorized transactions by requiring multiple forms of verification.

Question 74: Correct Answer: A) Adverse effect of Lisinopril

Rationale: Lisinopril, an ACE inhibitor, commonly causes a persistent dry cough as an adverse effect. Metformin typically does not cause this symptom; its side effects include gastrointestinal issues like diarrhea. While a persistent dry cough is an adverse effect, it is not a contra-indication for using Lisinopril; however, it may lead to discontinuation if intolerable. Therefore, option A is correct because it directly identifies the adverse effect associated with the medication prescribed.

Question 75: Correct Answer: A) Fifth intercostal space at the midclavicular line

Rationale: V4 is correctly placed in the fifth intercostal space at the midclavicular line. This specific location ensures accurate heart activity recording. Option B is incorrect because it places V4 one intercostal space higher. Option C is misleading as it shifts V4 laterally to the anterior axillary line, which is actually closer to V5's position. Option D combines both errors, placing it too high and too lateral. Proper electrode placement is crucial for accurate EKG interpretation and avoiding diagnostic errors.

Question 76: Correct Answer: C) Facing the patient and speaking clearly

Rationale: Facing the patient and speaking clearly ensures that they can read lips and see facial expressions, which aids in understanding. Speaking louder can distort speech sounds, making it harder to comprehend. Written communication is useful but may not convey tone or urgency effectively. Using complex medical terminology can confuse patients; simpler language is often more effective.

Question 77: Correct Answer: A) 6 months

Rationale: The influenza vaccine is recommended for infants starting at 6 months of age. This recommendation helps protect infants during flu season when they are most vulnerable. Option B (12 months) and Option D (18 months) are incorrect because they delay necessary protection. Option C (9 months) is also incorrect as it does not align with current guidelines which clearly state initiation at 6 months. Thus, administering the vaccine at 6 months ensures timely immunization against influenza.

Question 78: Correct Answer: A) Use technical jargon with Dr. Smith and simplify the language for Mr. Johnson.

Rationale: Using technical jargon with Dr. Smith ensures that the information is communicated efficiently and accurately, leveraging his medical expertise. Simplifying the language for Mr. Johnson makes the complex procedure understandable for someone without medical training, ensuring he can follow along and make informed decisions

about his care. - Option B is incorrect because it fails to account for the differing levels of medical knowledge between Dr. Smith and Mr. Johnson. - Option C is incorrect as it suggests inconsistent non-verbal communication strategies that can lead to misunderstandings. - Option D is incorrect because providing written instructions only to Dr. Smith may overlook his need for verbal clarification, while verbal instructions only to Mr. Johnson may not cater to his need for reference material. By comparing these options, it's clear that option A best addresses the need to tailor communication styles appropriately based on the audience's background and comprehension level.

Question 79: Correct Answer: A) Co-pay

Rationale: The $25 payment made at the time of the visit is known as a co-pay. This is a fixed amount paid by the patient for specific services. Co-insurance (Option B) refers to a percentage of costs that the patient must pay after meeting their deductible. A deductible (Option C) is an amount paid out-of-pocket before insurance coverage begins. Tier Level (Option D) pertains to different levels of medication coverage within an insurance plan. Understanding these distinctions ensures accurate comprehension of insurance terminology.

Question 80: Correct Answer: B) Discontinue using the disinfectant until you obtain the SDS from the manufacturer.

Rationale: According to OSHA guidelines, it is mandatory to have an SDS for every hazardous chemical used in a workplace. The correct action is to discontinue using any product without an SDS to ensure safety and compliance. Option A is incorrect as it continues usage without proper documentation. Option C suggests a viable alternative but does not address discontinuing use immediately. Option D proposes creating a temporary document, which is not compliant with OSHA standards. Therefore, option B is correct as it ensures safety by halting use until proper documentation is obtained.

Question 81: Correct Answer: A) Ensure the patient has been sitting quietly for at least 5 minutes before taking the measurement.

Rationale: Ensuring the patient has been sitting quietly for at least 5 minutes helps stabilize their blood pressure, providing a more accurate reading. Option B is incorrect because placing the cuff over clothing can lead to inaccurate readings due to interference. Option C is partially correct but not specific enough; while you do inflate until you no longer feel a pulse, it's not as crucial as ensuring proper rest beforehand. Option D is incorrect because taking multiple readings too quickly can cause variations due to stress or movement, leading to inaccurate results.

Question 82: Correct Answer: A) Clean the site with 70% isopropyl alcohol and allow it to air dry completely.

Rationale: The correct method involves cleaning the site with 70% isopropyl alcohol and allowing it to air dry completely. This ensures that the antiseptic effect of alcohol takes place, reducing microbial presence effectively. Blowing on the site (Option B) can introduce contaminants from breath. Using sterile water (Option C) does not provide adequate antisepsis compared to alcohol. Immediate venipuncture after using 90% isopropyl alcohol (Option D) does not allow sufficient contact time for disinfection and can cause more irritation.

Question 83: Correct Answer: C) Heparin, EDTA, Serum

Rationale: The correct order of draw for micro-tubes is Heparin first to prevent clotting in plasma samples, followed by EDTA which binds calcium to prevent coagulation in whole blood samples, and lastly Serum for tests requiring clotted blood. This sequence minimizes cross-contamination between additives. Options A), B), and D) mix up this sequence and could lead to inaccurate test results due to additive carryover. Understanding the rationale behind each tube's placement helps ensure sample integrity.

Question 84: Correct Answer: D) Annual review and update of the ECP

Rationale: The correct answer is D) Annual review and update of the ECP. OSHA's Bloodborne Pathogens Standard mandates that an Exposure Control Plan must be reviewed and updated at least annually to reflect new or modified tasks and procedures which affect occupational exposure, and to reflect new or revised employee positions with occupational exposure. While regular training (A), engineering controls (B), and PPE (C) are essential elements of an ECP, they do not specifically address the requirement for annual review and updates, which is crucial for compliance.

Question 85: Correct Answer: B) Apologize for the wait and provide an estimated wait time.

Rationale: Apologizing for the wait and providing an estimated wait time (Option B) addresses the patient's immediate concern while managing their expectations, which is crucial in customer service. Option A, while polite, may not address the patient's need to be seen promptly. Option C lacks empathy and could further frustrate the patient. Option D may seem like good customer service but does not address the immediate issue of uncertainty about how much longer they will have to wait.

Question 86: Correct Answer: A) Pharmacist

Rationale: The pharmacist is primarily responsible for medication review and reconciliation, ensuring that all medications are correctly documented and appropriate for the patient's condition. While a Registered Nurse (B) may assist in medication administration and monitoring, and a Primary Care Physician (C) oversees overall patient care, neither specializes in detailed medication management like a pharmacist. A Surgical Nurse (D) focuses on perioperative care but does not handle comprehensive medication reconciliation. - Pharmacist: Specializes in detailed medication management. - Registered Nurse: Assists in medication administration but not specialized in reconciliation. - Primary Care Physician: Oversees overall care but delegates specific tasks. - Surgical Nurse: Focuses on perioperative care, not comprehensive medication management.

Question 87: Correct Answer: C) Thyroxine (T4)

Rationale: John's symptoms are indicative of hypothyroidism, where there is a deficiency of thyroxine (T4). Insulin deficiency typically presents with hyperglycemia and other diabetic symptoms. Cortisol deficiency would lead to symptoms like muscle weakness and low blood pressure, commonly seen in Addison's disease. Adrenaline deficiency is rare and usually not associated with such systemic symptoms. Therefore, thyroxine (T4) deficiency aligns best with the presented symptoms. - Insulin (A): Incorrect because insulin deficiency primarily causes hyperglycemia rather than fatigue and cold intolerance. - Cortisol (B): Incorrect as cortisol deficiency leads to different symptoms such as muscle weakness. - Thyroxine (T4) (C): Correct; aligns with hypothyroidism symptoms. - Adrenaline (D): Incorrect since adrenaline deficiency does not typically present with these systemic signs. This question challenges test-takers by presenting conditions that have overlapping yet distinct symptomatology, requiring precise knowledge to differentiate between them.

Question 88: Correct Answer: A) Red top, Lavender top, Yellow top

Rationale: The red-top tube (no additive) is used for chemistry tests like CMP. The lavender-top tube contains EDTA and is used for hematology tests like CBC. The yellow-top tube contains SPS and is used for microbiology tests like blood cultures. Option B is incorrect because the blue-top tube (sodium citrate) is used for coagulation studies. Option C is incorrect because it includes the blue-top tube instead of the lavender-top tube required for CBC. Option D includes a gray-top tube (sodium fluoride/potassium oxalate), which is used for glucose testing but not needed here.

Question 89: Correct Answer: B) Dispose of them in a puncture-resistant sharps container.

Rationale: According to OSHA guidelines, used needles and other sharps must be disposed of in a puncture-resistant sharps container (Option B). This prevents needlestick injuries and reduces the risk of infection. Option A is incorrect because red biohazard bags are meant for non-sharp biohazardous waste. Option C is unsafe as it poses significant health risks. Option D does not provide adequate protection against punctures and is not compliant with OSHA standards.

Question 90: Correct Answer: C) Ophthalmology

Rationale: Sarah's symptoms of blurred vision and frequent headaches may indicate diabetic retinopathy, a common complication of diabetes. An ophthalmologist specializes in eye health and can provide the necessary evaluation and treatment. While endocrinology (A) focuses on hormone-related diseases like diabetes, it does not address eye-specific issues. Neurology (B) deals with nervous system disorders but is not directly related to diabetic eye complications. General Internal Medicine (D) provides broad medical care but lacks the specialized focus required for Sarah's specific symptoms.

Question 91: Correct Answer: B) Advanced Search Function

Rationale: The Advanced Search Function in EMR/EHR software allows users to quickly locate specific patient information, such as lab results, by using keywords or filters. The Patient Summary Dashboard provides an overview but may not offer detailed search capabilities. The Appointment Scheduling Module is used for managing patient appointments, not retrieving records. The Billing and Coding Section is focused on financial aspects and insurance claims, not clinical data retrieval. Thus, the Advanced Search Function is the most efficient tool for Emma's needs.

Question 92: Correct Answer: B) Conducting quarterly reviews of incident reports to identify common hazards.

Rationale: Conducting quarterly reviews of incident reports allows for the identification and mitigation of recurring hazards, making it a proactive strategy for risk management. While regular training (Option A) is essential, it may not address specific recurring issues. Annual inspections (Option C) are important but less frequent than quarterly reviews. Ergonomic furniture (Option D) helps reduce injuries but does not encompass a comprehensive risk management strategy like incident report reviews.

Question 93: Correct Answer: A) Automated Drug Interaction Alerts

Rationale: Automated Drug Interaction Alerts are a critical feature that enhances medication safety by notifying prescribers of potential adverse drug interactions. While real-time insurance verification (Option B) improves administrative efficiency and EHR integration (Option C) streamlines patient data access, neither directly targets prescription error reduction. Patient education resources (Option D), although valuable for patient engagement, do not primarily address medication safety. Thus, Option A is the most relevant to enhancing medication safety by reducing prescription errors through timely alerts.

Question 94: Correct Answer: D) Sprain

Rationale: A sprain involves the stretching or tearing of ligaments, typically due to a twisting motion. Swelling, bruising, and pain during weight-bearing are characteristic symptoms. Lacerations involve cuts in the skin, abrasions are superficial scrapes, and fractures involve broken bones. In this case, the mechanism of injury (twisting) and symptoms (swelling, bruising, pain with weight-bearing) align most closely with a sprain.

Question 95: Correct Answer: A) Ensure John understands his medication regimen, including dosages and times.

Rationale: Ensuring that John understands his medication regimen is the most critical task because it directly impacts his ability to manage his diabetes and recover from pneumonia. Mismanagement of medications can lead to severe complications. While providing dietary plans (B), scheduling follow-ups (C), and educating about pneumonia signs (D) are important, they are secondary to understanding medications. Medication adherence is fundamental in preventing readmissions and ensuring overall health stability.

Question 96: Correct Answer: B) Detailed patient history and reason for referral

Rationale: The most crucial piece of information in a referral is a detailed patient history and reason for referral. This ensures that the specialist understands the patient's medical background and specific needs. While insurance information (Option A), contact details of the primary care physician (Option C), and appointment availability (Option D) are important, they do not provide clinical context necessary for effective patient care. Accurate documentation helps avoid redundant tests and facilitates appropriate treatment planning.

Question 97: Correct Answer: D) Accessing a patient's medical records for personal curiosity without a legitimate reason.

Rationale: Option D is correct because accessing patient records without a legitimate reason violates HIPAA's minimum necessary standard. Option A is incorrect because sharing information with another provider involved in care is permissible under HIPAA. Option B is close but incorrect; while it poses a risk, it isn't an immediate breach unless accessed by unauthorized individuals. Option C is also tricky but incorrect as sharing with family members can be allowed if they are involved in the patient's care or with patient consent.

Question 98: Correct Answer: C) Ensuring inspections are performed by certified medical equipment servicers

Rationale: While recording inspections immediately (Option A), conducting bi-annual inspections (Option B), and maintaining records (Option D) are important, ensuring that inspections are performed by certified medical equipment servicers (Option C) is crucial for compliance. Certified servicers ensure that inspections meet regulatory standards and identify potential issues accurately. This is more critical than merely documenting or scheduling because it directly impacts the quality and reliability of the inspection process.

Question 99: Correct Answer: B) Leucine

Rationale: Leucine is an essential amino acid that must be obtained through diet as the body cannot synthesize it. Alanine (A), Glutamine (C), and Glycine (D) are non-essential amino acids that the body can produce. Alanine is involved in glucose metabolism, Glutamine supports immune function and intestinal health, and Glycine is important for collagen formation. The key difference lies in their classification; only Leucine is essential, highlighting its unique requirement for dietary intake. This distinction underscores the importance of understanding amino acid roles in nutrition.

Question 100: Correct Answer: A) Reducing medication errors by eliminating handwritten prescriptions

Rationale: The primary benefit of CPOE systems is reducing medication errors by eliminating handwritten prescriptions, which can be prone to misinterpretation due to poor handwriting or ambiguous abbreviations. While options B), C), and D) are related to potential benefits of health IT systems, they do not specifically capture the core advantage of CPOE in minimizing prescription-related errors. Option B) focuses on patient satisfaction rather than error reduction. Option C) pertains to data centralization but not directly to error reduction. Option D) involves administrative efficiency but does not address clinical safety directly.

Question 101: Correct Answer: B) Simplify the information using layman's terms.

Rationale: Simplifying complex medical information into layman's terms ensures that patients understand their diagnosis and treatment plans. This approach respects patient autonomy and fosters effective communication. While using medical jargon (Option A) maintains accuracy, it can confuse patients. Providing written materials (Option C)

without verbal explanation lacks personal interaction needed for clarification. Referring patients directly to physicians (Option D) may be necessary in some cases but does not develop the medical assistant's role in patient education. Therefore, Option B is the most appropriate action.

Question 102: Correct Answer: B) The intradermal allergy test is more sensitive than the scratch test.

Rationale: The intradermal allergy test is indeed more sensitive than the scratch test because it introduces allergens directly into the dermis, leading to a stronger immune response. Option A is incorrect because it describes the procedure for an intradermal test, not a scratch test. Option C is incorrect as both tests typically have similar observation periods. Option D is incorrect because placing allergens on the skin surface pertains to a patch or scratch test, not an intradermal one.

Question 103: Correct Answer: C) Family History

Rationale: Family history is essential for identifying genetic predispositions and hereditary conditions. Social history (A) focuses on lifestyle factors like occupation and substance use. Surgical history (B) details past surgeries but doesn't address genetics. Medical history (D) includes past medical conditions but isn't specifically focused on heredity. Thus, family history (C) provides critical insights into genetic risks and inherited diseases, making it the correct answer.

Question 104: Correct Answer: B) Holter Monitoring

Rationale: Holter Monitoring is the most appropriate test for continuous monitoring of heart rhythm over 24-48 hours, capturing intermittent arrhythmias. A Stress Test evaluates heart function under physical exertion, which is not continuous monitoring. Event Monitoring records only during symptomatic episodes and may miss asymptomatic arrhythmias. An Echocardiogram assesses heart structure and function but does not provide continuous rhythm data. - A) Stress Test: Incorrect because it evaluates heart function during physical stress rather than providing continuous monitoring. - B) Holter Monitoring: Correct as it provides continuous ECG monitoring for 24-48 hours, suitable for detecting intermittent arrhythmias. - C) Event Monitoring: Incorrect because it only records during symptomatic events, potentially missing asymptomatic issues. - D) Echocardiogram: Incorrect as it assesses heart structure and function but does not offer continuous rhythm monitoring. The correct answer (Holter Monitoring) is justified by its ability to continuously record heart rhythms over an extended period, essential for detecting intermittent arrhythmias that might not be captured by other tests like stress tests or event monitors.

Question 105: Correct Answer: D) Utilizing electronic health records (EHR) for seamless information sharing.

Rationale: Utilizing EHRs ensures that all healthcare providers have access to up-to-date patient information, facilitating coordinated care. While scheduling follow-ups (Option A), providing education materials (Option B), and using a multidisciplinary team approach (Option C) are important, they rely on accurate and accessible information, which EHRs provide. EHRs streamline communication and reduce errors, making them the most effective strategy for continuity of care.

Question 106: Correct Answer: A) Apply a warm compress to the area for several minutes.

Rationale: Applying a warm compress helps dilate the veins, making them more visible and easier to access. While asking Mr. Smith to clench his fist (Option B) can help, it is less effective than warmth for increasing vein visibility. Elevating the arm (Option C) would actually decrease venous return and make veins less prominent. Using a blood pressure cuff (Option D) can be an alternative but is typically not as effective as applying warmth.

Question 107: Correct Answer: C) Assertive

Rationale: Maria's approach exemplifies assertive communication, characterized by clear, respectful expression of thoughts and feelings while considering others' perspectives. Unlike passive communication (Option A), which avoids confrontation, assertiveness addresses issues directly. Aggressive communication (Option B) involves hostility or dominance, which Maria did not exhibit. Passive-aggressive communication (Option D) subtly expresses anger or resentment indirectly, unlike Maria's straightforward and respectful response.

Question 108: Correct Answer: B) The practice manager
Rationale: The practice manager is typically responsible for overseeing administrative operations, including authorizing payment processing. While the attending physician (Option A) may be involved in clinical decisions, they usually do not handle financial authorizations. The billing department supervisor (Option C) manages billing operations but does not have final approval authority for payments. The patient care coordinator (Option D) focuses on patient scheduling and coordination rather than financial matters. Thus, the practice manager (Option B) is the correct answer as they have comprehensive oversight over administrative and financial processes in a medical practice.

Question 109: Correct Answer: B) Alcohol-based hand sanitizers should contain at least 60% alcohol to be effective.
Rationale: Option B is correct because CDC guidelines state that alcohol-based hand sanitizers need at least 60% alcohol to effectively kill most pathogens. Option A is incorrect as alcohol-based sanitizers are not effective against Clostridioides difficile spores; soap and water are required. Option C is tricky but incorrect because while true for visible dirt, it is not always less effective overall. Option D is incorrect because handwashing with soap and water is necessary in certain situations, such as after using the restroom or when hands are visibly soiled.

Question 110: Correct Answer: B) Fever and chills
Rationale: Fever and chills are hallmark signs of a systemic infection, indicating the body's response to pathogens. Localized redness and swelling (Option A) are more indicative of localized infection or inflammation. Increased heart rate without fever (Option C) could be due to various conditions like anxiety or dehydration. Mild fatigue (Option D) is non-specific and can result from numerous causes, including poor sleep or chronic illness. Therefore, Option B is the most accurate indicator of a systemic infection.

Question 111: Correct Answer: B) Asking the patient directly how they are feeling about the procedure.
Rationale: Asking the patient directly how they are feeling about the procedure is considered the most effective method because it allows for clear communication and provides an opportunity for patients to express their concerns. While observing body language (Option A), noting changes in vital signs (Option C), and providing information (Option D) are important, they do not offer direct insight into the patient's emotional state. Direct questioning ensures that healthcare providers can address specific anxieties and provide appropriate support, making it superior in accurately assessing patient anxiety levels.

Question 112: Correct Answer: C) Verifying current medications with the patient
Rationale: Verifying current medications with the patient is crucial because it ensures that all information is accurate and up-to-date, which is essential for patient safety. While adding new medications (A), deleting old ones (B), and recording dosage and frequency (D) are important tasks, they rely on having accurate baseline information. Verification directly from the patient minimizes errors due to outdated or incorrect records, making it the most critical step in this process.

Question 113: Correct Answer: D) Wearing gloves, a gown, and using a sharps container
Rationale: The correct answer is D because an Exposure Control Plan requires comprehensive protective measures including gloves, gowns, and proper disposal of sharps to minimize risk. Option A is incorrect as it lacks full-body protection (gown). Option B is insufficient as it omits

additional protective gear. Option C suggests double-gloving but misses other essential protections like gowns and proper disposal methods. Therefore, D covers all necessary precautions according to contemporary research and recognized theories in infection control.

Question 114: Correct Answer: B) Instruct John to use his rescue inhaler and recheck his peak flow rate in 15 minutes.
Rationale: A drop in peak flow rate to 75% (450 L/min) of John's personal best (600 L/min) indicates a moderate asthma exacerbation. The appropriate initial response is to use a rescue inhaler (short-acting bronchodilator) and recheck the peak flow rate after 15 minutes. If there's no improvement or further decline, more aggressive management may be needed. - Option A is incorrect because continuing the current regimen without immediate intervention could worsen John's condition. - Option C is incorrect as increasing the maintenance inhaler dosage without addressing acute symptoms is not appropriate. - Option D is overly aggressive for a moderate exacerbation when initial management with a rescue inhaler is warranted first.

Question 115: Correct Answer: A) Vancomycin
Rationale: Vancomycin is an antibiotic with a narrow therapeutic index, requiring close monitoring of serum levels to avoid nephrotoxicity. Metronidazole, Ceftriaxone, and Amoxicillin are antibiotics but do not require such stringent monitoring for nephrotoxicity. Metronidazole is primarily used for anaerobic infections and does not have significant nephrotoxic risks. Ceftriaxone is a broad-spectrum antibiotic but does not typically require intensive monitoring for kidney function. Amoxicillin has a wide therapeutic index and minimal nephrotoxic risk, making it less likely to be the medication in question.

Question 116: Correct Answer: A) Bacteria
Rationale: The correct plural form of "bacterium" is "bacteria." Option B, "bacteriums," incorrectly adds an -s to form the plural. Option C, "bacterias," incorrectly adds an -s to an already pluralized term. Option D, "bacteri," is incorrect as it does not follow standard pluralization rules in medical terminology. Recognizing correct plural forms is essential for accurate communication in medical contexts.

Question 117: Correct Answer: B) Including detailed notes on the patient's progress, current medications, allergies, and any changes since the last visit.
Rationale: Option B is correct because comprehensive documentation including detailed notes on progress, medications, allergies, and changes ensures compliance with both government and insurance requirements. Option A is incorrect as it omits progress notes and changes since the last visit. Option C fails to include complete information about current medications and allergies. Option D lacks specificity required for compliance. Detailed records are essential for accurate billing and legal protection.

Question 118: Correct Answer: B) Patient's medical history
Rationale: The patient's medical history is a critical component of a medical record as it provides comprehensive information about past illnesses, treatments, surgeries, and family health history, which is essential for ensuring continuity and quality of care. While patient's insurance information (A), billing information (C), and consent forms (D) are important administrative elements, they do not directly impact clinical decision-making or continuity of care like the medical history does. Medical history directly influences diagnosis and treatment plans, making it indispensable for clinical patient care.

Question 119: Correct Answer: A) ST-segment elevation
Rationale: ST-segment elevation is a hallmark sign of an acute myocardial infarction (MI), indicating injury to the heart muscle. T-wave inversion (B) can suggest ischemia but is less specific for MI. A prolonged PR interval (C) indicates first-degree heart block, unrelated to acute MI. Sinus tachycardia (D) is a non-specific finding that can occur in various conditions, not specifically indicative of MI.

Understanding these differences is essential for accurate diagnosis and patient care.

Question 120: Correct Answer: B) Gastroscope
Rationale: A gastroscope is specifically designed for examining the upper gastrointestinal tract, including the esophagus, stomach, and duodenum. A colonoscope (Option A) is used for examining the colon and rectum, which is not relevant in this case. A bronchoscope (Option C) is intended for viewing the airways and lungs. A laryngoscope (Option D) is used primarily for visualizing the larynx and vocal cords. Hence, while all options are endoscopic instruments, only the gastroscope fits the specific scenario described.

Question 121: Correct Answer: B) At least 2 inches (5 cm)
Rationale: The American Heart Association recommends that chest compressions for an adult should be at least 2 inches (5 cm) deep to be effective. This depth ensures adequate blood flow during resuscitation efforts. Option A is too shallow to be effective, while Option C is closer but still insufficient. Option D exceeds the recommended depth and could cause injury to the patient. Understanding these precise measurements is critical for performing high-quality CPR and improving patient outcomes.

Question 122: Correct Answer: A) Radiology
Rationale: Radiology is the ancillary service responsible for providing diagnostic imaging, such as X-rays, CT scans, and MRIs, which are crucial for diagnosing various medical conditions. Pathology focuses on analyzing bodily fluids and tissues to diagnose diseases. Physical Therapy aims at rehabilitating patients through exercises and treatments to improve mobility and function. Respiratory Therapy specializes in treating patients with breathing disorders. While all these services are essential, Radiology specifically deals with diagnostic imaging, making it the correct answer.

Question 123: Correct Answer: C) Procedural
Rationale: Procedural records specifically document the details of medical procedures performed on a patient, including steps taken and outcomes. Administrative records (Option A) include patient demographics and scheduling information but not procedure details. Clinical records (Option B) cover overall patient health information but lack the specificity of procedural documentation. Consents (Option D) are legal documents authorizing treatments or procedures but do not detail the procedures themselves. Thus, procedural records are distinct in their focus on documenting specific medical interventions comprehensively.

Question 124: Correct Answer: B) Conducting a comprehensive initial inventory audit
Rationale: Conducting a comprehensive initial inventory audit is essential because it establishes a baseline for all subsequent inventory activities. This step ensures that all items are accounted for and accurately documented. While regularly updating the inventory list (Option A), setting minimum stock levels (Option C), and implementing an automated system (Option D) are important, they rely on having accurate initial data. Without a thorough initial audit, these subsequent steps may be ineffective or flawed.

Question 125: Correct Answer: C) Ventrogluteal site
Rationale: The ventrogluteal site is considered the safest and most appropriate site for intramuscular injections in adults due to its distance from major nerves and blood vessels, reducing the risk of injury. The vastus lateralis muscle (A) is often used in infants and children but can be less comfortable in adults. The deltoid muscle (B) is suitable for smaller volumes but may not be ideal for larger volumes or viscous medications. The dorsogluteal site (D), while historically common, carries a higher risk of sciatic nerve injury compared to the ventrogluteal site.

Question 126: Correct Answer: B) Label the specimen at the patient's bedside immediately after drawing.
Rationale: The correct procedure is to label the specimen at the patient's bedside immediately after drawing (Option B).

This ensures that there are no mix-ups or errors in patient identification. Option A is incorrect because placing it in a biohazard bag before labeling could lead to misidentification. Option C is incorrect as transporting without labeling increases error risk. Option D is incorrect because delaying labeling until reaching the lab can result in misidentification and contamination risks. Proper bedside labeling ensures accurate patient identification and sample integrity.

Question 127: Correct Answer: B) Detailed reason for referral
Rationale: The detailed reason for referral is crucial as it provides the receiving provider with specific information needed to continue care effectively. While patient's medical history (A), contact information of the referring provider (C), and patient's insurance information (D) are important, they do not directly address the immediate clinical needs and context that guide further diagnostic or therapeutic actions. The detailed reason for referral ensures that all necessary clinical information is conveyed accurately, facilitating appropriate and timely follow-up care.

Question 128: Correct Answer: A) Informed Consent Form
Rationale: The Informed Consent Form is required to ensure that Sarah understands the risks, benefits, and alternatives of the procedure. This form is essential for legal and ethical reasons. The HIPAA Privacy Notice (Option B) pertains to patient privacy rights and data handling but does not address specific medical procedures. An Advance Directive (Option C) outlines a patient's wishes for end-of-life care but is not specific to individual procedures. The Patient Bill of Rights (Option D) informs patients of their general rights within a healthcare setting but does not provide procedural consent.

Question 129: Correct Answer: B) Cholecystectomy
Rationale: A cholecystectomy is the surgical removal of the gallbladder, which is the standard treatment for cholecystitis. An appendectomy (A) involves removing the appendix and is unrelated to gallbladder issues. A colectomy (C) involves removing part or all of the colon, which does not address gallbladder inflammation. A hysterectomy (D) is the removal of the uterus and is unrelated to cholecystitis. The correct answer, cholecystectomy (B), directly addresses Sarah's condition by removing the inflamed gallbladder, providing relief from her symptoms.

Question 130: Correct Answer: B) Refuse to assist in ending John's life, as it contradicts the principle of "do no harm."
Rationale: The Hippocratic Oath emphasizes "do no harm," which traditionally prohibits physicians from participating in euthanasia or assisted suicide. Option A is incorrect because it focuses on patient autonomy, which, while important, does not override the oath's prohibition against causing harm. Option C is misleading because seeking a second opinion does not address the ethical dilemma directly tied to the oath's principles. Option D is close but incorrect; while referring to palliative care is appropriate, it doesn't directly answer what Dr. Smith should do according to the Hippocratic Oath.

Question 131: Correct Answer: C) "I can see you're worried. Let's discuss your symptoms in detail so I can inform the doctor."
Rationale: Option C is correct because it demonstrates empathy and active listening, essential components of patient-centered care. It acknowledges Mrs. Johnson's feelings and provides a platform for detailed discussion, ensuring accurate information is relayed to the physician. Option A offers an explanation but may come off as dismissive of her immediate concerns. Option B reassures but doesn't address her anxiety directly or gather detailed information. Option D could lead to non-compliance without proper medical advice, posing potential health risks.

Question 132: Correct Answer: A) Peanuts
Rationale: Peanuts are the most common food allergen responsible for severe allergic reactions, particularly

anaphylaxis, in children. While shellfish (B), eggs (C), and soy (D) are also significant allergens, they are not as frequently associated with severe reactions in children as peanuts. Shellfish allergies are more common in adults, while egg and soy allergies often present with milder symptoms compared to peanut allergies. Understanding these distinctions helps medical assistants prioritize patient education and emergency preparedness.

Question 133: Correct Answer: B) Sinoatrial (SA) node
Rationale: The sinoatrial (SA) node, located in the right atrium, is known as the heart's natural pacemaker because it initiates electrical impulses that regulate heartbeat. The atrioventricular (AV) node (A), while also part of the conduction system, primarily delays the impulse before it moves to the ventricles. The Bundle of His (C) and Purkinje fibers (D) are involved in conducting impulses through the ventricles but do not initiate them. Understanding these distinctions is crucial for accurately diagnosing and treating cardiac conditions.

Question 134: Correct Answer: B) Tonometer
Rationale: A tonometer is specifically designed to measure intraocular pressure, which is crucial in diagnosing and managing glaucoma. An ophthalmoscope (A) is used to examine the retina and other parts of the eye but does not measure pressure. A retinoscope (C) helps determine refractive errors by observing the reflection of light from the retina. A slit lamp (D) allows detailed examination of the anterior eye structures but does not measure intraocular pressure. Thus, understanding each instrument's specific function highlights why tonometer (B) is correct.

Question 135: Correct Answer: C) Use a gentle stream of solution at body temperature.
Rationale: Using a gentle stream of solution at body temperature is crucial to prevent injury to the tympanic membrane and avoid causing dizziness or discomfort. Cold water (Option A) can cause vertigo. Directing the solution towards the eardrum (Option B) risks perforation. Positioning the patient's head forward (Option D) is incorrect as it does not facilitate proper drainage; instead, tilting the head slightly toward the affected ear is recommended. Therefore, Option C is correct as it ensures safety and comfort during ear irrigation.

Question 136: Correct Answer: A) Labeling the specimen immediately after collection at the patient's bedside.
Rationale: Labeling specimens immediately at the patient's bedside ensures that each sample is correctly identified, minimizing risks of mislabeling and ensuring patient safety. Option B suggests labeling in the lab, which can lead to mix-ups. Option C involves labeling post-centrifugation, which delays identification. Option D involves labeling after refrigeration, which could compromise sample integrity due to potential mix-ups during storage. Immediate bedside labeling is vital for maintaining accurate patient records and reliable test results.

Question 137: Correct Answer: C) Consult with the physician or nurse practitioner about accommodating the patient.
Rationale: The correct answer is C) Consult with the physician or nurse practitioner about accommodating the patient. This ensures that Emily follows proper protocol by seeking guidance from a healthcare provider who can make an informed decision based on clinical judgment. Option A might be appropriate in some cases but bypasses internal protocols. Option B delays necessary care, and Option D may not be suitable if immediate medical attention is required. Consulting with a healthcare provider ensures appropriate triage and prioritization of care.

Question 138: Correct Answer: C) Open the sterile dressing package away from your body.
Rationale: Opening the sterile dressing package away from your body is crucial to avoid contamination from clothing or skin contact, maintaining sterility. While cleaning the wound with antiseptic (Option A) is essential, it does not directly address maintaining sterility of supplies. Wearing clean gloves (Option B) is important but does not guarantee sterility. Using non-sterile gloves (Option D) would compromise sterility when handling a new dressing. Thus, Option C ensures that sterility is maintained throughout the procedure.

Question 139: Correct Answer: B) Use sterile forceps to lift each suture knot and cut it close to the skin before pulling it out.
Rationale: Option B is correct because lifting the suture knot with sterile forceps ensures minimal tissue trauma by allowing precise cutting close to the skin. This technique reduces the risk of introducing bacteria into the wound. Options A and C involve cutting at the knot, which can leave a fragment of suture material in the tissue, increasing infection risk. Option D adds unnecessary steps that do not significantly enhance safety or efficacy compared to Option B. Proper technique is crucial for promoting optimal wound healing and preventing complications.

Question 140: Correct Answer: D) Shaving any hair at electrode sites if necessary
Rationale: Shaving any hair at electrode sites is crucial for proper electrode adhesion and accurate readings. Option A is incorrect because avoiding caffeine is more relevant to stress tests. Option B is partially correct but not as critical as ensuring proper electrode placement. Option C is misleading; while positioning is important, it does not address potential interference like hair removal does.

Question 141: Correct Answer: B) Use a bleach-based disinfectant to clean all high-touch surfaces.
Rationale: Bleach-based disinfectants are effective against C. diff spores, which are resistant to many other disinfectants. Alcohol-based products (Option A) are ineffective against C. diff spores. Quaternary ammonium compounds (Option C) are also ineffective against these spores. Hydrogen peroxide vapor (Option D) can be effective but is not practical for routine disinfection of high-touch surfaces in a clinical setting. Therefore, bleach-based disinfectants are the most appropriate choice for ensuring complete sanitization after treating a patient with C. diff infection.

Question 142: Correct Answer: A) Nodding occasionally and maintaining eye contact while the patient speaks.
Rationale: Option A is correct because it incorporates key components of active listening, including non-verbal cues (nodding) and maintaining eye contact, which demonstrate engagement and understanding. Option B is incorrect because interrupting disrupts the patient's flow and can hinder effective communication. Option C is tricky but incorrect; while taking notes is important, not maintaining consistent eye contact can make patients feel unheard. Option D, though valuable, focuses more on questioning rather than demonstrating continuous engagement through non-verbal behavior. Active listening emphasizes being fully present and responsive without interrupting or breaking eye contact.

Question 143: Correct Answer: D) Wear gloves, a gown, and a face shield.
Rationale: Universal Precautions require healthcare workers to treat all human blood and certain body fluids as if they were known to be infectious for HIV, HBV, and other bloodborne pathogens. Wearing gloves, a gown, and a face shield provides comprehensive protection against potential splashes or contact with infectious materials. Option A is incorrect because it omits the gown, which protects against contamination of clothing. Option B is incorrect because it omits the face shield, which protects mucous membranes from splashes. Option C is incorrect because it provides insufficient protection against potential splashes or sprays of infectious material.

Question 144: Correct Answer: A) Confirming the patient's insurance coverage and obtaining pre-authorization if required.

Rationale: Confirming the patient's insurance coverage and obtaining pre-authorization if required is crucial because it ensures that the services will be covered by insurance, preventing unexpected costs for the patient. Option B is incorrect because scheduling before verifying insurance can lead to denied claims. Option C is wrong as patient consent is necessary for referrals. Option D is incorrect because specific reasons for referral are needed to justify medical necessity and secure authorization.

Question 145: Correct Answer: A) Autoclaving

Rationale: Autoclaving is the most effective method for sterilizing surgical instruments because it uses saturated steam under pressure to achieve high temperatures (typically 121°C for 15-20 minutes), which ensures the complete elimination of all microorganisms, including spores. Boiling (B) does not reach temperatures high enough to kill all spores. Dry Heat Sterilization (C) requires much longer exposure times and higher temperatures, making it less efficient. Chemical Disinfection (D) may not effectively eliminate all spores and can be less reliable than autoclaving.

Question 146: Correct Answer: B) Referring provider's National Provider Identifier (NPI)

Rationale: The referring provider's National Provider Identifier (NPI) is crucial for proper processing as it uniquely identifies the healthcare provider in all transactions. While options A, C, and D contain important information, they do not serve as a unique identifier in electronic referrals. The insurance policy number helps with billing but is not essential for identifying the referring provider. The social security number is sensitive information but not necessary for referral processing. The office address provides location details but does not uniquely identify the provider.

Question 147: Correct Answer: A) Mitochondria

Rationale: Mitochondria are the powerhouse of the cell, responsible for producing ATP through oxidative phosphorylation. Ribosomes (Option B) are involved in protein synthesis, not energy production. Lysosomes (Option C) contain digestive enzymes for breaking down waste materials. The nucleus (Option D) houses genetic material and controls cellular activities but does not produce energy. Understanding these differences is crucial for recognizing the unique role of mitochondria in energy metabolism.

Question 148: Correct Answer: B) Consult with Dr. Smith about the alert before proceeding.

Rationale: Consulting with Dr. Smith about the alert ensures that any potential drug interactions are addressed before administering medication, prioritizing patient safety. Ignoring or overriding alerts can lead to adverse drug events (Options A and C), while documenting without consulting does not mitigate immediate risk (Option D).

Question 149: Correct Answer: B) Neurologist

Rationale: A neurologist is the most appropriate referral for managing John's peripheral neuropathy, a common complication of diabetes affecting the nervous system. While an endocrinologist (Option A) specializes in diabetes management, they may not be as equipped to handle neurological complications. A podiatrist (Option C) focuses on foot care but may not address systemic neuropathy comprehensively. A cardiologist (Option D) deals with heart-related issues and is not relevant to John's neuropathy symptoms.

Question 150: Correct Answer: A) Hydrocodone

Rationale: Hydrocodone is classified as a Schedule II controlled substance due to its high potential for abuse and dependence. Alprazolam (B) and Diazepam (D) are Schedule IV drugs with lower abuse potential. Tramadol (C), although used for pain, is classified as a Schedule IV drug as well. This distinction is crucial for understanding the regulatory controls and prescribing practices for these medications.

CCMA Exam Practice Questions [SET 4]

Question 1: Which of the following is the most critical precaution to take when handling hazardous chemicals in a clinical setting?
A) Always wear gloves and a face shield.
B) Ensure proper ventilation in the area.
C) Store chemicals in labeled containers.
D) Dispose of chemicals according to MSDS guidelines.

Question 2: Which of the following bacteria is a common pathogen responsible for causing strep throat?
A) Streptococcus pyogenes
B) Streptococcus pneumoniae
C) Staphylococcus aureus
D) Escherichia coli

Question 3: Which factor is most critical for ensuring the validity of patient satisfaction survey results?
A) Survey length
B) Anonymity of responses
C) Timing of survey administration
D) Question wording

Question 4: Which of the following terms refers to the surgical removal of the gallbladder?
A) Cholecystectomy
B) Cholelithiasis
C) Cholecystitis
D) Choledochotomy

Question 5: Which of the following substances requires storage in a dark, cool environment to maintain its stability and efficacy?
A) Insulin
B) Vitamin C
C) Nitroglycerin
D) Levothyroxine

Question 6: Maria, a CCMA at a busy clinic, is responsible for managing patient appointments. She notices that Mr. Thompson's insurance information needs updating before his next visit. Which of the following actions should Maria prioritize to ensure compliance with administrative protocols?
A) Call Mr. Thompson to remind him to bring his updated insurance card to his next appointment.
B) Update Mr. Thompson's insurance information in the system based on his last visit.
C) Verify Mr. Thompson's insurance details by contacting his insurance provider before his appointment.
D) Schedule an additional appointment solely for updating Mr. Thompson's insurance information.

Question 7: Which of the following is the most effective method for disinfecting surfaces contaminated with Clostridium difficile spores in a clinical setting?
A) Alcohol-based disinfectants
B) Quaternary ammonium compounds
C) Chlorine bleach solutions
D) Hydrogen peroxide vapor

Question 8: Which surgical intervention is most commonly performed to treat acute inflammation of the gallbladder?
A) Appendectomy
B) Cholecystectomy
C) Herniorrhaphy
D) Colectomy

Question 9: Which of the following actions is most effective in facilitating service recovery after a patient has experienced poor customer service?
A) Offering a discount on future services.
B) Providing immediate feedback to the staff involved.
C) Following up with the patient through a phone call.
D) Sending an apology email to the patient.

Question 10: Sarah, a medical assistant, needs to send an email to a patient, Mr. Johnson, regarding his upcoming appointment. Which of the following is the most appropriate way for Sarah to address Mr. Johnson in the email?
A) "Hey Mr. J,"
B) "Dear Mr. Johnson,"
C) "Hi there,"
D) "Hello John,"

Question 11: Which of the following scenarios best exemplifies a breach of patient confidentiality under HIPAA regulations?
A) A medical assistant discussing a patient's condition with another healthcare provider involved in the patient's care.
B) A medical assistant sharing patient information with a family member without the patient's consent.
C) A medical assistant accessing a patient's records to provide care during an emergency.
D) A medical assistant using de-identified patient data for research purposes.

Question 12: When reviewing a provider's discharge instructions with a patient, which of the following is most critical to ensure patient comprehension and adherence to the plan of care?
A) Providing written instructions only
B) Confirming patient understanding through teach-back method
C) Advising the patient to contact their provider if they have questions
D) Scheduling follow-up appointments before discharge

Question 13: A 45-year-old patient named John presents with a deep laceration on his forearm requiring suturing. Considering the need for strong tensile strength and minimal tissue reaction, which type and size of suture would be most appropriate?

A) 3-0 Vicryl
B) 4-0 Silk
C) 2-0 Nylon
D) 5-0 Chromic Gut

Question 14: Maria, a 45-year-old Hispanic woman with limited English proficiency and low socio-economic status, visits a clinic for her chronic diabetes management. Despite receiving educational pamphlets in English, she struggles to manage her condition. What is the most significant barrier to Maria's effective care?
A) Language barrier
B) Socio-economic status
C) Cultural differences
D) Education level

Question 15: Which of the following actions is most critical in ensuring accurate EKG readings during patient testing?
A) Verifying that all leads are securely attached to the patient.
B) Ensuring the EKG machine is properly calibrated before each use.
C) Checking that the patient remains still during the recording process.
D) Confirming that the EKG paper speed is set to 50 mm/sec.

Question 16: Which of the following steps is most critical when calibrating an EKG machine to ensure accurate patient readings?
A) Adjusting the paper speed to 25 mm/sec.
B) Verifying the voltage calibration signal is set at 1 mV.
C) Ensuring the electrodes are properly placed on the patient.
D) Checking that the machine is plugged into a grounded outlet.

Question 17: Which psychological approach is most effective in helping physically disabled individuals develop adaptive coping strategies?
A) Psychoanalytic Therapy
B) Cognitive Behavioral Therapy (CBT)
C) Humanistic Therapy
D) Psychodynamic Therapy

Question 18: Which instrument is specifically used for measuring intraocular pressure during an eye examination?
A) Tonometer
B) Ophthalmoscope
C) Retinoscope
D) Slit Lamp

Question 19: During the discharge process, Maria, a medical assistant, is reviewing Mr. Johnson's plan of care. Mr. Johnson has been prescribed a new medication and needs to follow specific dietary restrictions. Which of the following actions should Maria prioritize to ensure Mr. Johnson understands his discharge instructions?
A) Provide Mr. Johnson with written instructions and ask him to read them aloud.
B) Explain the medication dosage and dietary restrictions verbally while Mr. Johnson listens.
C) Ask Mr. Johnson to demonstrate how he will take his medication and explain his dietary plan.
D) Schedule a follow-up call to review the instructions with Mr. Johnson after he gets home.

Question 20: Which of the following drugs is classified as a Schedule II controlled substance under the Controlled Substances Act?

A) Alprazolam
B) Methadone
C) Diazepam
D) Tramadol

Question 21: Which task is most critical for a Clinical Medical Assistant when coordinating care for a patient with multiple chronic conditions?
A) Scheduling follow-up appointments
B) Documenting patient history accurately
C) Educating the patient about medication adherence
D) Communicating lab results to the healthcare team

Question 22: Sarah, a 45-year-old patient, calls the clinic complaining of severe chest pain radiating to her left arm and shortness of breath. As a Certified Clinical Medical Assistant (CCMA), how should you prioritize her need for an appointment?
A) Schedule an appointment for later in the week.
B) Advise her to come in first thing tomorrow morning.
C) Recommend she visit the nearest emergency room immediately.
D) Suggest she take over-the-counter pain medication and monitor her symptoms.

Question 23: Which type of healthcare delivery model emphasizes coordinated care across multiple healthcare providers to improve patient outcomes and reduce costs?
A) Accountable Care Organization (ACO)
B) Patient-Centered Medical Home (PCMH)
C) Health Maintenance Organization (HMO)
D) Preferred Provider Organization (PPO)

Question 24: Dr. Smith is ordering a complete blood count (CBC) for his patient, John Doe. Which of the following sets of information is most critical to include on the provider request or requisition form to ensure accurate processing?
A) Patient's full name, date of birth, test requested, and insurance information
B) Patient's full name, date of birth, test requested, and provider's contact information
C) Patient's full name, test requested, provider's contact information, and clinical diagnosis
D) Patient's full name, date of birth, test requested, and clinical diagnosis

Question 25: Which of the following is the most effective strategy for a Clinical Medical Assistant to ensure seamless patient care coordination among an interdisciplinary team?
A) Regularly updating patient records in the electronic health record (EHR) system.
B) Scheduling regular interdisciplinary team meetings to discuss patient care plans.
C) Ensuring all team members have access to the patient's treatment plan.
D) Providing patients with educational materials about their conditions and treatments.

Question 26: Which of the following practices ensures that medical documentation complies with both government and insurance requirements?
A) Including patient demographics and medical history in every note.
B) Ensuring all entries are signed and dated by the provider.
C) Using standardized medical terminology and abbreviations.
D) Documenting only significant changes in patient condition.

Question 27: Which of the following communication strategies is most effective for ensuring patient

understanding and compliance with medical instructions?
A) Using medical jargon to explain procedures in detail.
B) Speaking slowly and repeating key points multiple times.
C) Encouraging patients to ask questions and providing clear, simple answers.
D) Providing written instructions without verbal explanation.

Question 28: John, a 45-year-old male, presents with severe abdominal pain. Upon examination, the pain is localized in the right lower quadrant (RLQ). Which anatomical structure is most likely involved?
A) Cecum
B) Sigmoid colon
C) Spleen
D) Stomach

Question 29: During a routine check-up, Mr. Thompson, a diabetic patient, mentions feeling unusually dizzy and weak over the past few days. As a Certified Clinical Medical Assistant (CCMA), when should you escalate this situation to the supervising nurse or physician?
A) Immediately, as dizziness and weakness could indicate severe hypoglycemia.
B) After checking Mr. Thompson's blood sugar levels and finding them within normal range.
C) Only if Mr. Thompson's symptoms persist for more than 24 hours.
D) At the end of the day during your regular report to the supervising nurse.

Question 30: Sarah is a medical assistant working in a Patient-Centered Medical Home (PCMH) model. During a team meeting, the healthcare team discusses Mr. Johnson's chronic condition management plan. Which of the following actions should Sarah prioritize to effectively participate in this team-based care approach?
A) Ensuring Mr. Johnson's medication list is up-to-date and communicated to all team members.
B) Scheduling follow-up appointments with specialists for Mr. Johnson.
C) Conducting a patient education session on lifestyle modifications for chronic disease management.
D) Documenting Mr. Johnson's symptoms and vital signs accurately in his electronic health record (EHR).

Question 31: After completing a phlebotomy procedure, which of the following actions is most critical to perform immediately to ensure patient safety?
A) Apply a sterile bandage to the puncture site.
B) Instruct the patient to keep their arm elevated for 10 minutes.
C) Monitor the puncture site for signs of bleeding or hematoma.
D) Advise the patient to drink plenty of fluids.

Question 32: John is a newly hired healthcare worker at a large hospital. He is responsible for both administrative tasks and assisting with patient care under the supervision of a physician. John has completed a training program accredited by the Commission on Accreditation of Allied Health Education Programs (CAAHEP). What title should John use?
A) Certified Clinical Medical Assistant (CCMA)
B) Registered Medical Assistant (RMA)
C) Certified Medical Administrative Assistant (CMAA)
D) Licensed Practical Nurse (LPN)

Question 33: During a minor surgical procedure on Mr. Johnson, a medical assistant must ensure that the sterile field is maintained. Which of the following actions is most appropriate to maintain sterility?
A) The medical assistant should open sterile packages away

from the sterile field to avoid contamination.
B) The medical assistant should reach over the sterile field to adjust instruments as needed.
C) The medical assistant should wear non-sterile gloves when handling sterile instruments.
D) The medical assistant should ensure that all items introduced into the sterile field are sterile.

Question 34: Which of the following is considered the most reliable method for verifying a patient's identity before administering medication?
A) Asking the patient to state their full name and date of birth.
B) Checking the patient's wristband against the medical record.
C) Verifying the patient's room number and bed assignment.
D) Confirming with a family member or caregiver.

Question 35: When verifying a phlebotomy order, which step is most crucial to ensure patient safety and accuracy of the test results?
A) Confirming the patient's full name and date of birth with their ID band.
B) Verifying the test requisition form against the patient's medical record.
C) Ensuring that all tubes are correctly labeled before drawing blood.
D) Checking for any allergies or special instructions noted on the order.

Question 36: A patient named Mr. Johnson has been prescribed nitroglycerin tablets for his angina. As a Certified Clinical Medical Assistant, you need to ensure that these tablets are stored correctly to maintain their efficacy. Which of the following storage conditions is appropriate for nitroglycerin tablets?
A) Store in a clear glass bottle at room temperature.
B) Store in an amber glass bottle at room temperature.
C) Store in a plastic container in the refrigerator.
D) Store in an opaque container at room temperature.

Question 37: Which of the following tests is specifically designed to assess a patient's central visual acuity?
A) Snellen Chart Test
B) Ishihara Test
C) Amsler Grid Test
D) Confrontation Visual Field Test

Question 38: Sarah, a 45-year-old patient, presents with a urinary tract infection (UTI). Laboratory results indicate the presence of Gram-negative rods. The physician suspects an extended-spectrum beta-lactamase (ESBL) producing organism. Which of the following bacteria is most likely responsible for this infection?
A) Escherichia coli
B) Staphylococcus aureus
C) Streptococcus pyogenes
D) Clostridium difficile

Question 39: A 45-year-old patient presents with muscle weakness and arrhythmias. The patient's serum potassium level is reported as 6.2 mEq/L. Which of the following best describes this lab value?
A) Normal
B) Mildly elevated
C) Moderately elevated
D) Severely elevated

Question 40: During an EKG reading of a patient named John, you observe a prolonged PR interval. Which condition is most likely indicated by this finding?
A) First-degree AV block

B) Second-degree AV block
C) Third-degree AV block
D) Bundle branch block

Question 41: Which of the following is the most critical step in preventing hemolysis when collecting a blood sample?
A) Using a large-gauge needle
B) Allowing alcohol to dry completely before puncture
C) Filling tubes to their maximum capacity
D) Inverting tubes immediately after collection

Question 42: Which of the following actions is essential to maintain aseptic technique when preparing a sterile field for a minor surgical procedure?
A) Wearing non-sterile gloves before opening the sterile pack
B) Washing hands with soap and water before donning sterile gloves
C) Donning sterile gloves after setting up the sterile field
D) Using an alcohol-based hand rub before opening the sterile pack

Question 43: During a routine check, Maria, a CCMA, notices that the blood pressure monitor is giving inconsistent readings. What is the first step she should take to ensure accurate calibration of the equipment?
A) Replace the batteries and recheck the readings.
B) Adjust the monitor settings according to manufacturer guidelines.
C) Use a calibrated reference device to compare readings.
D) Clean all external parts of the monitor thoroughly.

Question 44: Mr. Johnson is prescribed an antibiotic that needs to be administered intravenously due to severe infection. The nurse prepares the medication in a small-volume parenteral (SVP) bag for administration. Which of the following best describes the correct route and form of administration for this medication?
A) Oral tablet
B) Intramuscular injection
C) Intravenous infusion
D) Subcutaneous injection

Question 45: In the communication cycle, which of the following is crucial for ensuring that the message relayed is clear and concise?
A) Using technical jargon to demonstrate expertise.
B) Providing detailed background information.
C) Ensuring feedback from the receiver.
D) Speaking at a slow pace to ensure understanding.

Question 46: When drafting a formal business email to inform a patient about a change in their appointment schedule, which of the following is the most appropriate closing line?
A) "Please let us know if this new time works for you."
B) "Feel free to reach out with any questions."
C) "Thank you for your understanding and cooperation."
D) "We apologize for any inconvenience this may cause."

Question 47: Which chamber of the heart receives oxygenated blood from the lungs?
A) Right Atrium
B) Left Atrium
C) Right Ventricle
D) Left Ventricle

Question 48: When answering a patient's call, which of the following is the most appropriate initial greeting?
A) "Hello, this is [Your Name], how can I help you today?"
B) "Good morning, you've reached [Medical Office Name], how may I assist you?"

C) "Hi there, what can I do for you?"
D) "This is [Medical Office Name], please hold."

Question 49: During a routine check-up, Sarah, a patient with a history of MRSA (Methicillin-resistant Staphylococcus aureus) infection, visits the clinic. As a Certified Clinical Medical Assistant (CCMA), what is the most appropriate action to prevent cross-contamination?
A) Wear gloves when drawing blood from Sarah.
B) Use hand sanitizer before and after contact with Sarah.
C) Don both gloves and a gown before entering Sarah's room.
D) Disinfect all surfaces in Sarah's room after she leaves.

Question 50: Which regulatory agency is primarily responsible for overseeing the safety and efficacy of medications and medical devices in the United States?
A) Centers for Disease Control and Prevention (CDC)
B) Food and Drug Administration (FDA)
C) National Institutes of Health (NIH)
D) Occupational Safety and Health Administration (OSHA)

Question 51: When is an Advanced Beneficiary Notice (ABN) required to be issued to a Medicare beneficiary?
A) When a service is not covered by Medicare and the provider expects denial of payment.
B) When a service is covered by Medicare but requires prior authorization.
C) When a service is covered by Medicare but might be deemed medically unnecessary.
D) When a service is covered by Medicare but performed out-of-network.

Question 52: John, a medical assistant, is processing blood samples for various tests. After drawing the blood, he needs to centrifuge the samples to separate the plasma. Which of the following actions should John take to ensure accurate results?
A) Centrifuge the blood samples immediately after drawing them.
B) Allow the blood samples to clot before centrifuging.
C) Use a high-speed setting on the centrifuge for faster separation.
D) Balance the centrifuge by placing tubes of equal volume opposite each other.

Question 53: Which of the following is the most effective method for preventing the spread of healthcare-associated infections (HAIs) in a clinical setting?
A) Regular use of alcohol-based hand sanitizers
B) Wearing gloves for all patient interactions
C) Proper handwashing with soap and water
D) Sterilizing medical instruments after each use

Question 54: Emily, a 35-year-old patient, presents with signs of anaphylaxis after being stung by a bee. As a Certified Clinical Medical Assistant (CCMA), which immediate intervention should you prioritize?
A) Administer oral antihistamines
B) Apply ice packs to the sting site
C) Administer intramuscular epinephrine
D) Provide oxygen therapy

Question 55: Which of the following is the most effective duration for hand-washing to ensure optimal removal of pathogens?
A) 10 seconds
B) 15 seconds
C) 20 seconds
D) 30 seconds

Question 56: When performing venipuncture, which of

the following steps is crucial to ensure accurate test results and patient safety?
A) Identifying the patient using two identifiers
B) Applying the tourniquet for more than 2 minutes
C) Using a needle with a gauge larger than recommended
D) Labeling the specimen tubes after leaving the patient's room

Question 57: Maria is a medical assistant reviewing the insurance policy of a patient, John, who recently underwent surgery. John's policy includes a deductible, co-insurance, and an out-of-pocket maximum. John has already paid his deductible for the year. His insurance covers 80% of the costs after the deductible is met. John's total surgery bill is $10,000. How much will John need to pay out-of-pocket for this surgery?
A) $2,000
B) $8,000
C) $1,500
D) $2,200

Question 58: Maria, a 65-year-old patient with diabetes, has difficulty understanding complex medical instructions. As a Certified Clinical Medical Assistant (CCMA), which educational delivery method would be most effective in ensuring Maria comprehends her care plan?
A) Written instructions with medical jargon
B) Verbal instructions using layman's terms
C) Interactive video demonstrations
D) Group education sessions

Question 59: During a busy shift, Medical Assistant Maria observes that patient John Doe experienced a sudden drop in blood pressure after receiving medication. Which of the following actions should Maria take to ensure accurate and effective documentation of this event?
A) Document the event immediately after her shift ends.
B) Record the event as soon as possible, including time, details of the medication, and patient's response.
C) Wait until she can consult with the attending physician before documenting.
D) Write a brief note about the event without specific details to save time.

Question 60: Sarah, a Certified Clinical Medical Assistant, notices that her colleague has been consistently arriving late to work and falsifying their time sheets to avoid reprimand. Sarah is aware that this behavior violates the clinic's professional code of ethics. What should Sarah do according to the professional codes of ethics?
A) Confront her colleague directly about their behavior.
B) Report her colleague's behavior to the clinic's supervisor.
C) Ignore the situation as it does not directly affect patient care.
D) Discuss the issue with other colleagues to gather more opinions.

Question 61: Mrs. Johnson, a 68-year-old patient with a history of hypertension, suddenly complains of severe chest pain radiating to her left arm and jaw while waiting for her routine check-up. As a Certified Clinical Medical Assistant (CCMA), what is your immediate priority action?
A) Administer aspirin and call for emergency medical services (EMS).
B) Provide oxygen via nasal cannula and monitor vital signs.
C) Position the patient in a semi-Fowler's position and start an IV line.
D) Obtain an ECG and prepare for possible defibrillation.

Question 62: After performing an EKG on Mr. Johnson, you need to transmit the results to his Electronic Medical Record (EMR) and inform the provider. Which of the following steps is MOST appropriate to ensure accuracy and confidentiality?
A) Enter the results directly into the EMR, then verbally inform the provider.
B) Print out the results, place them in Mr. Johnson's paper chart, and hand it to the provider.
C) Upload the results to the EMR, verify accuracy, and use secure messaging to notify the provider.
D) Email the results to the provider after entering them into Mr. Johnson's EMR.

Question 63: John, a 65-year-old patient with a history of anticoagulant therapy due to atrial fibrillation, is scheduled for a venipuncture procedure. Which tube should be drawn first to ensure accurate test results and minimize the risk of contamination?
A) Red-top tube
B) Light blue-top tube
C) Green-top tube
D) Lavender-top tube

Question 64: Sarah, a Certified Clinical Medical Assistant (CCMA), is asked by a colleague to share patient John Doe's medical records for a research study. What should Sarah do to ensure she adheres to medical law and ethics?
A) Share the records only after receiving verbal consent from John Doe.
B) Share the records only after obtaining written consent from John Doe.
C) Share the records if the research study is approved by an Institutional Review Board (IRB).
D) Share the records only if John Doe's primary care physician approves.

Question 65: Which of the following is the most critical component in ensuring a successful transition of care for patients being discharged from a hospital to home?
A) Providing the patient with detailed written discharge instructions.
B) Ensuring follow-up appointments are scheduled before discharge.
C) Conducting a thorough medication reconciliation process.
D) Educating the patient's family about post-discharge care.

Question 66: Mrs. Thompson, a 65-year-old patient with a history of chronic obstructive pulmonary disease (COPD), presents with shortness of breath. As a Certified Clinical Medical Assistant (CCMA), which method is most appropriate for accurately measuring her oxygen saturation level?
A) Using a standard digital thermometer
B) Using a pulse oximeter on her finger
C) Using an arterial blood gas (ABG) analysis
D) Using a sphygmomanometer

Question 67: Maria, a medical assistant, is communicating with Mr. Johnson about his upcoming surgical procedure. Mr. Johnson expresses concern about the potential side effects of anesthesia. What is the best approach for Maria to take in this situation?
A) Reassure Mr. Johnson that anesthesia is generally safe and there is nothing to worry about.
B) Provide Mr. Johnson with detailed medical literature on anesthesia and its side effects.
C) Listen to Mr. Johnson's concerns, clarify any misunderstandings, and relay his questions to the provider for further discussion.
D) Advise Mr. Johnson to discuss his concerns directly with the anesthesiologist during his pre-operative visit.

Question 68: You are a CCMA at a busy clinic. A patient named Mrs. Johnson calls to inquire about her lab results. What is the most appropriate way to handle this call?
A) Politely inform Mrs. Johnson that you will check her records and place her on hold.
B) Ask Mrs. Johnson for her date of birth and verify her identity before discussing any details.
C) Immediately provide Mrs. Johnson with her lab results over the phone.
D) Suggest Mrs. Johnson schedule an appointment with her physician to discuss the results.

Question 69: When performing charge reconciliation in an EHR system, which of the following steps is essential to ensure accurate financial reporting?
A) Verifying patient insurance information before entering charges
B) Entering all charges immediately after services are rendered
C) Regularly auditing and adjusting accounts receivable records
D) Ensuring that all staff are trained in using the EHR system

Question 70: John, a 45-year-old male, presents with fatigue, pallor, and shortness of breath. His complete blood count (CBC) results show the following values: - Hemoglobin: 10 g/dL - Hematocrit: 30% - Mean Corpuscular Volume (MCV): 70 fL - Red Blood Cell (RBC) count: 4.0 million cells/mcL Which of the following conditions is most likely indicated by these lab results?
A) Iron deficiency anemia
B) Vitamin B12 deficiency anemia
C) Chronic kidney disease
D) Thalassemia

Question 71: Maria, a 45-year-old patient with diabetes, is being discharged from an acute care hospital. As a Certified Clinical Medical Assistant (CCMA), you need to ensure continuity of care by coordinating with various healthcare services. Which of the following actions is most appropriate to facilitate her transition from hospital to home care?
A) Schedule a follow-up appointment with her primary care physician.
B) Arrange for home health nursing services to visit her at home.
C) Provide her with educational materials on diabetes management.
D) Refer her to a diabetes support group in her community.

Question 72: Which term describes a position closer to the point of attachment or origin of a structure?
A) Distal
B) Proximal
C) Medial
D) Lateral

Question 73: Which defense mechanism involves redirecting unacceptable impulses into socially acceptable activities?
A) Projection
B) Displacement
C) Sublimation
D) Reaction Formation

Question 74: John, a 55-year-old diabetic patient, often misses his follow-up appointments and struggles with medication adherence. As his Clinical Medical Assistant, what is the most effective strategy to facilitate John's compliance and optimize his health outcomes?
A) Schedule follow-up appointments during his initial visit and provide him with a printed reminder.
B) Educate John about the importance of medication adherence and provide him with a pill organizer.
C) Set up a system for regular phone calls to remind John of his appointments and assess any barriers he may face.
D) Provide John with educational brochures about diabetes management during each visit.

Question 75: During a routine check-up, Mr. Johnson's blood pressure readings appear unusually high. Upon investigation, you suspect that the sphygmomanometer might be improperly calibrated. What is the first step you should take to ensure accurate calibration?
A) Compare the device readings with a known standard.
B) Adjust the device settings to match previous patient records.
C) Replace the device with a new one immediately.
D) Consult the manufacturer's manual for specific calibration instructions.

Question 76: During an internal audit at a medical clinic, you are reviewing patient records for compliance with documentation standards. You notice that one of the patient records for Mr. John Doe is missing a physician's signature on a critical procedure note. What is the most appropriate next step to ensure compliance?
A) Sign the note yourself as an authorized medical assistant.
B) Notify the physician and request them to sign the note immediately.
C) Document the missing signature in your audit report and move on.
D) Add a note indicating that the signature was overlooked but approved verbally by the physician.

Question 77: Which of the following structures is unique to gram-negative bacteria and plays a crucial role in their pathogenicity?
A) Peptidoglycan layer
B) Lipopolysaccharide (LPS)
C) Teichoic acids
D) Capsule

Question 78: After performing a venipuncture on Mr. Johnson, a 65-year-old patient on anticoagulant therapy, what is the most appropriate post-procedural care step to ensure proper hemostasis and minimize complications?
A) Apply firm pressure to the puncture site for at least 1 minute.
B) Apply firm pressure to the puncture site for at least 5 minutes.
C) Apply a bandage immediately without applying pressure.
D) Elevate the arm above heart level and apply gentle pressure for 2 minutes.

Question 79: While performing an ear irrigation on Mr. Johnson, a 65-year-old patient with cerumen impaction, which of the following steps should be taken to ensure the procedure is performed safely and effectively?
A) Use cold water to avoid discomfort.
B) Direct the stream of water towards the eardrum.
C) Pull the auricle upward and backward before irrigating.
D) Use a high-pressure stream to ensure removal of cerumen.

Question 80: You are about to administer medication to Mr. John Smith, who is in room 102. Which of the following steps is the most accurate method to confirm his identity before proceeding?
A) Ask Mr. Smith to state his full name and date of birth.
B) Verify Mr. Smith's identity by checking his wristband and asking him to confirm his room number.
C) Confirm Mr. Smith's identity by asking him for his full

name and comparing it with the medication chart.
D) Check Mr. Smith's medical record number against the chart without disturbing him.

Question 81: When entering patient information into an Electronic Health Record (EHR) system, which of the following is the most critical step to ensure data integrity?
A) Verifying patient identity through multiple identifiers
B) Ensuring all fields are filled out completely
C) Regularly updating software to the latest version
D) Using standardized medical terminologies

Question 82: Sarah, a CCMA, is preparing to assist in a minor surgical procedure. She observes that the sterile field has been set up. During the procedure, she notices that a non-sterile item has come into contact with the sterile field. What should Sarah do next to maintain infection control?
A) Remove the non-sterile item and continue with the procedure.
B) Inform the physician and replace any contaminated sterile items.
C) Cover the contaminated area with a sterile drape and proceed.
D) Ignore it if no visible contamination is present.

Question 83: John, a 45-year-old male, visits the clinic complaining of persistent sadness, loss of interest in daily activities, and fatigue for the past six months. As a Clinical Medical Assistant, which initial screening tool should you use to assess John's mental health condition?
A) Generalized Anxiety Disorder 7 (GAD-7)
B) Patient Health Questionnaire-9 (PHQ-9)
C) Beck Depression Inventory (BDI)
D) Hamilton Depression Rating Scale (HDRS)

Question 84: Which of the following is the most critical step to ensure the integrity of a blood sample during transportation?
A) Maintaining the sample at room temperature.
B) Properly labeling the sample with patient information.
C) Using a biohazard bag for transportation.
D) Ensuring timely delivery within 24 hours.

Question 85: Maria, a medical assistant at a busy clinic, is reviewing an aging report to identify overdue patient accounts. She notices that several accounts are more than 90 days past due. What should be her first step in addressing these overdue accounts?
A) Send a final notice letter to the patients.
B) Call the patients to remind them of their overdue balance.
C) Write off the balances as bad debt.
D) Review the accounts for any possible billing errors or adjustments.

Question 86: John, a 35-year-old construction worker, presents with severe pain in his right ankle after falling from a ladder. The ankle is swollen, bruised, and he is unable to bear weight on it. An X-ray shows no bone displacement. What is the most likely diagnosis?
A) Grade II Ankle Sprain
B) Hairline Fracture
C) Severe Contusion
D) Achilles Tendon Rupture

Question 87: Which of the following is the most critical step in preventing the transmission of pathogens according to Universal Precautions?
A) Wearing gloves when handling bodily fluids
B) Using a face mask during patient interactions
C) Performing hand hygiene before and after patient contact
D) Disposing of needles in puncture-resistant containers

Question 88: Which additive is used in blood collection tubes to prevent coagulation by binding calcium ions?
A) Sodium Citrate
B) Heparin
C) EDTA
D) Potassium Oxalate

Question 89: A patient's blood test reveals a potassium level of 6.5 mEq/L. Which of the following is the most appropriate initial response by a Certified Clinical Medical Assistant (CCMA)?
A) Advise the patient to increase their water intake and re-test in 24 hours.
B) Immediately notify the supervising physician and prepare for an ECG.
C) Suggest dietary modifications to reduce potassium intake.
D) Schedule a follow-up appointment for further evaluation.

Question 90: Which auditing method is most effective for ensuring compliance and accuracy in medical record audits?
A) Concurrent Auditing
B) Retrospective Auditing
C) Random Sampling Auditing
D) Targeted Auditing

Question 91: Sarah, a 22-year-old female, presents with severe weight loss, amenorrhea, and an intense fear of gaining weight despite being underweight. She reports excessive exercise and a restrictive diet. Based on her symptoms and behavior, what is the most likely diagnosis?
A) Bulimia Nervosa
B) Anorexia Nervosa
C) Binge Eating Disorder
D) Avoidant/Restrictive Food Intake Disorder (ARFID)

Question 92: Mrs. Thompson, a 58-year-old woman, presents to your clinic for a routine check-up. During the history-taking process, she mentions that her father had heart disease and her mother had diabetes. She also reveals that she underwent gallbladder surgery five years ago and has been experiencing increased stress at work recently. Which element of Mrs. Thompson's history is most relevant for assessing her risk for cardiovascular disease?
A) Her father's history of heart disease
B) Her mother's history of diabetes
C) Her gallbladder surgery
D) Her increased stress at work

Question 93: Which of the following is a contraindication for the use of Warfarin in patients?
A) Active peptic ulcer disease
B) History of myocardial infarction
C) Controlled hypertension
D) Chronic atrial fibrillation

Question 94: Patient John Doe is scheduled for a blood draw. The physician has ordered a Complete Blood Count (CBC) test. As a clinical medical assistant, you are responsible for verifying the order details before proceeding with the blood draw. Which step is MOST critical in ensuring the accuracy of the order?
A) Confirming the patient's full name and date of birth against the order form.
B) Verifying the test type (CBC) with the laboratory requisition form.
C) Ensuring that the physician's signature is present on the order form.
D) Checking that the correct tube type for CBC is available.

Question 95: Which of the following tasks is primarily the responsibility of a Medical Assistant (MA) rather than other healthcare providers or allied health personnel?
A) Administering medication as directed by a physician.
B) Diagnosing patient conditions based on clinical assessments.
C) Developing treatment plans for chronic diseases.
D) Performing surgical procedures.

Question 96: Sarah, a 45-year-old female with a history of osteoporosis, is seeking advice on dietary changes to improve her bone health. Which nutrient is most critical for Sarah to include in her diet to enhance calcium absorption and support bone health?
A) Vitamin D
B) Magnesium
C) Vitamin K
D) Phosphorus

Question 97: Which of the following abbreviations stands for "as needed" in medical terminology?
A) PRN
B) BID
C) TID
D) QID

Question 98: Sarah, a 45-year-old patient with hypertension, was prescribed clonidine for blood pressure management. However, she accidentally received clozapine instead. What potential complication should the medical assistant be most concerned about?
A) Severe hypotension
B) Agranulocytosis
C) Bradycardia
D) Hyperglycemia

Question 99: Sarah, a 45-year-old patient, requires the administration of an antibiotic eye drop for conjunctivitis. Which of the following steps is crucial to ensure proper administration and avoid contamination?
A) Instruct Sarah to tilt her head back and pull down her lower eyelid to create a pocket.
B) Place the dropper tip directly on the surface of the eye for accurate application.
C) Advise Sarah to blink several times immediately after administering the drops.
D) Ensure Sarah closes her eyes gently for 1-2 minutes after instilling the drops.

Question 100: When explaining a blood pressure measurement to a 6-year-old child, which term is most appropriate to use?
A) "Blood pressure"
B) "Arm hug"
C) "Pressure reading"
D) "Squeeze test"

Question 101: During a routine eye examination, Mrs. Thompson reports difficulty distinguishing between red and green colors. Which test is most appropriate to assess her condition?
A) Snellen Chart Test
B) Ishihara Test
C) Confrontation Visual Field Test
D) Audiometry Test

Question 102: When transmitting results or reports to a patient's EMR or paper chart, which of the following is the most important step to ensure accuracy and confidentiality?
A) Verifying patient identifiers before entering data

B) Using generic identifiers for all patients
C) Entering data immediately without verification
D) Relying on memory for patient details

Question 103: When preparing to administer an intramuscular (IM) injection, which needle gauge and length are most appropriate for an average adult patient?
A) 25 gauge, 5/8 inch
B) 27 gauge, 1/2 inch
C) 22 gauge, 1.5 inches
D) 20 gauge, 2 inches

Question 104: Which medical condition or medication history most significantly impacts the order of draw for venipuncture?
A) Anticoagulation therapy
B) Recent surgery
C) Chemotherapy
D) Chronic kidney disease

Question 105: Which of the following medications is most commonly found in a crash cart for immediate use during cardiac arrest?
A) Epinephrine
B) Atropine
C) Amiodarone
D) Lidocaine

Question 106: Which of the following is considered one of the fundamental "Rights" of medication administration to ensure patient safety?
A) Right Diagnosis
B) Right Patient
C) Right Physician
D) Right Insurance

Question 107: Which of the following is the most critical step for a medical assistant when preparing a patient for cryosurgery?
A) Ensuring the patient has fasted for at least 8 hours before the procedure.
B) Applying a topical anesthetic to the area to be treated.
C) Verifying that informed consent has been obtained and documented.
D) Sterilizing all surgical instruments thoroughly.

Question 108: Which of the following actions best demonstrates a medical assistant's effective collaboration with community-based organizations to enhance patient care?
A) Referring patients to local food banks for nutritional support.
B) Coordinating with a patient's primary care physician for follow-up appointments.
C) Providing patients with information on local transportation services.
D) Facilitating patient enrollment in community health education programs.

Question 109: When preparing a patient for a thoracentesis procedure, which position is most appropriate to facilitate access to the pleural space?
A) Supine with arms at the sides
B) Sitting upright and leaning forward over a table
C) Lateral decubitus with the affected side up
D) Prone with arms extended

Question 110: A 45-year-old patient named Mr. Johnson presents with a fever, chills, and localized redness and swelling at the site of a recent surgical incision. He also reports feeling generally unwell. Which sign most definitively indicates an infection at the surgical site?

A) Increased pain at the surgical site
B) Purulent discharge from the incision
C) Elevated white blood cell count
D) General malaise

Question 111: Sarah, a Certified Clinical Medical Assistant, is responsible for managing medication storage in a busy clinic. She notices that a vial of insulin has been left out at room temperature for an unknown period. According to best practices for medication storage, what should Sarah do with the insulin vial?
A) Return it to the refrigerator immediately and use it within 28 days.
B) Discard the insulin vial immediately as it may have lost its efficacy.
C) Store it at room temperature and use it within 14 days.
D) Mark the vial with the date and time found and use it within 7 days.

Question 112: John, a 55-year-old male with a history of type 2 diabetes, presents for a routine check-up. His fasting blood glucose level is reported as 250 mg/dL. As a Certified Clinical Medical Assistant (CCMA), what is the most appropriate initial response?
A) Advise John to increase his insulin dose immediately.
B) Notify the supervising physician and prepare to recheck the blood glucose level.
C) Schedule an appointment with a dietitian for dietary adjustments.
D) Instruct John to monitor his blood glucose levels more frequently at home.

Question 113: Sarah, a 45-year-old patient, is scheduled for a surgical procedure. During her pre-operative consultation, she expresses concerns about potential complications and asks detailed questions about the risks involved. The physician explains the procedure and its risks but does not provide written documentation. What should the medical assistant do to ensure compliance with informed consent laws?
A) Reassure Sarah verbally that the physician has explained everything.
B) Provide Sarah with written documentation outlining the procedure and risks.
C) Document in Sarah's medical record that she verbally agreed to the procedure.
D) Ask Sarah to sign a consent form without further explanation.

Question 114: Jane, a 55-year-old patient with diabetes, has been experiencing difficulty managing her condition due to lack of access to nutritious food. As a Certified Clinical Medical Assistant (CCMA), which is the best approach to collaborate with healthcare providers and community-based organizations to address Jane's needs?
A) Refer Jane to a dietitian within the healthcare facility.
B) Coordinate with a local food bank that provides diabetic-friendly food options.
C) Schedule regular follow-up appointments with Jane's primary care physician.
D) Enroll Jane in an online diabetes management program.

Question 115: John Doe is scheduled for a minor surgical procedure. As a Certified Clinical Medical Assistant (CCMA), you are responsible for verifying his identity before proceeding. Which of the following methods provides the most accurate and comprehensive verification of John Doe's identity?
A) Asking John Doe to state his full name and date of birth.
B) Checking John Doe's wristband for his name and medical record number.
C) Verifying John Doe's full name, date of birth, and home

address.
D) Confirming John Doe's name and comparing it with his photograph in the medical record.

Question 116: Sarah is a newly graduated medical assistant looking to start her career in a clinical setting. She is aware that she needs to meet certain professional standards before she can begin working. Which of the following actions should Sarah prioritize to ensure she meets the necessary professional requirements?
A) Obtain state licensure specific to medical assistants.
B) Achieve certification through a recognized certifying body.
C) Complete a mandatory residency program in medical assistance.
D) Enroll in continuing education courses immediately after graduation.

Question 117: Which of the following actions best demonstrates compliance with the Health Insurance Portability and Accountability Act (HIPAA) regulations regarding patient confidentiality?
A) Sharing patient information only with family members who provide a written consent.
B) Discussing patient information in a private room with authorized healthcare providers.
C) Leaving detailed patient records on a desk in a restricted access area.
D) Providing patient information to insurance companies without verifying their request validity.

Question 118: You are assisting Dr. Smith in the emergency room when a patient named John suddenly collapses and becomes unresponsive. You immediately check for a pulse and find none. What is the correct depth of chest compressions you should perform during CPR for an adult?
A) At least 1 inch (2.5 cm)
B) At least 2 inches (5 cm)
C) At least 3 inches (7.5 cm)
D) At least 4 inches (10 cm)

Question 119: Which of the following drugs is primarily metabolized by cytochrome P450 enzymes in the liver?
A) Acetaminophen
B) Warfarin
C) Metformin
D) Furosemide

Question 120: Which form of medication is specifically designed to release its active ingredient slowly over an extended period?
A) Extended-release tablet
B) Immediate-release capsule
C) Enteric-coated pill
D) Transdermal patch

Question 121: Sarah, a 45-year-old woman with chronic lower back pain, is exploring alternative therapies to manage her symptoms. After consulting with her healthcare provider, which of the following therapies is most supported by contemporary research for effectively reducing chronic lower back pain?
A) Acupuncture
B) Aromatherapy
C) Homeopathy
D) Reflexology

Question 122: Which of the following is the most appropriate way to start a professional email to a patient regarding their upcoming appointment?
A) "Hey there, just a reminder about your appointment."
B) "Dear [Patient's Name], I hope this email finds you well."
C) "Hi [Patient's Name], your appointment is coming up

soon."
D) "Good day, please be reminded of your upcoming appointment."

Question 123: What is the most effective method for ensuring proper patient identification before administering medication in a clinical setting?
A) Asking the patient to state their full name and date of birth.
B) Checking the patient's wristband against the medical chart.
C) Verifying the patient's room number and bed assignment.
D) Confirming with a family member or caregiver.

Question 124: Mrs. Johnson, a 78-year-old frail patient with limited mobility, needs assistance transferring from her bed to a wheelchair. As a Clinical Medical Assistant, which of the following actions should you prioritize to ensure her safety during the transfer?
A) Use a gait belt to provide support and maintain balance.
B) Ask Mrs. Johnson to hold onto your shoulders while you lift her.
C) Position the wheelchair at a 45-degree angle to the bed.
D) Have Mrs. Johnson stand up quickly to minimize time spent transferring.

Question 125: Which community resource is specifically designed to provide supervised care and social activities for elderly individuals during daytime hours?
A) Adult Day Care
B) Home Health Care
C) Assisted Living Facility
D) Senior Community Center

Question 126: Sarah, a 55-year-old patient, is scheduled for an EKG test. As a Certified Clinical Medical Assistant, which of the following tasks is most crucial to ensure accurate results?
A) Ensuring Sarah has fasted for at least 8 hours before the test.
B) Instructing Sarah to avoid caffeine for 24 hours prior to the test.
C) Making sure Sarah's skin is clean and free from oils or lotions.
D) Advising Sarah to refrain from taking her morning medications.

Question 127: Maria, a Certified Clinical Medical Assistant (CCMA), needs to send a prescription refill request for a patient named John Doe. She decides to use email to communicate with the pharmacy. Which of the following actions should Maria take to ensure compliance with guidelines?
A) Include only the patient's first name and prescription details in the email.
B) Encrypt the email before sending it to protect patient information.
C) Send the email from her personal account to expedite the process.
D) Attach a scanned copy of John's medical record for reference.

Question 128: When communicating with a patient over the telephone regarding their medical condition, which of the following practices is MOST crucial to ensure effective and professional communication?
A) Using medical jargon to explain the condition clearly
B) Ensuring patient confidentiality by verifying their identity
C) Providing detailed personal opinions about the treatment options
D) Speaking quickly to cover more information in less time

Question 129: Which of the following is the most

appropriate method for ensuring that patient appointments are scheduled efficiently in a busy medical practice?
A) Scheduling patients back-to-back without breaks
B) Implementing an electronic health record (EHR) system with automated reminders
C) Allowing patients to self-schedule their appointments online
D) Scheduling longer appointment slots to accommodate potential delays

Question 130: Sarah, a 35-year-old single mother living in an urban area with high pollution levels, has been experiencing increased anxiety and depressive symptoms. Which of the following is the most likely primary environmental stressor contributing to her mental health issues?
A) Noise pollution from nearby traffic
B) Limited access to green spaces
C) Exposure to industrial air pollutants
D) Crowded living conditions

Question 131: Mrs. Johnson, a 55-year-old woman with chronic lower back pain, is considering alternative therapies after conventional treatments have provided limited relief. She asks you about the efficacy of different therapies based on current research. Which alternative therapy is most supported by contemporary research for managing chronic lower back pain?
A) Acupuncture
B) Homeopathy
C) Aromatherapy
D) Reflexology

Question 132: Mrs. Johnson received a denial for her recent medical procedure from her insurance company, citing "lack of medical necessity." As a Certified Clinical Medical Assistant (CCMA), what is the first step you should take to resolve this issue?
A) Immediately resubmit the claim with additional documentation.
B) Contact Mrs. Johnson's physician to obtain a letter of medical necessity.
C) File an appeal with the insurance company, including all relevant medical records.
D) Advise Mrs. Johnson to pay out-of-pocket and seek reimbursement later.

Question 133: Sarah, a Certified Clinical Medical Assistant, is helping her clinic transition to a new electronic health record (EHR) system. As part of this process, she needs to ensure that the clinic meets Meaningful Use criteria. Which of the following actions is most directly related to fulfilling Stage 2 Meaningful Use requirements?
A) Implementing a patient portal for secure online access to health information.
B) Conducting regular patient satisfaction surveys.
C) Increasing the number of paper-based patient records.
D) Providing printed educational materials during patient visits.

Question 134: Which communication style is characterized by expressing one's needs and desires clearly and respectfully without violating the rights of others?
A) Assertive
B) Passive
C) Aggressive
D) Passive-Aggressive

Question 135: During a routine check-up, Dr. Smith notes that patient John Doe has "bradycardia." What

does this term indicate about John's condition?
A) John has an abnormally slow heart rate.
B) John has an abnormally fast heart rate.
C) John has an irregular heart rhythm.
D) John has high blood pressure.

Question 136: Which of the following medical terms accurately describes the layman's term "heart attack"?
A) Myocarditis
B) Myocardial infarction
C) Angina pectoris
D) Cardiomyopathy

Question 137: Which section of the Safety Data Sheet (SDS) provides detailed information on the potential health effects of exposure to a chemical and the symptoms associated with exposure?
A) Section 2: Hazard Identification
B) Section 4: First-Aid Measures
C) Section 8: Exposure Controls/Personal Protection
D) Section 11: Toxicological Information

Question 138: John, a 45-year-old construction worker, arrives at the clinic with a deep laceration on his forearm caused by a sharp metal edge. As a Certified Clinical Medical Assistant, what is the most appropriate initial step in administering first aid to John?
A) Apply direct pressure to the wound with a sterile gauze pad.
B) Rinse the wound thoroughly with hydrogen peroxide.
C) Elevate the arm above heart level and apply ice directly to the wound.
D) Cover the wound with an adhesive bandage immediately.

Question 139: Sarah, a 65-year-old patient with a chronic illness, wants to ensure her healthcare decisions are respected if she becomes incapacitated. She asks her medical assistant to help her designate a healthcare proxy. Which step should the medical assistant take first to assist Sarah in this process?
A) Provide Sarah with a standard healthcare proxy form to fill out.
B) Explain the importance of discussing her wishes with her chosen proxy.
C) Verify that Sarah's chosen proxy meets legal requirements.
D) Document Sarah's verbal consent for her chosen proxy in her medical record.

Question 140: During a routine check-up, a Medical Assistant named Alex is tasked with disposing of used needles after administering vaccines to patients. Which is the most appropriate disposal method for these used needles?
A) Place them in a regular trash bin.
B) Dispose of them in a puncture-resistant sharps container.
C) Wrap them in gauze and place them in a biohazard bag.
D) Sterilize them and then dispose of them in a recycling bin.

Question 141: Sarah, a 45-year-old patient with Type 2 diabetes, presents with symptoms of dizziness, sweating, and confusion. As a medical assistant, you suspect hypoglycemia. What is the most appropriate immediate action?
A) Administer 15 grams of glucose orally.
B) Administer an insulin injection.
C) Provide a high-protein snack.
D) Advise the patient to rest and rehydrate.

Question 142: Which sterilization technique is most effective for ensuring complete elimination of all microorganisms, including spores, from surgical instruments?

A) Autoclave
B) Instrument Cleaner
C) Germicidal Disinfectants
D) Disposables

Question 143: Sarah, a medical assistant, is preparing to transport a blood specimen for a glucose tolerance test. Which of the following steps should she ensure to correctly follow the requirements for transportation, diagnosis, storage, and disposal of specimens?
A) Label the specimen with only the patient's initials and date of birth.
B) Store the specimen at room temperature until it is picked up by the lab courier.
C) Ensure that the specimen container is sealed properly and labeled with two patient identifiers.
D) Dispose of any unused portion of the specimen immediately after collection.

Question 144: Sarah, a 68-year-old patient with diabetes, has been admitted for a routine check-up. During her visit, she mentions feeling light-headed and dizzy. As a CCMA, what is the most appropriate initial action to take?
A) Administer oral glucose immediately.
B) Check her blood pressure and pulse.
C) Provide her with a glass of water and monitor her symptoms.
D) Notify the supervising physician immediately.

Question 145: A 45-year-old patient named John presents with symptoms of fever, chills, and a productive cough. His sputum culture reveals the presence of bacteria. Which of the following organisms is most likely responsible for John's symptoms?
A) Streptococcus pneumoniae
B) Staphylococcus epidermidis
C) Lactobacillus acidophilus
D) Escherichia coli

Question 146: Which of the following is the most secure method for a medical assistant to verify an electronic funds transfer (EFT) when using online banking?
A) Using a single-factor authentication method.
B) Relying on email notifications from the bank.
C) Implementing multi-factor authentication (MFA).
D) Checking the transaction status on the bank's website.

Question 147: When checking a patient in for an appointment, which step is crucial to ensure accurate patient identification?
A) Asking the patient to state their full name and date of birth.
B) Verifying the patient's insurance information first.
C) Confirming the patient's appointment time before anything else.
D) Collecting the patient's co-payment immediately upon arrival.

Question 148: What is the most effective strategy a medical assistant can use to ensure a patient's medication compliance?
A) Providing written instructions for medication use.
B) Scheduling regular follow-up appointments.
C) Educating the patient about the importance of their medication regimen.
D) Encouraging patients to use a pill organizer.

Question 149: When matching and labeling a specimen to a patient and completed requisition form, which of the following steps is most critical to ensure accuracy?
A) Verify the patient's identity by asking them to state their full name and date of birth.

B) Compare the specimen label with the patient's wristband only.
C) Ensure that the requisition form is signed by the physician before labeling.
D) Label the specimen immediately after collection in front of the patient.

Question 150: Maria, a patient with severe hearing impairment, visits the clinic for a routine check-up. Which is the most appropriate method for effectively communicating with her?
A) Speak loudly and exaggerate lip movements.
B) Use written notes or text messaging.
C) Rely solely on an interpreter.
D) Ensure face-to-face interaction and speak clearly.

ANSWER WITH DETAILED EXPLANATION SET [4]

Question 1: Correct Answer: B) Ensure proper ventilation in the area.
Rationale: Ensuring proper ventilation is crucial because it prevents the inhalation of harmful fumes, which can cause respiratory issues or other systemic effects. While wearing gloves and a face shield (Option A) is important for personal protection, it doesn't address airborne risks. Storing chemicals in labeled containers (Option C) ensures proper identification but doesn't mitigate immediate exposure risks. Disposing of chemicals according to MSDS guidelines (Option D) is essential for long-term safety but does not address immediate handling precautions. Therefore, ensuring proper ventilation (Option B) is the most critical precaution.

Question 2: Correct Answer: A) Streptococcus pyogenes
Rationale: Streptococcus pyogenes is the bacterium responsible for causing strep throat, a common infection of the throat and tonsils. Streptococcus pneumoniae, while also a pathogen, primarily causes pneumonia and meningitis. Staphylococcus aureus is known for causing skin infections and other conditions but not typically strep throat. Escherichia coli is generally associated with gastrointestinal infections and urinary tract infections. The key difference lies in their specific pathogenic roles, making Streptococcus pyogenes the correct answer due to its direct association with strep throat.

Question 3: Correct Answer: B) Anonymity of responses
Rationale: Anonymity of responses (B) is crucial for ensuring the validity of patient satisfaction survey results because it encourages honesty and reduces social desirability bias. Survey length (A), while important for response rates, does not directly impact the validity of responses. Timing of survey administration (C) can influence recall accuracy but isn't as critical as anonymity. Question wording (D) affects clarity and understanding but does not have as significant an impact on the honesty and validity of responses as anonymity does.

Question 4: Correct Answer: A) Cholecystectomy
Rationale: Cholecystectomy is the correct term for the surgical removal of the gallbladder. "Chole-" refers to bile or gall, and "-cyst" refers to a sac or bladder, while "-ectomy" means surgical removal. Cholelithiasis (B) refers to gallstones formation; "lithiasis" means stone formation. Cholecystitis (C) is inflammation of the gallbladder; "-itis" denotes inflammation. Choledochotomy (D) involves an incision into the common bile duct; "choledocho-" refers to the bile duct, and "-tomy" indicates cutting or incision. The key difference lies in understanding suffixes like "-ectomy," "-itis," and "-tomy," which denote different medical procedures or conditions.

Question 5: Correct Answer: C) Nitroglycerin
Rationale: Nitroglycerin is highly sensitive to light and heat, necessitating storage in a dark, cool environment to prevent degradation. Insulin also requires refrigeration but is less sensitive to light. Vitamin C is sensitive to light but more stable at room temperature. Levothyroxine should be stored away from light but does not specifically require a cool environment. Thus, Nitroglycerin's dual sensitivity makes it the correct answer.

Question 6: Correct Answer: C) Verify Mr. Thompson's insurance details by contacting his insurance provider before his appointment.
Rationale: The correct action is to verify Mr. Thompson's insurance details by contacting his insurance provider before his appointment (Option C). This ensures that the most accurate and current information is on file, which is crucial for billing and avoiding claim denials. Option A is incorrect because reminding the patient does not guarantee the update will be done timely or accurately. Option B is incorrect because using outdated information can lead to errors in billing and coverage issues. Option D is unnecessary and inefficient as it adds an extra step when verification can be done directly with the provider.

Question 7: Correct Answer: C) Chlorine bleach solutions
Rationale: Chlorine bleach solutions are recognized as the most effective method for disinfecting surfaces contaminated with Clostridium difficile spores due to their sporicidal properties. Alcohol-based disinfectants (A) and quaternary ammonium compounds (B) are ineffective against spores. Hydrogen peroxide vapor (D) can be effective but is less practical for routine surface disinfection compared to chlorine bleach solutions. This question tests the candidate's knowledge of specific pathogen control and appropriate disinfection methods in clinical settings.

Question 8: Correct Answer: B) Cholecystectomy
Rationale: A cholecystectomy is the surgical removal of the gallbladder, typically performed to treat acute cholecystitis (inflammation of the gallbladder). Appendectomy (A) is the removal of the appendix, usually due to appendicitis. Herniorrhaphy (C) is the surgical repair of a hernia. Colectomy (D) involves removing part or all of the colon, often for conditions like colorectal cancer or diverticulitis. The key difference lies in the specific anatomical targets and indications for each procedure, making cholecystectomy the correct answer for treating acute gallbladder inflammation.

Question 9: Correct Answer: C) Following up with the patient through a phone call.
Rationale: Following up with the patient through a phone call is most effective as it allows for personal interaction, immediate clarification of issues, and reassurance that their concerns are being addressed. Offering a discount (A) might not address the emotional aspect of the complaint. Providing immediate feedback to staff (B) is important internally but doesn't directly resolve the patient's dissatisfaction. Sending an apology email (D) lacks the personal touch and immediacy that a phone call provides.

Question 10: Correct Answer: B) "Dear Mr. Johnson,"
Rationale: Option B is correct because it maintains a professional tone and uses the patient's last name, which is appropriate for formal communication. Option A ("Hey Mr. J,") is too casual and informal. Option C ("Hi there,") lacks personalization and professionalism. Option D ("Hello John,") is overly familiar without permission to use the patient's first name. By addressing these nuances, we

ensure that test-takers understand the importance of maintaining professionalism in written communication with patients.

Question 11: Correct Answer: B) A medical assistant sharing patient information with a family member without the patient's consent.

Rationale: Option B is correct because sharing patient information without consent breaches HIPAA regulations. Option A is incorrect as it involves necessary communication for patient care. Option C is also incorrect because accessing records during an emergency is permissible under HIPAA. Option D is incorrect since de-identified data can be used for research without breaching confidentiality. The key difference lies in whether consent or necessity justifies the sharing of information, which makes option B the breach scenario.

Question 12: Correct Answer: B) Confirming patient understanding through teach-back method

Rationale: The teach-back method is crucial because it ensures that the patient comprehensively understands the discharge instructions by having them repeat the information in their own words. This technique helps identify any misunderstandings and allows for clarification. While providing written instructions (A), advising to contact their provider (C), and scheduling follow-up appointments (D) are important, they do not directly confirm patient comprehension at the time of discharge. Thus, option B is superior in ensuring immediate understanding and adherence.

Question 13: Correct Answer: C) 2-0 Nylon

Rationale: Nylon sutures (2-0) are non-absorbable and offer strong tensile strength with minimal tissue reaction, making them suitable for deep lacerations. Vicryl (A), while absorbable and strong, is not ideal for long-term tensile strength. Silk (B), though non-absorbable, has higher tissue reactivity. Chromic Gut (D), an absorbable suture, is less optimal for areas requiring prolonged support.

Question 14: Correct Answer: A) Language barrier

Rationale: The primary barrier in this scenario is the language barrier, as Maria's limited English proficiency prevents her from understanding educational materials provided in English. While socio-economic status, cultural differences, and education level are also significant barriers, they do not directly address the immediate issue of communication and comprehension critical for managing her diabetes effectively. Understanding contemporary research shows that language barriers often lead to miscommunication and misunderstanding in healthcare settings. - A) Language barrier - Correct because Maria's limited English proficiency directly impacts her ability to understand medical instructions. - B) Socio-economic status - Incorrect but plausible; while it affects access to resources, it doesn't directly hinder immediate comprehension of care instructions. - C) Cultural differences - Incorrect but relevant; cultural factors may influence health beliefs but are secondary to the immediate communication issue. - D) Education level - Incorrect but close; while low education can impact understanding health information, the key issue here is language comprehension. This analysis ensures that test-takers must discern between closely related barriers to identify the primary issue affecting patient care.

Question 15: Correct Answer: B) Ensuring the EKG machine is properly calibrated before each use.

Rationale: Proper calibration of the EKG machine is fundamental to obtaining accurate readings, as it ensures that electrical signals are correctly interpreted and displayed. While securing leads (A), maintaining patient stillness (C), and setting paper speed (D) are important, they do not directly address potential calibration errors that can significantly impact results. Calibration verifies machine accuracy, which is essential for reliable diagnostics.

Question 16: Correct Answer: B) Verifying the voltage calibration signal is set at 1 mV.

Rationale: Verifying that the voltage calibration signal is set at 1 mV is crucial because it ensures that the EKG machine accurately measures and displays electrical activity from the heart. Incorrectly calibrated voltage can lead to misinterpretation of cardiac conditions. - Option A, adjusting paper speed, while important for reading clarity, does not affect accuracy. - Option C, proper electrode placement, affects signal quality but not calibration. - Option D, plugging into a grounded outlet, prevents electrical interference but does not directly impact calibration accuracy. The correct step (B) directly impacts the machine's ability to produce reliable data.

Question 17: Correct Answer: B) Cognitive Behavioral Therapy (CBT)

Rationale: Cognitive Behavioral Therapy (CBT) is most effective because it focuses on altering dysfunctional thoughts and behaviors, promoting adaptive coping strategies. Psychoanalytic and psychodynamic therapies delve into unconscious processes but are less focused on immediate coping skills. Humanistic therapy emphasizes self-actualization rather than specific coping mechanisms. CBT's structured approach aligns well with contemporary research supporting its efficacy in managing chronic illness and disability. Each option analyzed: - A) Psychoanalytic Therapy: Focuses on unconscious processes and past experiences; less immediate impact on coping strategies. - C) Humanistic Therapy: Emphasizes personal growth and self-actualization; not specifically tailored for adaptive coping. - D) Psychodynamic Therapy: Similar to psychoanalytic but with more focus on emotional processes; still less effective for immediate coping needs.

Question 18: Correct Answer: A) Tonometer

Rationale: A tonometer is specifically used to measure intraocular pressure, which is crucial for diagnosing glaucoma. An ophthalmoscope is used to examine the interior structures of the eye, a retinoscope assesses refractive errors by observing reflections from the retina, and a slit lamp provides a magnified view of the eye's anterior segment. While all these instruments are used in ophthalmology, only the tonometer measures intraocular pressure directly, making it the correct answer.

Question 19: Correct Answer: C) Ask Mr. Johnson to demonstrate how he will take his medication and explain his dietary plan.

Rationale: Asking Mr. Johnson to demonstrate how he will take his medication and explain his dietary plan ensures that he comprehends the instructions through active participation, which is a key teaching strategy in patient education. This method allows Maria to identify any misunderstandings or gaps in knowledge immediately. - Option A is incorrect because reading aloud doesn't guarantee comprehension. - Option B is less effective as it relies solely on verbal communication without confirming understanding. - Option D is beneficial but doesn't provide immediate feedback on Mr. Johnson's understanding. By comparing these options, we see that option C actively involves the patient in demonstrating their understanding, making it the most effective approach for ensuring comprehension of discharge instructions.

Question 20: Correct Answer: B) Methadone

Rationale: Methadone is classified as a Schedule II controlled substance due to its high potential for abuse, which may lead to severe psychological or physical dependence. Alprazolam (Option A) and Diazepam (Option C) are both Schedule IV substances, which have a lower potential for abuse relative to Schedule II drugs. Tramadol (Option D), while often considered less dangerous, is classified as a Schedule IV drug due to its lower abuse potential compared to Schedule II substances. Understanding these classifications helps in recognizing the varying levels of control and regulation required for different medications.

Question 21: Correct Answer: C) Educating the patient

about medication adherence

Rationale: Educating the patient about medication adherence is crucial because it directly impacts their ability to manage multiple chronic conditions effectively. While scheduling follow-up appointments (A), documenting patient history (B), and communicating lab results (D) are important tasks, they do not have as immediate an effect on patient outcomes as ensuring that patients understand and adhere to their medication regimens. This education can prevent complications, reduce hospital readmissions, and improve overall health outcomes, making it the most critical task in this context.

Question 22: Correct Answer: C) Recommend she visit the nearest emergency room immediately.

Rationale: Severe chest pain radiating to the left arm and shortness of breath are classic signs of a potential heart attack, requiring immediate medical attention. Option A and B delay necessary care, increasing risk. Option D is inappropriate for potentially life-threatening symptoms.

Question 23: Correct Answer: A) Accountable Care Organization (ACO)

Rationale: An Accountable Care Organization (ACO) is a healthcare delivery model that emphasizes coordinated care among multiple providers to improve patient outcomes and reduce costs. While a Patient-Centered Medical Home (PCMH) also focuses on coordinated care, it is typically centered around primary care. Health Maintenance Organizations (HMOs) and Preferred Provider Organizations (PPOs) are insurance models that focus more on cost management rather than coordination across multiple providers. Thus, ACOs uniquely emphasize both coordination and cost reduction across various providers, making them distinct in this context.

Question 24: Correct Answer: B) Patient's full name, date of birth, test requested, and provider's contact information

Rationale: The most critical set of information includes the patient's full name and date of birth for accurate identification, the test requested to ensure proper processing in the lab, and the provider's contact information for any necessary follow-up or clarification. Option A omits the provider's contact information which is crucial for follow-up. Option C omits the date of birth which is essential for patient identification. Option D omits the provider's contact information which is necessary for any further communication regarding the test.

Question 25: Correct Answer: B) Scheduling regular interdisciplinary team meetings to discuss patient care plans.

Rationale: Scheduling regular interdisciplinary team meetings ensures that all healthcare providers are on the same page regarding patient care, which can significantly improve outcomes. While updating EHRs (Option A) and providing access to treatment plans (Option C) are important, they do not facilitate active communication and collaboration as effectively as regular meetings. Providing educational materials (Option D) is crucial for patient education but does not directly address coordination among healthcare providers.

Question 26: Correct Answer: B) Ensuring all entries are signed and dated by the provider.

Rationale: Ensuring all entries are signed and dated by the provider is crucial for compliance with government and insurance requirements, as it verifies authenticity and accountability. Option A is important but not as critical for compliance. Option C is good practice but not specifically required by regulations. Option D is incorrect because comprehensive documentation, not just significant changes, is necessary for compliance.

Question 27: Correct Answer: C) Encouraging patients to ask questions and providing clear, simple answers.

Rationale: Encouraging patients to ask questions and providing clear, simple answers (Option C) ensures that patients fully understand their medical instructions, which is crucial for compliance. Using medical jargon (Option A) can confuse patients, speaking slowly and repeating points (Option B) may not address specific patient concerns, and providing only written instructions (Option D) lacks the interactive component necessary for clarity. Effective communication involves active engagement with the patient to ensure they comprehend their care plan fully.

Question 28: Correct Answer: A) Cecum

Rationale: The cecum is located in the right lower quadrant (RLQ) of the abdomen and is often associated with conditions like appendicitis. The sigmoid colon is in the lower left quadrant (LLQ), making it an incorrect option. The spleen is situated in the left upper quadrant (LUQ), while the stomach primarily occupies the left upper quadrant (LUQ) and some of the epigastric region. Therefore, these options are incorrect due to their anatomical locations not aligning with RLQ pain.

Question 29: Correct Answer: A) Immediately, as dizziness and weakness could indicate severe hypoglycemia.

Rationale: The correct option is A because dizziness and weakness in a diabetic patient can be signs of severe hypoglycemia, which requires immediate attention to prevent serious complications. Option B is incorrect as normal blood sugar levels do not rule out other urgent issues. Option C is incorrect because waiting 24 hours could delay necessary treatment. Option D is incorrect as it postpones critical intervention that should occur immediately. Prompt escalation ensures timely assessment and management by healthcare providers.

Question 30: Correct Answer: A) Ensuring Mr. Johnson's medication list is up-to-date and communicated to all team members.

Rationale: In a PCMH model, ensuring accurate communication of Mr. Johnson's medication list among all team members is crucial for coordinated care and preventing medication errors. While scheduling follow-ups (B), conducting patient education (C), and documenting symptoms (D) are important tasks, they do not directly address the immediate need for comprehensive communication among the healthcare team, which is central to effective team-based care.

Question 31: Correct Answer: C) Monitor the puncture site for signs of bleeding or hematoma.

Rationale: Monitoring the puncture site for signs of bleeding or hematoma is crucial immediately after phlebotomy to prevent complications. While applying a sterile bandage (Option A) is important, it does not directly address monitoring for complications. Instructing the patient to keep their arm elevated (Option B) and advising them to drink plenty of fluids (Option D) are beneficial but are secondary actions compared to immediate monitoring. Monitoring ensures any adverse reactions are promptly identified and managed, ensuring patient safety.

Question 32: Correct Answer: A) Certified Clinical Medical Assistant (CCMA)

Rationale: The title "Certified Clinical Medical Assistant (CCMA)" is appropriate for John as he has completed a training program accredited by CAAHEP, which qualifies him to perform both administrative and clinical tasks under physician supervision. The RMA is also a credential for medical assistants but is typically awarded by a different accrediting body, the American Medical Technologists (AMT). The CMAA focuses more on administrative tasks alone, while the LPN is a nursing credential requiring different training and licensure.

Question 33: Correct Answer: D) The medical assistant should ensure that all items introduced into the sterile field are sterile.

Rationale: Ensuring that all items introduced into the sterile field are sterile is crucial for maintaining sterility and preventing infection. Option A, while partially correct, does not fully address maintaining sterility within the field itself. Option B is incorrect because reaching over the sterile field can lead to contamination. Option C is incorrect as non-sterile gloves can contaminate sterile instruments. Therefore, Option D is comprehensive and directly addresses maintaining a completely sterile environment during procedures.

Question 34: Correct Answer: B) Checking the patient's wristband against the medical record.

Rationale: The most reliable method for verifying a patient's identity is checking their wristband against the medical record. Wristbands contain critical identifiers like name, date of birth, and medical record number, ensuring accurate patient identification. Option A is less reliable because patients may provide incorrect information. Option C is not recommended as room numbers can change. Option D can be unreliable due to potential miscommunication or lack of familiarity with medical details. Thus, option B ensures accuracy by cross-referencing directly with documented records.

Question 35: Correct Answer: A) Confirming the patient's full name and date of birth with their ID band.

Rationale: Confirming the patient's full name and date of birth with their ID band is crucial as it directly ensures that the correct patient is being tested, which is fundamental for patient safety and accurate results. While verifying the test requisition form (B), labeling tubes (C), and checking for allergies or special instructions (D) are important steps, they come after ensuring patient identification. Misidentification can lead to severe errors, making option A paramount.

Question 36: Correct Answer: B) Store in an amber glass bottle at room temperature.

Rationale: Nitroglycerin tablets are highly sensitive to light and moisture, which can degrade their potency. Storing them in an amber glass bottle protects them from light exposure while maintaining room temperature, which is crucial for their stability. Option A is incorrect because clear glass does not protect from light. Option C is incorrect because refrigeration is unnecessary and may cause condensation. Option D is incorrect as "opaque" does not specify material type; amber glass is specifically recommended for light protection.

Question 37: Correct Answer: A) Snellen Chart Test

Rationale: The Snellen Chart Test is specifically designed to measure central visual acuity by determining the smallest letters a person can read on a standardized chart at a specified distance. The Ishihara Test assesses color vision deficiencies, not acuity. The Amsler Grid Test is used to detect problems in the central visual field, such as macular degeneration, rather than overall visual acuity. The Confrontation Visual Field Test evaluates peripheral vision. Thus, while all options are related to vision testing, only the Snellen Chart directly measures central visual acuity.

Question 38: Correct Answer: A) Escherichia coli

Rationale: Escherichia coli is a common Gram-negative rod known to produce extended-spectrum beta-lactamases (ESBLs), which confer resistance to many beta-lactam antibiotics. Staphylococcus aureus is Gram-positive and not typically associated with ESBL production. Streptococcus pyogenes is also Gram-positive and not known for ESBL production. Clostridium difficile is a Gram-positive rod associated with antibiotic-associated diarrhea but not ESBL production. This detailed differentiation helps identify E. coli as the correct answer due to its specific resistance mechanism and common association with UTIs.

Question 39: Correct Answer: C) Moderately elevated

Rationale: Normal serum potassium levels range from 3.5 to 5.0 mEq/L. A level of 6.2 mEq/L is considered moderately elevated, indicating hyperkalemia, which can cause muscle weakness and arrhythmias. Option A (Normal) is incorrect as it falls outside the normal range. Option B (Mildly elevated) would apply to levels between 5.1-5.5 mEq/L. Option D (Severely elevated) typically refers to levels above 7.0 mEq/L, where immediate intervention is required.

Question 40: Correct Answer: A) First-degree AV block

Rationale: A prolonged PR interval typically indicates a first-degree AV block, where there is a delay in the conduction from the atria to the ventricles but all impulses eventually reach the ventricles. Second-degree AV block (B) involves some impulses not reaching the ventricles. Third-degree AV block (C) is a complete disconnection between atrial and ventricular activity. A bundle branch block (D) affects the electrical conduction through one of the bundle branches but does not specifically prolong the PR interval.

Question 41: Correct Answer: B) Allowing alcohol to dry completely before puncture

Rationale: Allowing alcohol to dry completely before puncture is crucial to prevent hemolysis, as residual alcohol can cause red blood cells to rupture. Using a large-gauge needle (Option A) can also prevent hemolysis but is not as critical as ensuring the site is dry. Filling tubes to their maximum capacity (Option C) is unrelated to hemolysis and more about ensuring sufficient sample volume. Inverting tubes immediately after collection (Option D) prevents clotting and ensures proper mixing with additives but does not directly prevent hemolysis. Therefore, Option B is the most critical step in this context.

Question 42: Correct Answer: B) Washing hands with soap and water before donning sterile gloves

Rationale: Washing hands with soap and water before donning sterile gloves is crucial to eliminate transient flora and reduce the risk of contamination. This step ensures that even if there is an inadvertent breach in glove integrity, the risk of infection is minimized. Option A is incorrect because non-sterile gloves can contaminate the sterile pack. Option C is wrong as it increases contamination risk; setting up a sterile field should be done with sterile gloves. Option D, while good practice, does not replace handwashing before donning sterile gloves. Each option challenges understanding by being partially correct but missing critical steps in maintaining aseptic technique.

Question 43: Correct Answer: C) Use a calibrated reference device to compare readings.

Rationale: The first step in ensuring accurate calibration is to use a calibrated reference device to compare readings (Option C). This ensures that any discrepancies are identified accurately. Replacing batteries (Option A) or adjusting settings (Option B) might be necessary steps but come after confirming inconsistency with a reference device. Cleaning external parts (Option D) is essential for maintenance but not directly related to calibration accuracy.

Question 44: Correct Answer: C) Intravenous infusion

Rationale: Intravenous infusion (C) is the correct answer as it aligns with the need for rapid drug delivery directly into the bloodstream for severe infections, which is achieved through an SVP bag. Oral tablets (A) are not suitable for immediate systemic effects required in severe infections. Intramuscular injections (B) and subcutaneous injections (D), while parenteral routes, do not provide as quick or direct access to the bloodstream as intravenous infusion, making them less ideal for this scenario.

Question 45: Correct Answer: C) Ensuring feedback from the receiver.

Rationale: Ensuring feedback from the receiver is crucial as it confirms that the message has been understood correctly and allows for any necessary clarifications. Option A is incorrect because using technical jargon can confuse the receiver. Option B is incorrect because while background information can be helpful, too much detail can overwhelm and obscure the main message. Option D is incorrect because speaking slowly does not necessarily guarantee understanding; it's more important to confirm comprehension through feedback.

Question 46: Correct Answer: C) "Thank you for your understanding and cooperation."

Rationale: Option C is the most appropriate because it acknowledges the patient's flexibility and fosters a positive relationship. Option A is polite but less formal. Option B invites further questions but does not close the communication effectively. Option D focuses on the negative aspect (inconvenience), which is less ideal in maintaining a positive tone. Therefore, option C best aligns with professional standards for business correspondence in medical settings.

Question 47: Correct Answer: B) Left Atrium
Rationale: The left atrium receives oxygenated blood from the lungs via the pulmonary veins, making it distinct from other heart chambers. The right atrium receives deoxygenated blood from systemic circulation, while the right ventricle pumps deoxygenated blood to the lungs. The left ventricle pumps oxygenated blood into systemic circulation. This question tests detailed knowledge of cardiac anatomy and physiology, specifically distinguishing between the functions and locations of each chamber.

Question 48: Correct Answer: B) "Good morning, you've reached [Medical Office Name], how may I assist you?"
Rationale: The correct answer B) demonstrates professionalism by including a greeting ("Good morning"), identifying the medical office, and offering assistance. Option A), while polite and personal, lacks the identification of the medical office. Option C) is too informal for a professional medical setting. Option D) immediately places the caller on hold without any initial interaction, which is not courteous or helpful. Proper telephone etiquette involves a balance of politeness, professionalism, and clear communication.

Question 49: Correct Answer: C) Don both gloves and a gown before entering Sarah's room.
Rationale: The correct action is to don both gloves and a gown before entering Sarah's room to prevent cross-contamination. While wearing gloves (Option A) and using hand sanitizer (Option B) are important, they alone do not provide sufficient protection against MRSA. Disinfecting surfaces (Option D) is necessary but does not address immediate personal protective equipment needs. Therefore, Option C is the most comprehensive approach in accordance with infection control guidelines for MRSA.

Question 50: Correct Answer: B) Food and Drug Administration (FDA)
Rationale: The FDA is responsible for ensuring the safety, efficacy, and security of drugs, biological products, and medical devices. The CDC focuses on public health and disease prevention. The NIH conducts medical research but does not regulate drugs or devices. OSHA is concerned with workplace safety, not specifically with medications or medical devices. Understanding these distinctions helps clarify why the FDA is the correct answer. - A) CDC: Incorrect because it focuses on public health, not drug/device regulation. - B) FDA: Correct as it oversees drug/device safety and efficacy. - C) NIH: Incorrect since it conducts research rather than regulatory oversight. - D) OSHA: Incorrect because it deals with workplace safety rather than drug/device regulation.

Question 51: Correct Answer: A) When a service is not covered by Medicare and the provider expects denial of payment.
Rationale: An ABN must be issued when a provider believes that Medicare may not cover a service, allowing the beneficiary to decide whether to proceed with the service knowing they may have to pay out-of-pocket. Option B is incorrect because prior authorization does not necessitate an ABN. Option C is close but incorrect; while medical necessity can trigger an ABN, it specifically refers to services expected to be denied. Option D is irrelevant as network status does not affect ABN issuance. Thus, A accurately captures the requirement for issuing an ABN.

Question 52: Correct Answer: D) Balance the centrifuge by placing tubes of equal volume opposite each other.
Rationale: Balancing the centrifuge by placing tubes of equal volume opposite each other is crucial to prevent mechanical failure and ensure even separation of components. Incorrect options: A) Centrifuging immediately can cause incomplete separation if clotting hasn't occurred. B) Allowing blood samples to clot is necessary before

centrifuging serum but not plasma. C) High-speed settings can cause hemolysis, leading to inaccurate results. The correct procedure ensures both safety and accuracy in sample processing.

Question 53: Correct Answer: C) Proper handwashing with soap and water
Rationale: Proper handwashing with soap and water is the most effective method for preventing the spread of HAIs because it removes pathogens that may not be eliminated by alcohol-based sanitizers. While alcohol-based hand sanitizers (Option A) are useful, they are not effective against all types of germs. Wearing gloves (Option B) is important but does not replace the need for proper hand hygiene. Sterilizing medical instruments (Option D) is crucial for invasive procedures but does not address direct person-to-person transmission as effectively as proper handwashing.

Question 54: Correct Answer: C) Administer intramuscular epinephrine
Rationale: Intramuscular epinephrine is the first-line treatment for anaphylaxis due to its rapid action in reversing severe allergic reactions. Oral antihistamines (A) are too slow for acute anaphylaxis. Ice packs (B) can help reduce localized swelling but do not address systemic symptoms. Oxygen therapy (D) may be necessary if respiratory distress occurs but is secondary to administering epinephrine. The key difference lies in the immediacy and efficacy of epinephrine in treating life-threatening symptoms compared to other supportive measures.

Question 55: Correct Answer: C) 20 seconds
Rationale: The CDC recommends washing hands with soap and water for at least 20 seconds to effectively remove pathogens. While options A (10 seconds) and B (15 seconds) are shorter than recommended and less effective, option D (30 seconds) exceeds the necessary duration without providing additional benefit. The correct answer, C (20 seconds), aligns with evidence-based guidelines ensuring thorough cleaning without unnecessary excess.

Question 56: Correct Answer: A) Identifying the patient using two identifiers
Rationale: Identifying the patient using two identifiers is critical to ensure that the correct patient is being tested and treated, which directly impacts test accuracy and patient safety. Option B is incorrect as applying the tourniquet for too long can cause hemoconcentration. Option C is incorrect because using an inappropriate needle gauge can cause hemolysis or injury. Option D is incorrect because labeling should be done in the presence of the patient to prevent mislabeling errors.

Question 57: Correct Answer: A) $2,000
Rationale: After meeting his deductible, John's insurance covers 80% of his surgery costs. Therefore, he is responsible for 20% of the $10,000 bill. This means John will pay $2,000 out-of-pocket (20% of $10,000). The other options are incorrect because: - B) assumes John pays the entire amount without considering insurance coverage. - C) miscalculates the percentage John needs to cover. - D) overestimates John's share by not correctly applying the 20% co-insurance rate. In summary, understanding how deductibles and co-insurance work in conjunction with total costs is crucial in determining out-of-pocket expenses accurately.

Question 58: Correct Answer: C) Interactive video demonstrations
Rationale: Interactive video demonstrations are effective because they cater to visual and auditory learning styles, which can enhance comprehension for patients like Maria who may struggle with complex instructions. Written instructions with medical jargon (Option A) can be confusing for patients without medical background. Verbal instructions using layman's terms (Option B) may not be as effective without visual support. Group education sessions (Option D) might not address individual comprehension issues

effectively. Each option analysis: - Option A: Written instructions with medical jargon may overwhelm Maria due to complexity. - Option B: While using layman's terms is helpful, verbal-only instruction lacks visual reinforcement. - Option C: Interactive video demonstrations provide both visual and auditory learning aids, enhancing comprehension. - Option D: Group sessions might not offer personalized attention needed for Maria's understanding. This thorough analysis ensures that test-takers must deeply understand educational methods and their effectiveness in patient care coordination and education.

Question 59: Correct Answer: B) Record the event as soon as possible, including time, details of the medication, and patient's response.

Rationale: The correct action is to document the event promptly with all relevant details. Immediate documentation ensures accuracy and provides a clear timeline of events, which is crucial for patient safety and legal purposes. Option A is incorrect because delaying documentation can lead to inaccuracies. Option C is not ideal since waiting for consultation might cause delays in critical information being recorded. Option D lacks sufficient detail necessary for comprehensive medical records. Proper documentation includes specifics like time, medication details, and patient response to ensure thorough communication among healthcare providers.

Question 60: Correct Answer: B) Report her colleague's behavior to the clinic's supervisor.

Rationale: According to professional codes of ethics, it is Sarah's duty to report unethical behavior, such as falsifying time sheets, to a supervisor rather than confronting the colleague directly or ignoring it. This ensures that appropriate actions can be taken by those in authority. Confronting a colleague (Option A) could lead to conflict without resolving the issue through proper channels. Ignoring the situation (Option C) is unethical as it allows misconduct to continue unchecked. Discussing with other colleagues (Option D) could lead to gossip and does not ensure resolution through official procedures.

Question 61: Correct Answer: A) Administer aspirin and call for emergency medical services (EMS).

Rationale: Administering aspirin helps inhibit platelet aggregation, which can reduce clot formation during a myocardial infarction. Calling EMS ensures that advanced care is on the way. Providing oxygen (B) is important but not the immediate priority over initiating EMS contact. Positioning the patient (C) and starting an IV line are secondary actions after contacting EMS. Obtaining an ECG (D) is critical but should follow after ensuring EMS has been contacted and initial treatment with aspirin has been administered.

Question 62: Correct Answer: C) Upload the results to the EMR, verify accuracy, and use secure messaging to notify the provider.

Rationale: Option C is correct because it ensures that results are accurately recorded in Mr. Johnson's EMR and maintains confidentiality by using secure messaging for notification. Option A lacks verification of accuracy and verbal communication may not be secure. Option B involves paper charts which are less secure and can lead to misplacement. Option D involves email, which may not be secure for transmitting sensitive health information. Thus, option C is aligned with best practices for security and accuracy in healthcare data management.

Question 63: Correct Answer: B) Light blue-top tube

Rationale: The light blue-top tube, containing sodium citrate, is used for coagulation studies and must be drawn first to avoid contamination from other additives that could affect clotting tests. The red-top (serum), green-top (heparin), and lavender-top (EDTA) tubes follow in the standard order of draw but are not prioritized in this scenario due to their lesser impact on coagulation results. - Option A (Red-top tube): Used for serum tests; drawing it first could lead to

contamination affecting coagulation studies. - Option C (Green-top tube): Contains heparin which can alter coagulation results if drawn before the light blue-top tube. - Option D (Lavender-top tube): Contains EDTA which can interfere with calcium-dependent clotting tests if drawn before the light blue-top tube. The rationale emphasizes the need for proper order of draw to prevent cross-contamination and ensure accurate test results, especially critical for patients on anticoagulant therapy.

Question 64: Correct Answer: B) Share the records only after obtaining written consent from John Doe.

Rationale: According to HIPAA regulations and ethical guidelines, patient information can only be shared for research purposes with explicit written consent from the patient. Verbal consent (Option A) is not legally sufficient. While IRB approval (Option C) is necessary for research, it does not replace the need for patient consent. Approval from John Doe's primary care physician (Option D) does not override the requirement for written patient consent. Thus, Option B ensures compliance with both legal and ethical standards.

Question 65: Correct Answer: C) Conducting a thorough medication reconciliation process.

Rationale: Conducting a thorough medication reconciliation process is crucial as it ensures that all medications are correctly documented and any discrepancies between pre-admission and discharge medications are resolved. This reduces the risk of adverse drug events, which are common during transitions of care. While providing detailed discharge instructions (A), scheduling follow-up appointments (B), and educating the family (D) are important, they do not directly address potential medication errors, making option C the most critical.

Question 66: Correct Answer: B) Using a pulse oximeter on her finger

Rationale: The pulse oximeter is the most appropriate tool for measuring oxygen saturation non-invasively and quickly in patients like Mrs. Thompson with COPD. While ABG analysis (Option C) provides detailed information, it is invasive and not typically the first step in routine monitoring. A digital thermometer (Option A) measures body temperature, not oxygen saturation. A sphygmomanometer (Option D) measures blood pressure, not oxygen levels. Thus, Option B is correct as it aligns with best practices for assessing oxygen saturation in clinical settings.

Question 67: Correct Answer: C) Listen to Mr. Johnson's concerns, clarify any misunderstandings, and relay his questions to the provider for further discussion.

Rationale: The correct approach is to actively listen to Mr. Johnson's concerns, ensure he understands the information correctly, and communicate his questions to the provider for detailed discussion (Option C). This ensures that Mr. Johnson's concerns are addressed comprehensively by a qualified professional while maintaining clear communication lines. - Option A is incorrect because it dismisses Mr. Johnson's concerns without addressing them specifically. - Option B is incorrect as it might overwhelm him with technical details rather than providing personalized clarification. - Option D is partially correct but does not facilitate immediate clarification or address current anxieties effectively. This question tests understanding of effective communication strategies and emphasizes the importance of active listening and accurate information relay in a clinical setting.

Question 68: Correct Answer: B) Ask Mrs. Johnson for her date of birth and verify her identity before discussing any details.

Rationale: The correct answer is B because verifying the patient's identity ensures confidentiality and complies with HIPAA regulations. Option A is incorrect as placing the patient on hold without verification can lead to potential privacy breaches. Option C is incorrect because providing results without verification may violate confidentiality policies.

Option D, while cautious, is not necessary if proper identification procedures are followed, making it less efficient in addressing patient concerns promptly.

Question 69: Correct Answer: C) Regularly auditing and adjusting accounts receivable records

Rationale: Regularly auditing and adjusting accounts receivable records is essential for accurate financial reporting as it ensures that all transactions are correctly recorded and discrepancies are identified and rectified. While verifying patient insurance information (A), entering charges promptly (B), and training staff (D) are important, they do not directly address the accuracy of financial reporting through reconciliation processes. Option C specifically targets the core activity of charge reconciliation by focusing on continuous monitoring and adjustment of financial records. - Option A is incorrect because it focuses on pre-service verification rather than post-service reconciliation. - Option B is incorrect as timely entry is important but does not directly ensure accuracy in financial reporting. - Option D is incorrect since training staff is a preparatory step rather than an ongoing reconciliation activity. This analysis ensures that the question tests knowledge of specific tasks within charge reconciliation, emphasizing continuous auditing and adjustments as critical for accurate financial management in a medical setting.

Question 70: Correct Answer: A) Iron deficiency anemia

Rationale: John's CBC results show low hemoglobin and hematocrit levels, along with a low MCV, which indicates microcytic anemia. The most common cause of microcytic anemia is iron deficiency anemia. Vitamin B12 deficiency anemia typically presents with macrocytic (high MCV) anemia. Chronic kidney disease can cause normocytic or slightly microcytic anemia but usually has additional indicators like elevated creatinine levels. Thalassemia also causes microcytic anemia but often presents with more severe RBC abnormalities and a family history of the condition. Thus, iron deficiency anemia is the most likely diagnosis.

Question 71: Correct Answer: B) Arrange for home health nursing services to visit her at home.

Rationale: Arranging for home health nursing services ensures that Maria receives professional medical care and monitoring in her home environment, which is crucial immediately after discharge. While scheduling a follow-up appointment (Option A) and providing educational materials (Option C) are important, they do not address the immediate need for professional medical supervision at home. Referring her to a support group (Option D) is beneficial for long-term support but not as critical as ensuring immediate post-discharge care. Home health nursing services provide comprehensive, ongoing medical support that bridges the gap between hospital discharge and independent living.

Question 72: Correct Answer: B) Proximal

Rationale: The term "proximal" refers to a position closer to the point of attachment or origin of a structure, such as the shoulder being proximal to the elbow. This contrasts with "distal," which means farther from the point of attachment (e.g., the hand is distal to the elbow). "Medial" and "lateral" describe positions relative to the midline of the body, with medial being closer and lateral being farther away. Understanding these distinctions is crucial for accurate anatomical descriptions.

Question 73: Correct Answer: C) Sublimation

Rationale: Sublimation is a defense mechanism where unacceptable impulses are transformed into socially acceptable actions or behaviors. For example, someone with aggressive tendencies might take up a sport like boxing. Projection involves attributing one's own unacceptable thoughts to others. Displacement redirects emotions from a threatening target to a safer one. Reaction formation involves converting unwanted thoughts or feelings into their opposites. While all options involve handling unacceptable impulses, only sublimation channels them into positive

activities, making it the correct answer.

Question 74: Correct Answer: C) Set up a system for regular phone calls to remind John of his appointments and assess any barriers he may face.

Rationale: Regular phone calls offer personalized reminders and allow for real-time assessment of barriers to compliance, promoting continuity of care. Option A is less effective as printed reminders can be easily forgotten or misplaced. Option B is helpful but does not address appointment adherence. Option D provides valuable information but lacks the personalized follow-up necessary for ensuring compliance.

Question 75: Correct Answer: A) Compare the device readings with a known standard.

Rationale: The first step in ensuring accurate calibration of a sphygmomanometer is to compare its readings with a known standard (Option A). This establishes whether there is a discrepancy. Adjusting device settings based on previous records (Option B) is unreliable as past records may also be inaccurate. Replacing the device immediately (Option C) is premature without confirming if recalibration can solve the issue. Consulting the manufacturer's manual (Option D) is important but comes after identifying if there's an issue by comparison. Thus, Option A is correct as it directly addresses verification of accuracy against a known standard.

Question 76: Correct Answer: B) Notify the physician and request them to sign the note immediately.

Rationale: The correct step in this scenario is to notify the physician and request them to sign the note immediately (Option B). This ensures that all documentation is completed accurately and legally, maintaining compliance with medical record-keeping standards. Option A is incorrect because only authorized personnel can sign off on their own notes. Option C fails to rectify the immediate issue of missing documentation. Option D is inappropriate as verbal approval does not meet legal requirements for medical documentation.

Question 77: Correct Answer: B) Lipopolysaccharide (LPS)

Rationale: Lipopolysaccharide (LPS) is unique to gram-negative bacteria and is a key factor in their pathogenicity due to its endotoxic properties. The peptidoglycan layer (A) is present in both gram-positive and gram-negative bacteria but is thicker in gram-positive. Teichoic acids (C) are found only in gram-positive bacteria. The capsule (D), while contributing to pathogenicity, is not unique to gram-negative bacteria. Thus, LPS's uniqueness and role in immune response make it the correct answer.

Question 78: Correct Answer: B) Apply firm pressure to the puncture site for at least 5 minutes.

Rationale: For patients on anticoagulant therapy, it is crucial to apply firm pressure for at least 5 minutes to ensure proper hemostasis and prevent hematoma formation. Option A is incorrect because 1 minute is insufficient for patients on anticoagulants. Option C skips the essential step of applying pressure, increasing the risk of bleeding. Option D's elevation and gentle pressure may not provide adequate hemostasis in anticoagulated patients. Hence, option B is correct due to its adequacy in ensuring proper clot formation and preventing complications.

Question 79: Correct Answer: C) Pull the auricle upward and backward before irrigating.

Rationale: Pulling the auricle upward and backward helps straighten the ear canal, facilitating effective irrigation. Using cold water (Option A) can cause dizziness; directing water towards the eardrum (Option B) risks injury; using high pressure (Option D) can damage delicate structures within the ear. Therefore, Option C is correct as it aligns with best practices for safe and effective ear irrigation.

Question 80: Correct Answer: A) Ask Mr. Smith to state his full name and date of birth.

Rationale: The most accurate method for confirming a patient's identity involves using two identifiers, such as asking for the patient's full name and date of birth (Option A).

This practice aligns with contemporary research and recognized theories on patient safety, reducing the risk of misidentification errors. Option B is incorrect because room numbers can change and should not be used as an identifier. Option C lacks a second identifier, which is crucial for accuracy. Option D fails to involve direct patient confirmation, increasing the risk of error.

Question 81: Correct Answer: A) Verifying patient identity through multiple identifiers

Rationale: Verifying patient identity through multiple identifiers is crucial to ensure data integrity by preventing mix-ups and ensuring that all information entered corresponds to the correct patient. While ensuring all fields are filled out (Option B), updating software (Option C), and using standardized terminologies (Option D) are important, they do not directly address the core issue of data integrity related to patient identity verification.

Question 82: Correct Answer: B) Inform the physician and replace any contaminated sterile items.

Rationale: The correct action is to inform the physician and replace any contaminated sterile items to maintain a sterile field and prevent infection. Removing only the non-sterile item (Option A) or covering it (Option C) does not ensure sterility. Ignoring potential contamination (Option D) compromises patient safety. Thus, Option B adheres to strict aseptic protocols.

Question 83: Correct Answer: B) Patient Health Questionnaire-9 (PHQ-9)

Rationale: The PHQ-9 is specifically designed for screening depression in primary care settings and is validated for identifying depressive symptoms. The GAD-7 focuses on anxiety disorders, making it less suitable for John's presenting symptoms. The BDI is also used for depression but is more detailed and typically administered by mental health professionals rather than in an initial screening by medical assistants. The HDRS is a clinician-administered scale requiring more time and expertise than typically available in primary care settings.

Question 84: Correct Answer: B) Properly labeling the sample with patient information.

Rationale: Proper labeling of a blood sample with patient information is crucial because it ensures accurate diagnosis and treatment by preventing mix-ups. While maintaining temperature (A), using biohazard bags (C), and timely delivery (D) are important, they are secondary to proper identification. Mislabeling can lead to significant errors in patient care. Temperature control is necessary for certain tests, biohazard bags ensure safety, and timely delivery preserves sample integrity, but none are as fundamental as correct identification.

Question 85: Correct Answer: D) Review the accounts for any possible billing errors or adjustments.

Rationale: Reviewing the accounts for possible billing errors or adjustments should be Maria's first step. This ensures that all charges are accurate before proceeding with collection actions. Sending a final notice (A) or calling patients (B) should follow only if no errors are found. Writing off balances as bad debt (C) is premature and should only be done after exhausting all collection efforts and verifying account accuracy.

Question 86: Correct Answer: A) Grade II Ankle Sprain

Rationale: A Grade II ankle sprain involves partial tearing of the ligament, causing significant pain, swelling, and bruising but no bone displacement on X-ray. A hairline fracture would show a slight crack in the bone on X-ray. A severe contusion would not typically cause such inability to bear weight without visible tissue damage. An Achilles tendon rupture would present with difficulty or inability to push off the foot rather than general ankle swelling.

Rationale: - Option A (Correct): Fits the symptoms of pain, swelling, bruising, and inability to bear weight without bone displacement. - Option B (Incorrect): Hairline fractures show up as cracks on X-rays; John's X-ray showed no bone displacement. - Option C (Incorrect): Severe contusions are marked by tissue damage without ligament involvement; John's symptoms suggest ligament injury. - Option D (Incorrect): Achilles tendon rupture affects movement differently and usually involves a palpable gap above the heel. Each option is crafted to be clinically relevant but distinct upon deeper analysis of symptoms and diagnostic imaging results.

Question 87: Correct Answer: C) Performing hand hygiene before and after patient contact

Rationale: Hand hygiene is universally recognized as the single most effective measure to prevent pathogen transmission. While wearing gloves (Option A), using face masks (Option B), and disposing of needles properly (Option D) are essential components of Universal Precautions, they do not replace the critical role of hand hygiene. Gloves can have micro-tears, masks may not cover all routes of transmission, and improper needle disposal poses risks; however, thorough hand washing or sanitizing disrupts the chain of infection effectively.

Question 88: Correct Answer: C) EDTA

Rationale: EDTA (Ethylenediaminetetraacetic acid) prevents blood coagulation by binding calcium ions, which are essential for clotting. Sodium Citrate also binds calcium but is primarily used for coagulation studies as it preserves clotting factors. Heparin inhibits thrombin and other clotting factors directly, making it unsuitable for hematology tests due to cell morphology alterations. Potassium Oxalate binds calcium but is typically used in glucose testing tubes, not general anticoagulation. Thus, EDTA is specifically chosen for its effectiveness in preventing coagulation without affecting cell morphology, crucial for hematology tests.

Question 89: Correct Answer: B) Immediately notify the supervising physician and prepare for an ECG.

Rationale: Hyperkalemia (potassium level >5.0 mEq/L) can cause life-threatening cardiac arrhythmias. Immediate notification of the physician and preparation for an ECG are critical steps. Option A is incorrect because it delays necessary intervention. Option C, while relevant, is not an immediate response to severe hyperkalemia. Option D also delays urgent care needed for this critical condition.

Question 90: Correct Answer: A) Concurrent Auditing

Rationale: Concurrent auditing involves reviewing records in real-time as patient care is provided, allowing immediate identification and correction of errors. This method ensures high compliance and accuracy by addressing issues promptly. Retrospective auditing (B) reviews records after care, which can delay error correction. Random sampling auditing (C) reviews a random selection of records, which might miss systematic issues. Targeted auditing (D) focuses on specific areas or issues but may overlook broader compliance concerns. Thus, concurrent auditing is the most effective for real-time compliance and accuracy.

Question 91: Correct Answer: B) Anorexia Nervosa

Rationale: Anorexia Nervosa is characterized by severe weight loss, amenorrhea, intense fear of gaining weight, and restrictive eating behaviors. Sarah's symptoms align closely with this diagnosis. - Option A (Bulimia Nervosa) involves binge eating followed by compensatory behaviors like vomiting or laxative use, which Sarah does not report. - Option C (Binge Eating Disorder) involves recurrent episodes of binge eating without compensatory behaviors. - Option D (Avoidant/Restrictive Food Intake Disorder) involves restrictive eating but not necessarily due to fear of gaining weight or body image issues. Thus, Anorexia Nervosa is the most fitting diagnosis based on Sarah's presentation.

Question 92: Correct Answer: A) Her father's history of heart disease

Rationale: Mrs. Thompson's father's history of heart disease is most relevant for assessing her risk for cardiovascular disease due to genetic predisposition. While her mother's diabetes can also contribute to her overall health risk, it is less directly related to cardiovascular issues compared to heart disease. Gallbladder surgery is a past surgical event and not directly linked to cardiovascular risk. Increased stress at work can impact heart health but is not as significant as a direct familial history of heart disease in this context. - Option A is correct because familial history, particularly immediate family with heart disease, significantly raises one's risk for similar conditions. - Option B is incorrect because while diabetes can influence cardiovascular health, it's less directly indicative than a direct family history of heart disease. - Option C is incorrect because past gallbladder surgery does not directly impact cardiovascular risk. - Option D is incorrect as increased stress, although relevant, does not weigh as heavily as a genetic predisposition from an immediate family member with heart disease. This question challenges the test-taker's ability to discern between different elements of patient history and understand their relative significance in assessing specific health risks.

Question 93: Correct Answer: A) Active peptic ulcer disease
Rationale: Warfarin is an anticoagulant used to prevent thromboembolic events. It is contraindicated in patients with active peptic ulcer disease due to the increased risk of severe bleeding. While a history of myocardial infarction (B), controlled hypertension (C), and chronic atrial fibrillation (D) are conditions that may warrant anticoagulation therapy, they do not serve as contraindications for Warfarin use. This distinction requires understanding both the therapeutic uses and risks associated with Warfarin.

Question 94: Correct Answer: A) Confirming the patient's full name and date of birth against the order form.
Rationale: Confirming the patient's full name and date of birth against the order form is crucial to prevent any potential mix-up or error in patient identification. This step ensures that you are drawing blood from the correct patient, which is fundamental to patient safety. While verifying the test type (B), ensuring physician's signature (C), and checking tube type (D) are also important steps, they come after confirming patient identity. Misidentification can lead to serious consequences, including incorrect diagnosis or treatment. - Option A is correct because it directly addresses patient safety by confirming identity. - Option B is incorrect because although verifying test type is essential, it does not address patient identification. - Option C is incorrect because while a physician's signature validates an order, it does not ensure you have identified the correct patient. - Option D is incorrect because having the correct tube type is necessary but secondary to confirming patient identity.

Question 95: Correct Answer: A) Administering medication as directed by a physician.
Rationale: Administering medication as directed by a physician is a key responsibility of Medical Assistants, who work under the supervision of healthcare providers. Option B (Diagnosing patient conditions) is typically the role of physicians or nurse practitioners. Option C (Developing treatment plans) falls under the purview of physicians or specialized nurses. Option D (Performing surgical procedures) is reserved for surgeons and not within an MA's scope of practice. This distinction underscores the collaborative yet specific roles within healthcare teams.

Question 96: Correct Answer: A) Vitamin D
Rationale: Vitamin D is essential for calcium absorption in the intestines and plays a crucial role in bone health. While magnesium, vitamin K, and phosphorus are also important for bone health, they do not directly enhance calcium absorption like vitamin D. Magnesium helps with bone mineralization, vitamin K supports bone protein synthesis, and phosphorus is a component of bone mineral content. However, without adequate vitamin D, calcium absorption is significantly impaired, making it the most critical nutrient for Sarah's condition.

Question 97: Correct Answer: A) PRN
Rationale: PRN stands for "pro re nata," which means "as needed" in medical terminology. BID (twice a day), TID

(three times a day), and QID (four times a day) are all related to the frequency of medication administration, but do not mean "as needed." This distinction is crucial for correct medication scheduling and patient care.

Question 98: Correct Answer: B) Agranulocytosis
Rationale: Clozapine is an antipsychotic medication known for its risk of causing agranulocytosis, a potentially life-threatening condition characterized by extremely low white blood cell counts. While clonidine is used for hypertension and can cause bradycardia (option C) and severe hypotension (option A), these are not relevant to clozapine's primary risks. Hyperglycemia (option D) is also incorrect as it is not a primary concern with either medication in this context. Thus, recognizing the severe hematologic risk associated with clozapine is crucial.

Question 99: Correct Answer: A) Instruct Sarah to tilt her head back and pull down her lower eyelid to create a pocket.
Rationale: Option A is correct because creating a pocket in the lower eyelid ensures that the medication is administered correctly without contaminating the dropper. Option B is incorrect as placing the dropper tip on the eye can cause contamination and injury. Option C is misleading because blinking immediately can cause medication loss. Option D, while partially correct, does not address contamination prevention as effectively as option A. Proper technique minimizes infection risk and ensures medication efficacy.

Question 100: Correct Answer: B) "Arm hug"
Rationale: The term "arm hug" is simple and familiar, making it more understandable and less intimidating for a young child. "Blood pressure" (Option A) and "pressure reading" (Option C) are more technical terms that may confuse a child. "Squeeze test" (Option D), while somewhat relatable, might still evoke anxiety as it implies discomfort. Using child-friendly language like "arm hug" helps in reducing fear and improving cooperation during medical procedures.

Question 101: Correct Answer: B) Ishihara Test
Rationale: The Ishihara Test is specifically designed to assess color vision deficiencies, particularly red-green color blindness. The Snellen Chart Test (Option A) measures visual acuity/distance, not color vision. The Confrontation Visual Field Test (Option C) evaluates peripheral vision fields, not color perception. Audiometry Test (Option D) assesses hearing ability, unrelated to color vision. Thus, only the Ishihara Test directly addresses Mrs. Thompson's reported issue with distinguishing red and green colors.

Question 102: Correct Answer: A) Verifying patient identifiers before entering data
Rationale: Verifying patient identifiers before entering data is crucial to ensure that the information is accurately attributed to the correct patient, maintaining both accuracy and confidentiality. Generic identifiers (Option B) can lead to confusion and errors. Entering data immediately without verification (Option C) risks inaccuracies. Relying on memory (Option D) is unreliable and prone to error. Proper verification aligns with best practices and regulatory requirements, ensuring that sensitive health information is correctly recorded in the patient's medical record.

Question 103: Correct Answer: C) 22 gauge, 1.5 inches
Rationale: For an intramuscular (IM) injection in an average adult patient, a needle gauge of 22 and a length of 1.5 inches are typically recommended to ensure the medication is delivered deep into the muscle tissue. Option A (25 gauge, 5/8 inch) and Option B (27 gauge, 1/2 inch) are generally used for subcutaneous or intradermal injections due to their smaller size and shorter length. Option D (20 gauge, 2 inches) is often used for larger muscles or specific clinical scenarios but is less common for routine IM injections in average adults.

Question 104: Correct Answer: A) Anticoagulation therapy
Rationale: Anticoagulation therapy significantly impacts the order of draw for venipuncture due to the increased risk of bleeding and hematoma formation. This necessitates

prioritizing certain tubes to minimize clotting risks. Recent surgery (B), chemotherapy (C), and chronic kidney disease (D) can affect blood collection, but they do not specifically alter the order of draw as critically as anticoagulation therapy. For example, recent surgery might increase bleeding risk, but it doesn't change the tube sequence. Chemotherapy affects blood cell counts but not draw order directly. Chronic kidney disease affects electrolyte balance but not venipuncture sequence.

Question 105: Correct Answer: A) Epinephrine
Rationale: Epinephrine is the first-line medication used in cardiac arrest situations due to its potent vasoconstrictive properties, which help to increase coronary perfusion pressure and improve the chances of successful resuscitation. While atropine (B) may be used in specific cases such as bradycardia, it is not the primary drug for cardiac arrest. Amiodarone (C) and lidocaine (D) are antiarrhythmic agents used for ventricular arrhythmias but are not considered first-line treatments for cardiac arrest. This differentiation requires knowledge of ACLS protocols and medication indications within emergency action plans.

Question 106: Correct Answer: B) Right Patient
Rationale: The "Right Patient" is a fundamental principle in medication administration to ensure that the correct medication is given to the correct individual. This reduces the risk of medication errors and enhances patient safety. While "Right Diagnosis" (A), "Right Physician" (C), and "Right Insurance" (D) are important in healthcare, they are not part of the core rights of medication administration. The primary focus is on ensuring accuracy in identifying the patient before administering any drug.

Question 107: Correct Answer: C) Verifying that informed consent has been obtained and documented.
Rationale: Verifying informed consent is crucial as it ensures that the patient understands the procedure, risks, and benefits. While fasting (A) may be necessary for some surgeries, it is not typically required for cryosurgery. Applying a topical anesthetic (B) can be important but is secondary to legal and ethical requirements. Sterilizing instruments (D) is vital but usually falls under general preparation rather than being specific to cryosurgery.

Question 108: Correct Answer: D) Facilitating patient enrollment in community health education programs.
Rationale: Facilitating patient enrollment in community health education programs best exemplifies active collaboration with community-based organizations, directly impacting patient care by enhancing their knowledge and self-management skills. While referring patients to food banks (A), coordinating follow-up appointments (B), and providing transportation information (C) are important, they do not specifically demonstrate collaboration with community organizations to improve patient care comprehensively. Option D encompasses broader engagement, aligning with contemporary research emphasizing the importance of educational interventions in community health.

Question 109: Correct Answer: B) Sitting upright and leaning forward over a table
Rationale: The sitting upright and leaning forward over a table position is ideal for thoracentesis as it allows optimal access to the pleural space between the ribs. This position helps in expanding the intercostal spaces and makes it easier for the clinician to insert the needle safely. - Option A (Supine with arms at the sides): Incorrect because this position limits access to the pleural space. - Option C (Lateral decubitus with the affected side up): Incorrect as this may compress the lung on that side, complicating needle insertion. - Option D (Prone with arms extended): Incorrect since this position does not provide adequate access to the pleural space. Each incorrect option was crafted considering common clinical practices but lacks key aspects needed for optimal thoracentesis positioning.

Question 110: Correct Answer: B) Purulent discharge from the incision

Rationale: Purulent discharge is a definitive sign of infection, indicating bacterial activity at the surgical site. Increased pain (A), elevated white blood cell count (C), and general malaise (D) are also associated with infections but can occur in other conditions as well. The presence of purulent discharge specifically points to an infectious process, distinguishing it from other potential causes of these symptoms. Elevated white blood cell count is a systemic response and not specific to the surgical site, while increased pain and general malaise are non-specific symptoms that could result from various conditions.

Question 111: Correct Answer: B) Discard the insulin vial immediately as it may have lost its efficacy.
Rationale: Insulin that has been left out at room temperature for an unknown period should be discarded immediately due to potential loss of efficacy. Unlike other medications, insulin's stability is highly sensitive to temperature variations. Options A), C), and D) are incorrect because they involve using potentially compromised insulin, which could jeopardize patient safety. Option A) is incorrect because once insulin has been exposed to room temperature for an unknown duration, returning it to refrigeration does not guarantee its stability. Option C) assumes a safe room temperature storage period without knowing prior exposure time. Option D) suggests using compromised insulin within 7 days, which is unsafe without knowing exact exposure details.

Question 112: Correct Answer: B) Notify the supervising physician and prepare to recheck the blood glucose level.
Rationale: The correct response is to notify the supervising physician and prepare to recheck the blood glucose level. This ensures that the elevated reading is accurate and allows for timely medical intervention. Option A is incorrect because increasing insulin without physician oversight can be dangerous. Option C is premature; dietary adjustments may be needed but are not the immediate priority. Option D, while useful, does not address the immediate concern of verifying and responding to an acute abnormal result.

Question 113: Correct Answer: B) Provide Sarah with written documentation outlining the procedure and risks.
Rationale: Informed consent requires that patients receive comprehensive information about their treatment, including written documentation of risks and benefits. Option B ensures compliance by providing tangible evidence that Sarah was fully informed. Option A lacks written proof, Option C is insufficient without written documentation, and Option D bypasses proper patient education.

Question 114: Correct Answer: B) Coordinate with a local food bank that provides diabetic-friendly food options.
Rationale: Option B is correct because it directly addresses Jane's immediate need for access to nutritious food, which is critical for managing her diabetes. This approach involves collaboration with community resources tailored to her specific dietary requirements. Option A, while helpful, does not solve the issue of food access. Option C ensures medical oversight but doesn't address the root cause of her problem. Option D offers educational support but lacks the immediate practical solution needed for dietary management.

Question 115: Correct Answer: C) Verifying John Doe's full name, date of birth, and home address.
Rationale: Option C is the correct answer because it uses three distinct identifiers (full name, date of birth, and home address), which significantly reduces the risk of misidentification. Option A is incorrect because it uses only two identifiers, which may not be sufficient in all cases. Option B is close but relies solely on information from the wristband, which could be inaccurate if not updated correctly. Option D involves visual confirmation with a photograph but lacks multiple data points for verification. Comprehensive identification requires multiple identifiers to ensure accuracy and patient safety.

Question 116: Correct Answer: B) Achieve certification

through a recognized certifying body.

Rationale: Certification through a recognized certifying body (such as the CCMA by MSNCB) is crucial for medical assistants to validate their skills and knowledge. Unlike state licensure, which is not typically required for medical assistants, certification ensures they meet industry standards. Residency programs are not standard for medical assistants, and while continuing education is beneficial, it is not an immediate requirement post-graduation. Certification serves as the primary credential confirming their competency. - Option A (Obtain state licensure specific to medical assistants): Incorrect because most states do not require licensure specifically for medical assistants. - Option C (Complete a mandatory residency program in medical assistance): Incorrect because there are no mandatory residency programs for medical assistants; such programs are more common for physicians and nurses. - Option D (Enroll in continuing education courses immediately after graduation): Incorrect because while beneficial, continuing education is not an immediate requirement compared to certification. Each option was crafted considering common misconceptions about the professional requirements for medical assistants. The correct answer focuses on certification, which directly aligns with industry standards and expectations for entry-level practice.

Question 117: Correct Answer: B) Discussing patient information in a private room with authorized healthcare providers.

Rationale: Option B is correct because it ensures that patient information is discussed privately and only with authorized personnel, which aligns with HIPAA's privacy rules. Option A is incorrect because family members must have explicit authorization from the patient, not just written consent. Option C is incorrect as leaving records unattended, even in restricted areas, poses a risk of unauthorized access. Option D is incorrect because it fails to ensure the legitimacy of the request from insurance companies, which could lead to unauthorized disclosure.

Question 118: Correct Answer: B) At least 2 inches (5 cm)

Rationale: The American Heart Association (AHA) guidelines recommend that chest compressions for an adult should be at least 2 inches (5 cm) deep but not more than 2.4 inches (6 cm). This ensures adequate perfusion without causing excessive injury. Option A is incorrect as it is too shallow to be effective. Option C exceeds the recommended depth, increasing the risk of injury, while Option D is excessively deep and highly likely to cause significant harm.

Question 119: Correct Answer: B) Warfarin

Rationale: Warfarin is primarily metabolized by cytochrome P450 enzymes in the liver, specifically CYP2C9. Acetaminophen is also metabolized in the liver but mainly through conjugation reactions and minorly by CYP2E1. Metformin is minimally metabolized and excreted unchanged in urine. Furosemide undergoes minimal hepatic metabolism and is primarily excreted unchanged in urine. Understanding these differences helps in managing potential drug interactions and individualizing patient care.

Question 120: Correct Answer: A) Extended-release tablet

Rationale: Extended-release tablets are formulated to release the active ingredient slowly over time, ensuring a prolonged therapeutic effect. Immediate-release capsules provide rapid drug release, making option B incorrect. Enteric-coated pills protect the stomach lining but do not control the release rate (option C). Transdermal patches deliver medication through the skin over time but differ from oral extended-release forms (option D). This question requires a nuanced understanding of pharmacological formulations and their specific purposes.

Question 121: Correct Answer: A) Acupuncture

Rationale: Contemporary research supports acupuncture as an effective alternative therapy for managing chronic lower back pain. Studies have shown that acupuncture can reduce pain and improve function in patients with chronic lower back

issues. Aromatherapy, homeopathy, and reflexology, while beneficial for other conditions or symptoms, do not have as strong evidence supporting their effectiveness specifically for chronic lower back pain. Aromatherapy is more commonly used for stress relief and mood enhancement, homeopathy lacks robust clinical evidence for pain management, and reflexology is generally used for overall relaxation rather than targeted pain relief.

Question 122: Correct Answer: B) "Dear [Patient's Name], I hope this email finds you well."

Rationale: Option B is the correct answer because it combines a formal salutation ("Dear") with a polite and professional opening phrase. Option A is too informal for professional communication with patients. Option C, while polite, lacks the formality expected in medical settings. Option D, although formal, lacks personalization and warmth. The correct option balances professionalism and courtesy, which is essential in patient communication.

Question 123: Correct Answer: B) Checking the patient's wristband against the medical chart.

Rationale: The most effective method for ensuring proper patient identification is checking the patient's wristband against the medical chart. This practice is recommended by organizations such as The Joint Commission to prevent medication errors. While asking patients to state their name and date of birth (Option A) is also important, it can be unreliable if patients are confused or unable to communicate. Verifying room numbers (Option C) can lead to errors due to room changes. Confirming with family members (Option D) may not always be accurate or feasible, especially in busy clinical settings.

Question 124: Correct Answer: A) Use a gait belt to provide support and maintain balance.

Rationale: Using a gait belt (Option A) is the safest method as it provides additional support and helps maintain balance during transfers. Option B is incorrect because having Mrs. Johnson hold onto your shoulders can lead to instability and potential injury for both parties. Option C, while partially correct in positioning the wheelchair, does not address safety measures directly. Option D is incorrect as standing up quickly can cause dizziness or falls in frail patients. The correct answer ensures stability and minimizes risk of injury.

Question 125: Correct Answer: A) Adult Day Care

Rationale: Adult Day Care centers are specifically designed to offer supervised care, social activities, and sometimes health-related services for elderly individuals during daytime hours. This helps relieve caregivers while ensuring that seniors have a safe and engaging environment. Home Health Care (B) provides medical and personal care at home, which differs from the group setting of adult day care. Assisted Living Facilities (C) offer residential living with personal care services but do not cater specifically to daytime-only needs. Senior Community Centers (D) provide recreational activities but do not offer the level of supervision or structured care found in adult day care centers.

Question 126: Correct Answer: C) Making sure Sarah's skin is clean and free from oils or lotions.

Rationale: Ensuring the patient's skin is clean and free from oils or lotions is crucial because it helps improve electrode adhesion and reduces artifacts in the EKG reading. - Option A is incorrect because fasting is not typically required for an EKG. - Option B is tricky but incorrect as avoiding caffeine can help reduce heart rate variability but isn't as critical as proper skin preparation. - Option D might be relevant in some contexts but generally, patients should follow their usual medication regimen unless specifically instructed otherwise by their physician.

Question 127: Correct Answer: B) Encrypt the email before sending it to protect patient information.

Rationale: Encrypting the email ensures that sensitive patient information is protected during transmission, complying with HIPAA regulations. Option A is incorrect because including only partial patient information still poses a risk if not encrypted. Option C is incorrect as using a personal account does not comply with professional standards and security protocols. Option D is incorrect because attaching full medical records can lead to unnecessary exposure of sensitive data and is not typically required for prescription refills.

Question 128: Correct Answer: B) Ensuring patient confidentiality by verifying their identity

Rationale: Ensuring patient confidentiality by verifying their identity is crucial to maintaining privacy and trust in healthcare communications. Medical jargon (Option A) can confuse patients; providing personal opinions (Option C) is unprofessional and potentially misleading; speaking quickly (Option D) can lead to misunderstandings. Verifying identity ensures that sensitive information is shared only with authorized individuals, adhering to HIPAA regulations and ethical standards.

Question 129: Correct Answer: B) Implementing an electronic health record (EHR) system with automated reminders

Rationale: Implementing an EHR system with automated reminders ensures efficiency by reducing no-shows and optimizing appointment slots. Option A is incorrect because back-to-back scheduling can lead to burnout and inefficiency. Option C, while convenient, may not always result in optimal scheduling due to lack of oversight. Option D, though it accommodates delays, can reduce the number of patients seen. Therefore, option B is the most efficient method for managing appointments in a busy practice.

Question 130: Correct Answer: C) Exposure to industrial air pollutants

Rationale: Exposure to industrial air pollutants is a significant environmental stressor that can exacerbate anxiety and depressive symptoms due to its impact on respiratory health and overall well-being. While noise pollution (Option A), limited access to green spaces (Option B), and crowded living conditions (Option D) are also relevant stressors, contemporary research highlights that chronic exposure to industrial pollutants has a more direct and severe impact on mental health. This differentiation is crucial for understanding the primary contributors to Sarah's condition in an urban environment.

Question 131: Correct Answer: A) Acupuncture

Rationale: Acupuncture is supported by contemporary research as an effective alternative therapy for managing chronic lower back pain. Studies have shown that acupuncture can help reduce pain and improve function in patients with chronic lower back pain. Homeopathy, while popular, lacks strong scientific evidence for this condition. Aromatherapy may provide relaxation but has not been proven effective for chronic pain management specifically. Reflexology, like aromatherapy, lacks substantial evidence supporting its efficacy in treating chronic lower back pain. - Option A (Correct): Acupuncture has been extensively studied and shown to reduce pain and improve function in chronic lower back pain patients. - Option B (Incorrect): Homeopathy lacks robust scientific evidence supporting its effectiveness in managing chronic lower back pain. - Option C (Incorrect): Aromatherapy may aid relaxation but does not have strong evidence for effectively managing chronic lower back pain. - Option D (Incorrect): Reflexology has limited scientific support for its use in treating chronic lower back pain compared to acupuncture. This question tests the candidate's understanding of contemporary research and recognized theories regarding alternative therapies for specific conditions, making it challenging and relevant to their certification exam preparation.

Question 132: Correct Answer: B) Contact Mrs. Johnson's physician to obtain a letter of medical necessity.

Rationale: The first step in resolving a denial due to "lack of medical necessity" is obtaining a letter of medical necessity from Mrs. Johnson's physician, as this document provides essential support for the appeal. Option A is incorrect

because resubmitting without proper documentation may lead to another denial. Option C, while necessary, should follow after gathering all required documents. Option D is not advisable as it places financial burden on the patient and does not address the denial effectively.

Question 133: Correct Answer: A) Implementing a patient portal for secure online access to health information.

Rationale: Implementing a patient portal for secure online access to health information directly addresses Stage 2 Meaningful Use requirements, which emphasize patient engagement through electronic means. Option B is incorrect because while patient satisfaction surveys are important, they are not specifically required by Meaningful Use. Option C is incorrect as it contradicts the goal of digital records. Option D, although useful for patient education, does not fulfill the electronic engagement criteria central to Stage 2 Meaningful Use.

Question 134: Correct Answer: A) Assertive

Rationale: Assertive communication involves expressing one's needs and desires clearly and respectfully without violating the rights of others. It balances self-expression with respect for others, which is crucial in medical settings for effective patient care and team collaboration. Passive communication avoids confrontation but often leads to unmet needs. Aggressive communication involves expressing needs at the expense of others' rights, leading to conflict. Passive-aggressive communication indirectly expresses negative feelings instead of addressing them openly, causing misunderstandings and tension. Thus, assertive communication is the correct answer due to its balance of clarity and respect.

Question 135: Correct Answer: A) John has an abnormally slow heart rate.

Rationale: The term "bradycardia" is derived from the prefix "brady-" meaning slow, and the root word "cardia" meaning heart. Therefore, bradycardia refers to an abnormally slow heart rate. Option B is incorrect because "tachycardia" refers to an abnormally fast heart rate. Option C is incorrect because "arrhythmia" refers to an irregular heart rhythm. Option D is incorrect because high blood pressure is termed "hypertension." Understanding these prefixes and root words is crucial for accurately interpreting medical terminology.

Question 136: Correct Answer: B) Myocardial infarction

Rationale: The correct answer is B) Myocardial infarction. This term specifically refers to a heart attack, which occurs when blood flow to a part of the heart is blocked for a long enough time that part of the heart muscle is damaged or dies. - A) Myocarditis refers to inflammation of the heart muscle, not a heart attack. - C) Angina pectoris describes chest pain due to reduced blood flow to the heart but does not necessarily indicate a heart attack. - D) Cardiomyopathy refers to diseases of the heart muscle that affect its size, shape, and structure but do not specifically denote a heart attack. This question challenges candidates by including terms that are closely related but have distinct meanings in medical terminology.

Question 137: Correct Answer: D) Section 11: Toxicological Information

Rationale: Section 11 of the SDS specifically details the toxicological information, including potential health effects and symptoms associated with chemical exposure. While Section 2 outlines hazards and classifications, it does not provide detailed health effect information. Section 4 describes first-aid measures but not comprehensive toxicological data. Section 8 focuses on exposure controls and personal protection rather than health effects. This distinction is crucial for understanding SDS structure and content.

Question 138: Correct Answer: A) Apply direct pressure to the wound with a sterile gauze pad.

Rationale: The most appropriate initial step in administering first aid for a deep laceration is to apply direct pressure with a sterile gauze pad (Option A). This helps control bleeding and reduces the risk of infection. Rinsing with hydrogen peroxide (Option B) can damage tissue and delay healing. Elevating the arm and applying ice directly (Option C) does not address immediate bleeding control and can cause further tissue damage. Covering the wound with an adhesive bandage immediately (Option D) without addressing bleeding is inadequate for proper initial care.

Question 139: Correct Answer: C) Verify that Sarah's chosen proxy meets legal requirements.

Rationale: The first step in assisting Sarah is to verify that her chosen proxy meets legal requirements (Option C). This ensures that the designated person is legally eligible to act on Sarah's behalf. While providing a form (Option A) and explaining the importance of discussion (Option B) are essential steps, they come after verifying eligibility. Documenting verbal consent (Option D) is necessary but not the initial step. Ensuring legal compliance first prevents potential issues later in the process.

Question 140: Correct Answer: B) Dispose of them in a puncture-resistant sharps container.

Rationale: Used needles should always be disposed of in a puncture-resistant sharps container to prevent needlestick injuries and reduce the risk of infection. Option A is incorrect as regular trash bins do not offer protection against needle sticks. Option C is misleading because wrapping needles in gauze does not provide adequate protection, and biohazard bags are not designed for sharps. Option D is incorrect because sterilizing needles before disposal does not eliminate the need for proper sharps containers. The correct method ensures safety and compliance with infection control standards.

Question 141: Correct Answer: A) Administer 15 grams of glucose orally.

Rationale: Administering 15 grams of glucose orally is the most appropriate immediate action for suspected hypoglycemia, as it quickly raises blood sugar levels. Insulin injection (Option B) would worsen hypoglycemia by further lowering blood sugar. Providing a high-protein snack (Option C) does not address the immediate need for rapid glucose increase. Advising rest and rehydration (Option D) may help with general well-being but does not address acute hypoglycemia directly. Thus, Option A is correct due to its immediate effectiveness in raising blood glucose levels.

Question 142: Correct Answer: A) Autoclave

Rationale: An autoclave uses steam under pressure to achieve high temperatures, effectively killing all microorganisms and spores. Instrument cleaners and germicidal disinfectants are effective but may not eliminate all spores. Disposables are single-use items and do not undergo sterilization. Thus, autoclaving is the most reliable method for complete sterilization of surgical instruments.

Question 143: Correct Answer: C) Ensure that the specimen container is sealed properly and labeled with two patient identifiers.

Rationale: Proper labeling with two patient identifiers (e.g., full name and date of birth) ensures accurate identification and reduces errors. Sealing the container prevents contamination or spillage. Option A is incorrect because using only initials can lead to misidentification. Option B is incorrect because certain specimens require specific storage conditions, such as refrigeration. Option D is incorrect because unused portions might need to be retained for further testing or verification.

Question 144: Correct Answer: B) Check her blood pressure and pulse.

Rationale: Checking Sarah's blood pressure and pulse is the most appropriate initial action to assess her cardiovascular status, which could be contributing to her symptoms of light-headedness and dizziness. Administering oral glucose (Option A) is not appropriate without confirming hypoglycemia. Providing water (Option C) may not address the underlying cause. Notifying the physician (Option D) is important but should follow an initial assessment to provide accurate information.

Question 145: Correct Answer: A) Streptococcus pneumoniae

Rationale: Streptococcus pneumoniae is a common pathogen known to cause pneumonia, presenting with symptoms like fever, chills, and productive cough. Staphylococcus epidermidis is typically non-pathogenic and part of normal skin flora but can cause infections in immunocompromised patients or those with indwelling devices. Lactobacillus acidophilus is generally non-pathogenic and found in the gut, aiding digestion. Escherichia coli can be pathogenic but usually causes gastrointestinal issues rather than respiratory symptoms. Thus, Streptococcus pneumoniae is the most likely cause given John's respiratory symptoms.

Question 146: Correct Answer: C) Implementing multi-factor authentication (MFA).

Rationale: Implementing multi-factor authentication (MFA) is considered the most secure method for verifying an electronic funds transfer (EFT). MFA requires two or more verification methods, which significantly reduces the risk of unauthorized access. Single-factor authentication (Option A) is less secure as it relies on one form of verification. Email notifications (Option B) can be intercepted or spoofed. Checking the transaction status on the bank's website (Option D) is important but does not provide additional security layers like MFA. Therefore, Option C is correct due to its enhanced security measures.

Question 147: Correct Answer: A) Asking the patient to state their full name and date of birth.

Rationale: The correct answer is A) Asking the patient to state their full name and date of birth. This step is crucial for accurate patient identification as it ensures that the correct patient's records are accessed and updated. Option B, while important, does not directly verify identity. Option C is procedural but not focused on identification. Option D is also procedural but secondary to ensuring accurate identification first. Accurate identification minimizes errors in medical records and enhances patient safety.

Question 148: Correct Answer: C) Educating the patient about the importance of their medication regimen.

Rationale: Educating the patient about the importance of their medication regimen is crucial because it empowers them with knowledge about how their medications work and why adherence is essential. While providing written instructions (Option A), scheduling follow-ups (Option B), and using a pill organizer (Option D) are helpful, they do not address the underlying issue of understanding and motivation that education provides. Education helps patients internalize the necessity of compliance, leading to better health outcomes.

Question 149: Correct Answer: D) Label the specimen immediately after collection in front of the patient.

Rationale: Labeling the specimen immediately after collection in front of the patient ensures that there is no mix-up or misidentification between patients. This step is crucial for maintaining accuracy and patient safety. Option A is important but incomplete without immediate labeling. Option B overlooks verifying against other identifiers like date of birth. Option C, while necessary for documentation, does not directly prevent mislabeling at the point of collection.

Question 150: Correct Answer: D) Ensure face-to-face interaction and speak clearly.

Rationale: Ensuring face-to-face interaction and speaking clearly allows Maria to read lips and see facial expressions, which are crucial for understanding. Speaking loudly (A) can distort lip movements, making it harder to read lips. Written notes or text messaging (B) may not convey tone or urgency effectively. Relying solely on an interpreter (C) can impede direct communication and rapport-building between Maria and the medical assistant. Therefore, option D is the best practice supported by contemporary research on effective communication with hearing-impaired individuals.

CCMA Exam Practice Questions [SET 5]

Question 1: Mrs. Thompson, an 82-year-old woman with advanced osteoarthritis and moderate dementia, visits the clinic for a routine check-up. She lives alone but receives daily assistance from a home health aide. Which of the following is the most appropriate consideration for her care plan?
A) Encourage independent activities to promote autonomy.
B) Schedule regular physical therapy sessions to maintain mobility.
C) Ensure medication adherence through a pill organizer.
D) Coordinate with her home health aide to monitor her daily activities.

Question 2: Patient Maria, a 45-year-old woman, presents with symptoms consistent with a highly contagious respiratory infection during a local outbreak. As a medical assistant, you need to understand which measures are most effective in controlling such an epidemic. Which of the following is the most critical initial step in managing an epidemic?
A) Administering antiviral medications to all symptomatic patients
B) Isolating infected individuals to prevent further spread
C) Distributing personal protective equipment (PPE) to healthcare workers
D) Conducting mass vaccination campaigns

Question 3: Which of the following is the most critical step to prevent hemolysis when processing blood specimens for laboratory analysis?
A) Using a needle with a larger gauge size
B) Inverting the collection tube gently after drawing blood
C) Allowing the blood specimen to clot before centrifugation
D) Storing the blood specimen at room temperature immediately after collection

Question 4: Which of the following is the most crucial step in ensuring accurate calibration of clinical equipment?
A) Using manufacturer-specified calibration standards
B) Performing calibration checks biannually
C) Documenting calibration results in patient records
D) Cleaning equipment before each use

Question 5: A patient's complete blood count (CBC) reveals a hemoglobin level of 11.0 g/dL. Which of the following statements is correct regarding this value for an adult female?
A) This value is within the normal range.
B) This value indicates mild anemia.
C) This value suggests polycythemia.
D) This value requires immediate medical intervention.

Question 6: During a busy day at the clinic, Dr. Smith asks Maria, a Certified Clinical Medical Assistant (CCMA), to assist with patient documentation. Which credential would indicate that Maria is qualified to perform clinical tasks as well as administrative duties?
A) CMA (Certified Medical Assistant)
B) RMA (Registered Medical Assistant)
C) CCMA (Certified Clinical Medical Assistant)
D) CMRS (Certified Medical Reimbursement Specialist)

Question 7: When collecting a timed blood specimen for glucose tolerance testing, which of the following is the most crucial step to ensure accurate results?
A) Ensuring the patient has fasted for at least 8 hours before the test
B) Drawing the first blood sample exactly 30 minutes after glucose ingestion
C) Labeling each specimen with the exact time of collection
D) Using a tourniquet during every blood draw to ensure consistent venous pressure

Question 8: Which of the following is the most effective method for preventing the transmission of blood-borne pathogens in a clinical setting?
A) Using personal protective equipment (PPE) consistently
B) Practicing proper hand hygiene before and after patient contact
C) Disposing of needles and sharps in designated containers
D) Implementing standard precautions with all patients

Question 9: Mrs. Thompson, a 65-year-old patient, is prescribed an antibiotic ointment for her bacterial conjunctivitis. As a Certified Clinical Medical Assistant (CCMA), what is the correct method for administering the eye ointment?
A) Apply a thin line of ointment along the inner corner of the lower eyelid.
B) Apply a thin line of ointment along the outer edge of the lower eyelid.
C) Apply a thin line of ointment inside the lower eyelid from inner to outer corner.
D) Apply a thick layer of ointment across the entire surface of the eye.

Question 10: Sarah, a 45-year-old woman, presents with severe pain in her lower right abdomen, nausea, and fever. Upon physical examination, she has tenderness at McBurney's point. Which organ is most likely affected?
A) Gallbladder
B) Appendix
C) Pancreas
D) Kidney

Question 11: Which of the following resources is primarily known for providing comprehensive drug information including FDA-approved indications, dosages, and side effects, and is traditionally used by healthcare professionals in a physical format but now also available online?
A) Physicians' Desk Reference (PDR)
B) UpToDate
C) MedlinePlus
D) PubMed

Question 12: During a routine check-up, Maria, a 45-year-old patient, is scheduled for a fasting blood glucose test. As her medical assistant, what is the most

crucial instruction you should give her regarding the preparation for this test?
A) Do not eat or drink anything except water for at least 8 hours before the test.
B) Avoid only sugary foods and drinks for at least 8 hours before the test.
C) Do not eat anything but drinking tea or coffee without sugar is allowed.
D) Fast completely for 12 hours before the test.

Question 13: Maria, a 35-year-old woman, recently lost her job and has been experiencing significant stress. Instead of acknowledging her feelings of inadequacy, she begins to excessively criticize her colleagues who are still employed, accusing them of being incompetent. Which defense mechanism is Maria most likely exhibiting?
A) Projection
B) Displacement
C) Rationalization
D) Reaction Formation

Question 14: During a routine check-up, Dr. Smith asks Medical Assistant Emma to administer an intramuscular (IM) injection to a patient named John, who is due for his annual flu vaccine. Which of the following actions should Emma take next?
A) Administer the IM injection as instructed by Dr. Smith.
B) Prepare the IM injection but ask Dr. Smith to administer it.
C) Document the need for the IM injection and inform John about it.
D) Explain to John that she cannot administer injections and call a registered nurse (RN).

Question 15: During a cardiovascular examination, the medical assistant needs to position Mr. Johnson for an EKG. Which of the following positions is most appropriate to ensure accurate results?
A) Supine with arms at sides
B) Supine with arms above head
C) Semi-Fowler's position with arms at sides
D) Prone with arms at sides

Question 16: During a general physical examination of Mr. Smith, a 45-year-old male presenting with hypertension, which piece of equipment is essential for accurately measuring his blood pressure?
A) Stethoscope
B) Sphygmomanometer
C) Otoscope
D) Thermometer

Question 17: During a laboratory experiment, Maria is investigating the optimal conditions for the growth of Escherichia coli (E. coli). She observes that the bacteria thrive best at a specific temperature range. What is this optimal temperature range for E. coli growth?
A) 15-20°C
B) 20-25°C
C) 35-37°C
D) 45-50°C

Question 18: When measuring a patient's height accurately using a stadiometer, which of the following steps is crucial to ensure precision?
A) Ensuring the patient stands with feet flat and heels together.
B) Asking the patient to look down slightly during measurement.
C) Measuring height while the patient is wearing shoes.
D) Recording the height to the nearest half-inch.

Question 19: During a routine audit, it was found that several pieces of medical equipment at Dr. Smith's clinic had not been inspected according to the required schedule. As a Certified Clinical Medical Assistant (CCMA), what is the most appropriate immediate action to ensure compliance with equipment inspection regulations?
A) Immediately notify the medical equipment servicer and schedule an urgent inspection.
B) Document the missed inspections in the equipment log and inform the clinic manager.
C) Perform a preliminary check on all affected equipment and then notify the clinic manager.
D) Update the inspection logs to reflect current dates and plan for future compliance.

Question 20: Mrs. Johnson, an elderly patient with a history of frequent falls, is admitted to the clinic for observation. As her assigned medical assistant, what is the most appropriate action to ensure her safety within the clinical setting?
A) Place a "Fall Risk" sign above her bed and inform the nursing staff.
B) Ensure she has non-slip socks and keep her call light within reach.
C) Conduct hourly rounds to check on her and assist with mobility if needed.
D) Lower the bed to its lowest position and ensure side rails are up.

Question 21: When reviewing a patient's record prior to their visit, which of the following actions is most critical to ensure comprehensive healthcare delivery?
A) Reviewing the patient's current medication list for potential interactions.
B) Checking for any recent changes in the patient's insurance information.
C) Ensuring all previous visit notes are accurately documented.
D) Verifying the patient's contact information for appointment reminders.

Question 22: During a routine blood draw on Mr. Johnson, a 45-year-old diabetic patient, you notice that he has a history of difficult venous access. Which of the following actions should you take to ensure a successful blood draw while minimizing patient discomfort?
A) Use a butterfly needle and choose a dorsal hand vein.
B) Apply a tourniquet for an extended period to engorge the veins.
C) Ask the patient to make a fist and pump it repeatedly.
D) Select the median cubital vein using a straight needle.

Question 23: When billing for services performed, which document is crucial for ensuring accurate reimbursement from insurers and third-party payers?
A) Explanation of Benefits (EOB)
B) Superbill
C) Claim Form (CMS-1500)
D) Patient Ledger

Question 24: Which type of allergy test involves introducing small amounts of allergens into the skin to observe for a reaction?
A) Patch Testing
B) Intradermal Testing
C) Scratch Testing
D) Radioallergosorbent Test (RAST)

Question 25: Which feature of scheduling software is most critical for reducing patient wait times in a busy medical practice?
A) Automated Appointment Reminders

B) Real-Time Availability Updates
C) Multiple Provider Scheduling
D) Integrated Billing System

Question 26: Which of the following best describes the primary purpose of standardizing data fields in electronic health records (EHR)?
A) To ensure consistency and accuracy across patient records
B) To facilitate faster data entry by medical assistants
C) To reduce the need for patient consent for data sharing
D) To increase the storage capacity of EHR systems

Question 27: Which of the following individuals is typically authorized to approve payment processing in a medical practice?
A) Medical Assistant
B) Office Manager
C) Registered Nurse (RN)
D) Billing Specialist

Question 28: During a chart review, which of the following is the most crucial step to ensure accurate medication administration?
A) Verifying patient demographics
B) Checking for allergies and adverse reactions
C) Reviewing current medications and dosages
D) Confirming upcoming appointments

Question 29: John Doe visits a clinic for a routine check-up. The medical assistant is responsible for ensuring all required components of John Doe's medical record are complete. Which of the following is NOT considered a required component of medical records?
A) Patient demographics
B) Progress notes
C) Billing information
D) Consent forms

Question 30: Sarah, a Certified Clinical Medical Assistant (CCMA), is working in a multi-specialty clinic. She is tasked with coordinating patient care among various departments. Which of the following actions best demonstrates her understanding of the health care system and her role within it?
A) Scheduling patient appointments with specialists as needed.
B) Educating patients on their treatment plans and medication.
C) Communicating patient test results to primary care physicians.
D) Ensuring all patient records are updated and accurately filed.

Question 31: Mrs. Johnson, a 78-year-old woman with limited mobility, needs assistance with daily activities while her primary caregiver is at work. Which community resource would be most appropriate for her situation?
A) Home health aide services
B) Adult day care
C) Senior transportation services
D) Meals on Wheels

Question 32: Which of the following specialty resources is most appropriate for a family needing comprehensive support for both medical and mental health needs of a patient with chronic illness?
A) Social Worker
B) Psychiatrist
C) Integrated Care Team
D) Case Manager

Question 33: A patient named John is scheduled for a blood draw using micro-tubes. After selecting the appropriate site, which of the following steps should be performed to ensure proper site preparation and adherence to the correct order of draw?
A) Cleanse the site with iodine, apply a tourniquet, perform venipuncture, and then use a red-top micro-tube first.
B) Cleanse the site with alcohol, allow it to air dry, apply a tourniquet, perform venipuncture, and then use an EDTA micro-tube first.
C) Cleanse the site with alcohol, allow it to air dry, apply a tourniquet, perform venipuncture, and then use a light blue-top micro-tube first.
D) Cleanse the site with chlorhexidine, allow it to air dry, apply a tourniquet, perform venipuncture, and then use a yellow-top micro-tube first.

Question 34: When managing both electronic and paper medical records, which practice is essential to ensure compliance with HIPAA regulations?
A) Encrypting electronic records but not paper records
B) Regularly auditing both electronic and paper records for accuracy
C) Storing paper records in a locked cabinet but not encrypting electronic records
D) Shredding outdated paper records but keeping outdated electronic records

Question 35: While performing an EKG on Mr. Johnson, you notice that the baseline is wandering. Which of the following actions should you take to ensure proper functioning of the EKG equipment?
A) Reapply the electrodes and ensure they are securely attached.
B) Increase the paper speed to 50 mm/sec.
C) Ask Mr. Johnson to hold his breath during the recording.
D) Replace the EKG machine's battery.

Question 36: Sarah, a Certified Clinical Medical Assistant, is performing a CLIA-waived glucose test on a patient named John. She realizes that the test strips have expired by one day. According to CLIA-waived testing regulations, what should Sarah do next?
A) Proceed with the test since it is only one day past expiration.
B) Use a new batch of test strips and document the incident.
C) Perform the test and report the result with a disclaimer.
D) Discard the expired strips and reschedule John's test for another day.

Question 37: Which screening tool is most commonly used for initial assessment of depression in primary care settings?
A) Generalized Anxiety Disorder 7 (GAD-7)
B) Patient Health Questionnaire-9 (PHQ-9)
C) Beck Depression Inventory (BDI)
D) Hamilton Depression Rating Scale (HDRS)

Question 38: Mr. Smith is scheduled for a fasting blood glucose test at 8 AM. He mentions he last ate at 10 PM the previous night. What should the medical assistant do next?
A) Proceed with the blood draw as scheduled.
B) Ask Mr. Smith to return after fasting for at least 12 hours.
C) Reschedule the test for another day.
D) Check if Mr. Smith drank any water during the fasting period.

Question 39: Mrs. Johnson, a 65-year-old patient with severe arthritis, has been prescribed medication for pain management. Given her difficulty swallowing pills and her need for quick pain relief, which route of administration would be most appropriate?

A) Oral
B) Intravenous
C) Transdermal
D) Sublingual

Question 40: Which of the following strategies is most effective in promoting teamwork and team engagement among clinical medical assistants?
A) Encouraging open communication through regular team meetings.
B) Implementing a reward system based on individual performance.
C) Assigning clear, individual roles without overlap.
D) Fostering a competitive environment to motivate team members.

Question 41: During a routine check-up, the medical assistant notes in the patient's chart that Mr. Johnson has "HTN." Which of the following conditions is being referred to?
A) Hyperthyroidism
B) Hypertension
C) Hypotension
D) Hyperthermia

Question 42: John, a 35-year-old construction worker, has sustained a minor ankle sprain while working. As a Certified Clinical Medical Assistant (CCMA), which of the following is the most appropriate initial treatment step to minimize swelling and pain?
A) Apply heat immediately to increase blood flow.
B) Elevate the ankle above heart level.
C) Massage the area to reduce stiffness.
D) Apply a tight bandage to restrict movement.

Question 43: Maria, a 58-year-old patient with a history of hypertension and diabetes, is scheduled for her quarterly check-up. As a CCMA, what is the most crucial aspect to review in her patient record prior to her visit to ensure comprehensive healthcare?
A) Review her medication list for any potential drug interactions.
B) Check her latest lab results for any abnormal values.
C) Verify her allergy list to ensure no new allergies have been reported.
D) Assess her past medical history for any changes or updates.

Question 44: Which of the following is the most critical aspect of maintaining accurate temperature logs for medical refrigerators?
A) Recording temperatures at the end of each day
B) Ensuring logs are updated immediately after each temperature check
C) Conducting weekly reviews of temperature logs
D) Using automated systems to record temperatures

Question 45: Which of the following factors is most critical for the optimal growth of aerobic bacteria?
A) Oxygen availability
B) Carbon dioxide concentration
C) Light exposure
D) High salt concentration

Question 46: Sarah, a 55-year-old woman with chronic liver disease, is prescribed a new medication. Considering her condition, which pharmacokinetic process is most likely to be significantly altered in Sarah?
A) Absorption
B) Distribution
C) Metabolism
D) Excretion

Question 47: Maria, a 65-year-old patient with hypertension, is prescribed Metoprolol. As a Certified Clinical Medical Assistant (CCMA), which of the following actions best demonstrates adherence to the "Rights of Medication Administration"?
A) Administering Metoprolol to Maria after confirming her identity using her medical record number.
B) Administering Metoprolol to Maria based on the nurse's verbal order.
C) Administering Metoprolol to Maria after checking her blood pressure and confirming it is within the normal range.
D) Administering Metoprolol to Maria at any time during your shift as long as it is given within the same day.

Question 48: During a pelvic examination for a female patient named Maria, which positioning and draping technique is most appropriate to ensure both comfort and proper access for the clinician?
A) Position Maria in the supine position with her legs straight and drape only her lower abdomen.
B) Position Maria in the dorsal recumbent position with her knees bent and drape from her waist down to her knees.
C) Position Maria in the lithotomy position with her feet in stirrups and drape from her waist down, including over her legs.
D) Position Maria in the Trendelenburg position with her feet elevated above her head and drape from her shoulders down to her feet.

Question 49: Which of the following bacterial structures is primarily responsible for adherence to host tissues?
A) Flagella
B) Pili
C) Capsule
D) Endospore

Question 50: Which of the following best describes a sliding scale fee structure in a healthcare setting?
A) A fixed fee that all patients must pay regardless of income.
B) A fee structure where patients are charged based on their ability to pay.
C) A government-funded program providing free care to all indigent patients.
D) A discount program available only to patients with insurance.

Question 51: Maria, a CCMA, is tasked with scheduling follow-up appointments for patients after their initial consultation using both electronic and paper-based systems. Which of the following actions best ensures that no appointments are missed or double-booked?
A) Cross-referencing the electronic schedule with the paper-based log at the end of each day.
B) Relying solely on automated reminders from the electronic system.
C) Updating the paper-based log immediately after entering appointments into the electronic system.
D) Checking for appointment conflicts only when patients call to confirm.

Question 52: Which of the following is a primary function of a Patient-Centered Medical Home (PCMH) within healthcare systems?
A) Coordinating specialty care for patients
B) Providing comprehensive primary care
C) Managing hospital admissions and discharges
D) Offering emergency medical services

Question 53: During a routine blood draw for Mr. Johnson, a patient with suspected diabetes, you need to ensure that the blood sample is handled correctly for

glucose testing. Which of the following steps is crucial to prevent glycolysis and ensure accurate results?
A) Store the blood sample at room temperature.
B) Centrifuge the blood sample immediately after collection.
C) Use a gray-top tube containing sodium fluoride.
D) Collect the sample in a red-top tube without additives.

Question 54: When obtaining anthropometric measurements to calculate Body Mass Index (BMI), which of the following steps is most critical to ensure accuracy?
A) Ensuring the patient is wearing light clothing and no shoes during the measurement
B) Measuring the patient's height with their back against the wall and head level
C) Recording weight in kilograms and height in centimeters for accurate BMI calculation
D) Using a calibrated scale for weighing the patient

Question 55: Which of the following is the most appropriate action for a Certified Clinical Medical Assistant (CCMA) when storing medical records to ensure compliance with federal regulations?
A) Store all medical records in a locked filing cabinet accessible only to authorized personnel.
B) Keep digital medical records on a password-protected computer system with regular backups.
C) Maintain both paper and digital records indefinitely to avoid any potential legal issues.
D) Store sensitive patient information in a secure cloud storage service with encrypted access.

Question 56: Maria, a Certified Clinical Medical Assistant (CCMA), is preparing to greet a new patient who appears anxious. Which of the following approaches best demonstrates professional presence?
A) Greet the patient with a warm smile and maintain eye contact.
B) Use a calm and soothing tone while explaining procedures.
C) Wear clean, pressed scrubs and ensure personal hygiene.
D) Maintain a neutral expression to avoid overwhelming the patient.

Question 57: Which of the following laboratory tests is most appropriate for diagnosing a bacterial infection?
A) Complete Blood Count (CBC)
B) Blood Culture
C) Basic Metabolic Panel (BMP)
D) Urinalysis

Question 58: Which environmental and socio-economic stressor is most strongly associated with increased rates of anxiety disorders in urban populations?
A) Air pollution
B) Noise pollution
C) Lack of green spaces
D) High housing costs

Question 59: During a routine blood draw from Mr. Smith, a 45-year-old patient with a history of difficult venous access, you notice that blood flow into the tube is slow and intermittent. Which of the following actions should you take to ensure a successful blood draw?
A) Reposition the needle slightly by withdrawing it partially and then advancing it.
B) Apply more pressure to the tourniquet to increase venous pressure.
C) Use a smaller gauge needle to improve blood flow.
D) Release the tourniquet and try another vein.

Question 60: Maria, a medical assistant, is preparing to
administer a flu vaccine to Mr. Ahmed, who expresses concern about receiving the vaccine due to his religious beliefs. How should Maria proceed to ensure she provides unbiased care while respecting Mr. Ahmed's beliefs?
A) Explain the importance of the flu vaccine and insist on administering it.
B) Document Mr. Ahmed's refusal and notify the healthcare provider without further discussion.
C) Respectfully discuss alternative preventive measures with Mr. Ahmed and document his decision.
D) Schedule another appointment to give Mr. Ahmed more time to reconsider.

Question 61: Emily, a Certified Clinical Medical Assistant (CCMA), is responsible for ensuring that patient records are properly managed and compliant with regulatory standards. Which action should she prioritize to ensure compliance with the Health Insurance Portability and Accountability Act (HIPAA)?
A) Ensuring all electronic health records (EHRs) are password-protected.
B) Regularly updating patient consent forms.
C) Implementing encryption for all transmitted patient data.
D) Conducting annual staff training on HIPAA regulations.

Question 62: John, a 55-year-old male, presents with chest pain and shortness of breath. Upon examination, his physician suspects an issue with blood flow through the heart. Which structure is most likely compromised if there is a significant reduction in oxygenated blood being pumped into systemic circulation?
A) Right atrium
B) Left ventricle
C) Right ventricle
D) Left atrium

Question 63: When performing venipuncture on a patient with fragile veins, which method is most appropriate to minimize vein collapse?
A) Evacuated Tube Method
B) Syringe Method
C) Butterfly Method
D) Capillary Puncture

Question 64: Which of the following is the most appropriate technique for performing an ear irrigation procedure?
A) Use a steady stream of cold water aimed directly at the eardrum.
B) Use a gentle stream of warm water directed towards the upper wall of the ear canal.
C) Use a steady stream of warm water aimed directly at the eardrum.
D) Use a gentle stream of cold water directed towards the upper wall of the ear canal.

Question 65: Which of the following is a critical piece of information required on a provider request or requisition form to ensure accurate patient identification?
A) Patient's full name
B) Patient's insurance number
C) Patient's address
D) Patient's phone number

Question 66: During a physical examination, Dr. Smith asks Medical Assistant Jane to position Mr. Johnson in a way that his body is lying flat on his back with arms at his sides. What is the correct term for this position?
A) Prone
B) Supine
C) Lateral
D) Fowler's

Question 67: A patient in the clinic suddenly collapses and is unresponsive. What is the most appropriate first step a medical assistant should take?
A) Begin chest compressions immediately.
B) Check for a pulse and breathing.
C) Call for help and retrieve an AED (Automated External Defibrillator).
D) Administer rescue breaths.

Question 68: Which of the following best describes the primary physiological mechanism by which anxiety increases blood pressure?
A) Activation of the sympathetic nervous system
B) Increased release of acetylcholine
C) Stimulation of the parasympathetic nervous system
D) Decreased production of cortisol

Question 69: Which of the following services is most commonly associated with a specialty clinic rather than a general practice?
A) Immunizations
B) Routine physical exams
C) Chemotherapy administration
D) Blood pressure monitoring

Question 70: During a routine audit for COLA accreditation, it was noted that the laboratory's quality control (QC) procedures for hematology tests were not consistently documented. Which of the following actions is most aligned with COLA Accreditation Standards to address this issue?
A) Implementing a new QC protocol and training staff on it immediately.
B) Conducting a thorough review of current QC procedures and updating them as needed.
C) Ensuring all QC procedures are documented retrospectively for the past six months.
D) Assigning a dedicated staff member to oversee QC documentation going forward.

Question 71: Which of the following supplies is most appropriate for performing a blood culture test?
A) Lavender-top tube
B) Light blue-top tube
C) Blood culture bottles
D) Red-top tube

Question 72: Sarah, a certified clinical medical assistant, is preparing to perform a venipuncture on a patient. Before starting, she checks the calibration of her electronic blood pressure monitor. Which of the following steps should she take to ensure accurate calibration?
A) Compare the monitor's readings with a known standard pressure.
B) Calibrate using an arbitrary pressure value.
C) Check for any visible damage to the monitor.
D) Ensure that the monitor is fully charged before use.

Question 73: Which of the following is a crucial element that must be included in an informed consent form for it to be legally valid?
A) The patient's full medical history
B) A detailed description of the procedure
C) The names of all healthcare providers involved
D) Information on alternative treatments

Question 74: During a busy clinic day, a patient named Mr. Johnson becomes increasingly agitated because he has been waiting for over an hour past his appointment time. He starts raising his voice and demands to see the doctor immediately. As a Certified Clinical Medical

Assistant (CCMA), what is the most appropriate initial response to de-escalate the situation?
A) Apologize for the delay and assure him that he will be seen next.
B) Explain the reasons for the delay and provide an estimated wait time.
C) Acknowledge his frustration and offer to reschedule his appointment.
D) Remain calm, listen actively, and validate his feelings before providing any information.

Question 75: Which of the following is the most appropriate method for collecting a blood specimen to ensure accurate potassium levels?
A) Using a tourniquet for less than one minute before drawing blood
B) Drawing blood from an intravenous line
C) Collecting the sample in a lavender-top tube
D) Allowing the patient to make a fist tightly during the draw

Question 76: Sarah, a medical assistant, is discussing with a patient named Mr. Thompson about his upcoming surgery. Mr. Thompson mentions that he has given his daughter a Power of Attorney (POA) to make medical decisions on his behalf if he becomes incapacitated. Which type of POA is Mr. Thompson referring to?
A) General Power of Attorney
B) Durable Power of Attorney
C) Limited Power of Attorney
D) Springing Power of Attorney

Question 77: During an EKG test, a patient named Mr. Smith begins to exhibit signs of distress. Which of the following signs is most indicative of an adverse reaction that requires immediate attention?
A) Mild pallor
B) Slight increase in respiration rate
C) Elevated blood pressure and rapid breathing
D) Sweating

Question 78: You are a CCMA at a busy clinic when an irate patient named Mr. Johnson demands to see the doctor immediately, despite not having an appointment. How should you handle this situation to de-escalate his anger while maintaining professionalism?
A) Firmly tell Mr. Johnson that he must wait his turn like everyone else.
B) Listen actively to Mr. Johnson's concerns and acknowledge his frustration before explaining the scheduling policy.
C) Immediately call security to handle the situation as Mr. Johnson is becoming disruptive.
D) Allow Mr. Johnson to see the doctor immediately to avoid further conflict.

Question 79: During a busy clinic day, Dr. Smith asks Maria, a Certified Clinical Medical Assistant (CCMA), to perform tasks that include patient intake, administering injections, and documenting patient information in the Electronic Health Record (EHR). Which task is outside Maria's scope of practice as a CCMA?
A) Administering injections
B) Documenting patient information in the EHR
C) Interpreting lab results for patients
D) Conducting patient intake

Question 80: When administering ear drops to a patient, which of the following steps is crucial to ensure proper absorption and prevent complications?
A) Pull the earlobe down and back for adults.
B) Keep the ear drop bottle in the refrigerator before use.
C) Have the patient lie on their side with the affected ear facing up.

D) Apply pressure to the tragus after instilling drops.

Question 81: When measuring a patient's blood pressure, which of the following steps is most critical to ensure an accurate reading?
A) Ensuring the patient has not consumed caffeine within 30 minutes before the measurement.
B) Positioning the patient's arm at heart level.
C) Using a cuff that is appropriately sized for the patient's arm.
D) Having the patient sit quietly for at least 5 minutes before taking the measurement.

Question 82: Emily, a 35-year-old patient with a known latex allergy and sensitive skin, needs a bandage applied after a minor surgical procedure. Which type of bandage should the medical assistant use to prevent an allergic reaction and minimize skin irritation?
A) Latex-free adhesive bandage
B) Standard elastic bandage
C) Cotton gauze with hypoallergenic tape
D) Self-adherent cohesive wrap

Question 83: During a routine check-up, Mr. Johnson suddenly collapses and exhibits no pulse or breathing. As a Certified Clinical Medical Assistant (CCMA), which immediate action should you take according to the emergency action plan?
A) Administer epinephrine from the crash cart.
B) Start chest compressions immediately.
C) Call for help and retrieve the AED (Automated External Defibrillator).
D) Check for airway obstruction before starting CPR.

Question 84: Which of the following is the most appropriate action when performing venipuncture on a patient with a history of difficult veins?
A) Use a larger gauge needle to ensure successful blood draw.
B) Apply the tourniquet for more than 2 minutes to locate the vein.
C) Opt for a butterfly needle and use a smaller gauge.
D) Insert the needle at a 45-degree angle for better access.

Question 85: Which of the following is the most crucial element to include when labeling a patient's specimen for laboratory analysis?
A) Patient's full name
B) Date and time of collection
C) Type of specimen
D) Patient's medical record number

Question 86: Sarah, a medical assistant, is preparing to collect a blood sample from a patient for a fasting glucose test. Which of the following pre-analytical considerations is most critical to ensure the accuracy of the test results?
A) Ensuring the patient has fasted for at least 8 hours before the test
B) Collecting the sample in an EDTA tube
C) Transporting the sample on ice immediately after collection
D) Instructing the patient to avoid strenuous exercise prior to the test

Question 87: At what age is the first dose of the MMR vaccine recommended according to the CDC immunization schedule?
A) 6 months
B) 12 months
C) 15 months
D) 18 months

Question 88: Sarah, a 45-year-old woman with a family history of cardiovascular disease, visits her clinic for a routine check-up. She is concerned about her risk factors for developing coronary artery disease (CAD). Which of the following factors is most strongly associated with an increased incidence and prevalence of CAD in individuals like Sarah?
A) High LDL cholesterol levels
B) Regular physical activity
C) Low HDL cholesterol levels
D) Moderate alcohol consumption

Question 89: Mr. Johnson, a 65-year-old male with diabetes and hypertension, has been recently discharged from the hospital after an episode of heart failure. As a Clinical Medical Assistant, which strategy should you prioritize to ensure effective care coordination and education for Mr. Johnson?
A) Schedule regular follow-up appointments with his primary care physician.
B) Educate Mr. Johnson on recognizing early signs of heart failure.
C) Coordinate with a dietitian to develop a heart-healthy meal plan.
D) Arrange for home health visits to monitor his vital signs.

Question 90: During the end-of-day reconciliation process, Maria, a Certified Clinical Medical Assistant (CCMA), notices that several patient charges have not been entered into the Electronic Health Record (EHR) system. Which of the following steps should she take first to ensure accurate charge reconciliation?
A) Review the appointment schedule to verify all patients seen have corresponding charges.
B) Immediately enter any missing charges based on memory.
C) Contact each patient for confirmation of services received.
D) Adjust accounts receivable balances based on estimated charges.

Question 91: Which principle primarily ensures that a patient is fully informed about the potential risks and benefits before undergoing a medical procedure?
A) Autonomy
B) Beneficence
C) Informed Consent
D) Confidentiality

Question 92: During a comprehensive clinical intake process for a new patient named John Doe, which of the following steps is most crucial to accurately determine the primary purpose of his visit?
A) Reviewing John Doe's past medical history in detail.
B) Asking John Doe to describe his current symptoms and concerns.
C) Conducting a thorough medication reconciliation.
D) Measuring John Doe's vital signs accurately.

Question 93: Which of the following routes of administration is most appropriate for a medication that must bypass the gastrointestinal tract and provide rapid onset of action?
A) Oral
B) Intravenous (IV)
C) Subcutaneous (SC)
D) Intramuscular (IM)

Question 94: When reviewing a patient's advanced directive, which of the following actions should a Certified Clinical Medical Assistant (CCMA) take to ensure compliance with the patient's wishes?
A) Verify the directive with the patient's family members.

B) Consult the physician for interpretation and guidance.
C) Ensure that the directive is documented in the patient's medical record.
D) Follow the standard hospital protocol regardless of the directive.

Question 95: Mr. Johnson, a 65-year-old patient with severe rheumatoid arthritis, requires immediate pain relief. Due to his condition, he has difficulty swallowing and has recently undergone gastrointestinal surgery. Which route of administration would be most appropriate for administering his pain medication?
A) Oral
B) Intravenous
C) Subcutaneous
D) Rectal

Question 96: During a patient interview, which type of question is most effective for gathering detailed information about the patient's symptoms?
A) Open-ended question
B) Closed-ended question
C) Screening question
D) Leading question

Question 97: When matching and labeling a specimen to a patient and completing the requisition form, which step is crucial to ensure accuracy?
A) Labeling the specimen immediately after collection, before leaving the patient's side.
B) Verifying patient information on the requisition form after labeling the specimen.
C) Using pre-printed labels from the requisition form for labeling specimens.
D) Labeling specimens in bulk after collecting multiple samples from different patients.

Question 98: Sarah, a 45-year-old female patient with a history of hypertension and diabetes, presents with sudden onset chest pain and shortness of breath. Which ancillary service should be prioritized to assist in her immediate diagnosis?
A) Radiology
B) Cardiology
C) Laboratory Services
D) Physical Therapy

Question 99: Which of the following organ systems primarily regulates acid-base balance in the body?
A) Respiratory system
B) Digestive system
C) Integumentary system
D) Nervous system

Question 100: When documenting relevant aspects of patient care in a patient's record, which of the following is the most accurate and comprehensive practice?
A) Record only the medications administered and their dosages.
B) Document all patient interactions, including subjective complaints and objective findings.
C) Note only significant changes in the patient's condition.
D) Include only physician's orders and treatment plans.

Question 101: During a routine check-up, you notice that Patient John Doe's examination room needs cleaning after a minor surgical procedure. What is the correct order of cleaning and type of cleaning product to use for ensuring optimal infection control?
A) Clean high-touch surfaces first using a disinfectant, then clean floors with a detergent solution.
B) Clean floors first using a detergent solution, then clean high-touch surfaces with a disinfectant.

C) Clean high-touch surfaces first using a detergent solution, then clean floors with a disinfectant.
D) Clean floors first using a disinfectant, then clean high-touch surfaces with a detergent solution.

Question 102: Which of the following conditions is a contraindication for performing a venipuncture on a patient's arm?
A) Presence of a hemodialysis fistula
B) Recent surgical incision on the arm
C) Mild edema in the arm
D) Previous history of phlebitis in the arm

Question 103: Sarah, a Certified Clinical Medical Assistant (CCMA), is reviewing patient satisfaction surveys to identify areas for improvement in their clinic's communication strategies. One survey indicates that patients feel their concerns are not being adequately addressed during consultations. Which of the following actions should Sarah prioritize to enhance patient satisfaction?
A) Implementing a standardized script for all patient interactions.
B) Providing additional training for staff on active listening techniques.
C) Increasing the frequency of follow-up calls after appointments.
D) Reducing the duration of each consultation to increase efficiency.

Question 104: What is the primary purpose of obtaining pre-authorization from an insurance company before a medical procedure?
A) To ensure the patient's eligibility for coverage
B) To determine the exact cost of the procedure
C) To verify that the procedure is medically necessary
D) To confirm the patient's co-payment amount

Question 105: During a safety evaluation, which of the following actions is most critical for a Certified Clinical Medical Assistant (CCMA) to ensure accurate reporting of safety concerns?
A) Documenting all observed hazards in a detailed report.
B) Discussing observed hazards with colleagues before reporting.
C) Reporting observed hazards directly to the patient.
D) Waiting until the end of the shift to report observed hazards.

Question 106: Patient John is taking warfarin for anticoagulation therapy. He has been prescribed ciprofloxacin for a urinary tract infection. Which of the following actions should the medical assistant take?
A) Advise John to continue both medications as prescribed without any changes.
B) Inform John that he should increase his intake of green leafy vegetables.
C) Notify the healthcare provider about the potential interaction between warfarin and ciprofloxacin.
D) Suggest that John take an over-the-counter antacid to prevent gastrointestinal upset from ciprofloxacin.

Question 107: Which of the following scenarios requires the use of an N95 respirator rather than a standard surgical mask?
A) Assisting a patient with suspected tuberculosis during an aerosol-generating procedure.
B) Administering routine vaccinations in a primary care setting.
C) Providing care for a patient with confirmed influenza in a non-isolation room.
D) Conducting a routine physical examination on an asymptomatic patient.

Question 108: When measuring a patient's blood pressure, which of the following techniques ensures the most accurate reading?
A) Using a cuff that covers 40% of the patient's arm circumference
B) Measuring blood pressure immediately after the patient has climbed stairs
C) Positioning the patient's arm at heart level while seated
D) Taking the measurement with the patient lying down

Question 109: A 45-year-old patient named John presents with chronic inflammation of the liver. Which term best describes his condition?
A) Hepatitis
B) Hepatomegaly
C) Hepatosis
D) Hepatopathy

Question 110: During a routine check-up, Medical Assistant Sarah is responsible for updating patient John Doe's electronic health record. She needs to enter John's new insurance information, which includes his policy number, provider name, and coverage details. Which of the following is the most critical step Sarah should take to ensure data accuracy in this scenario?
A) Verifying the policy number with the insurance card
B) Entering the provider name exactly as it appears on the card
C) Double-checking the coverage details with John verbally
D) Cross-referencing the entered data with a secondary source

Question 111: In a Patient-centered Medical Home (PCMH), which team member is primarily responsible for coordinating patient care and ensuring that all aspects of the patient's health are managed comprehensively?
A) Physician
B) Nurse Practitioner
C) Clinical Medical Assistant
D) Care Coordinator

Question 112: When scheduling and monitoring patient appointments, which of the following methods ensures the highest level of efficiency and accuracy in managing patient data?
A) Using a fully integrated Electronic Health Record (EHR) system
B) Maintaining a detailed paper-based appointment ledger
C) Combining electronic scheduling with manual backup
D) Utilizing standalone electronic scheduling software without integration

Question 113: When preparing a blood sample for transportation to an outside reference laboratory, which of the following steps is most crucial to ensure sample integrity and accurate results?
A) Ensure the sample is placed in a biohazard bag with an ice pack.
B) Label the sample with the patient's name, date of birth, and collection date.
C) Use a transport container that maintains room temperature.
D) Document the sample collection details in the patient's medical record.

Question 114: When administering eye drops to a patient, which of the following steps is essential to prevent contamination of the medication?
A) Instruct the patient to blink rapidly after administration.
B) Place the dropper tip directly onto the sclera.
C) Avoid touching the dropper tip to any part of the eye or face.

D) Administer drops while the patient is lying flat.

Question 115: Patient John Doe has fragile veins that tend to collapse easily during blood draws. Which method would be most appropriate for obtaining a blood sample from him?
A) Using an evacuated tube system
B) Using a syringe with a straight needle
C) Using a butterfly needle with an evacuated tube system
D) Using a butterfly needle with a syringe

Question 116: During a routine cardiovascular test, Mr. Johnson's EKG shows an irregularly irregular rhythm without distinct P waves and a variable ventricular rate. Which dysrhythmia is most likely present?
A) Atrial Fibrillation
B) Ventricular Tachycardia
C) Supraventricular Tachycardia
D) Sinus Bradycardia

Question 117: A patient calls the clinic complaining of severe chest pain radiating to the left arm and shortness of breath. Which action should the medical assistant take first?
A) Schedule an appointment for later in the day.
B) Advise the patient to take an aspirin and wait for symptoms to improve.
C) Instruct the patient to call 911 immediately.
D) Suggest the patient come into the clinic as soon as possible.

Question 118: During a routine visit, a patient named John Doe needs to update his insurance information and sign a consent form for an upcoming procedure. Which category of the medical record will primarily include this updated insurance information?
A) Administrative
B) Clinical
C) Billing
D) Procedural

Question 119: Jane, a Certified Clinical Medical Assistant (CCMA), is responsible for storing patient medical records at her clinic. Which of the following actions best aligns with contemporary legal and ethical standards for the storage of medical records?
A) Storing records in a locked cabinet accessible only to authorized personnel.
B) Keeping records on an open shelf in a restricted area of the clinic.
C) Digitizing records and storing them on a password-protected computer accessible to all clinic staff.
D) Storing paper records in a locked cabinet but keeping digital records on an open-access network.

Question 120: When handling a difficult patient who is upset about a delayed appointment, which communication technique is most effective for a Certified Clinical Medical Assistant (CCMA) to use?
A) Empathizing with the patient's frustration and apologizing for the delay.
B) Explaining the reasons for the delay in detail to justify the situation.
C) Redirecting the conversation to focus on upcoming procedures.
D) Offering a rescheduled appointment as compensation for the inconvenience.

Question 121: Mrs. Johnson, a 68-year-old patient with a history of chronic obstructive pulmonary disease (COPD), is admitted with shortness of breath and increased sputum production. As her clinical medical assistant, you are responsible for monitoring her

oxygen saturation levels. During your assessment, you notice her oxygen saturation has dropped to 88%. What is the most appropriate immediate action?
A) Increase the oxygen flow rate.
B) Notify the attending physician immediately.
C) Encourage Mrs. Johnson to perform deep breathing exercises.
D) Reposition Mrs. Johnson to a semi-Fowler's position.

Question 122: When evaluating a food label, which component provides the most accurate measure of how much energy you will get from a serving of the product?
A) Total Carbohydrates
B) Calories
C) Total Fat
D) Protein

Question 123: Which alternative therapy primarily focuses on the manipulation of the body's soft tissues to enhance physical health and well-being?
A) Acupuncture
B) Chiropractic Care
C) Massage Therapy
D) Aromatherapy

Question 124: Which type of Power of Attorney specifically grants authority to make healthcare decisions on behalf of the principal when they are incapacitated?
A) General Power of Attorney
B) Durable Power of Attorney
C) Medical Power of Attorney
D) Springing Power of Attorney

Question 125: When preparing documentation and billing requests using current coding guidelines, which code set is primarily used for reporting outpatient procedures?
A) ICD-10-CM
B) CPT
C) HCPCS Level II
D) ICD-10-PCS

Question 126: During an EKG test, which of the following signs is most indicative of an adverse reaction requiring immediate intervention?
A) Elevated blood pressure
B) Increased respiratory rate
C) Sudden onset of chest pain
D) Mild dizziness

Question 127: When collecting a blood culture specimen, which of the following steps is crucial to avoid contamination?
A) Disinfecting the puncture site with alcohol only
B) Using a sterile technique and disinfecting with chlorhexidine
C) Filling the anaerobic bottle first before the aerobic bottle
D) Drawing blood directly into culture bottles without using a syringe

Question 128: Which of the following is the correct disposal method for a used needle in a clinical setting?
A) Dispose of it in a biohazard bag.
B) Place it in a sharps container.
C) Discard it in regular trash after capping.
D) Place it in a pharmaceutical waste container.

Question 129: Sarah, a 45-year-old woman, presents with symptoms of rapid heart rate and shortness of breath. Upon examination, her physician diagnoses her with tachycardia. Which medical term correctly describes Sarah's condition?

A) Bradycardia
B) Tachypnea
C) Tachycardia
D) Dyspnea

Question 130: Patient John Doe presents with symptoms of fatigue and pallor. His Complete Blood Count (CBC) reveals the following values: Hemoglobin (Hb) 10 g/dL, Hematocrit (Hct) 30%, Mean Corpuscular Volume (MCV) 70 fL, and Red Blood Cell (RBC) count 4.5 million cells/µL. Which of the following is the most likely diagnosis based on these lab results?
A) Iron deficiency anemia
B) Vitamin B12 deficiency anemia
C) Thalassemia minor
D) Anemia of chronic disease

Question 131: Which of the following factors is most likely to cause a significant decrease in a patient's peak flow rate?
A) Age
B) Asthma exacerbation
C) Recent physical exercise
D) Adequate hydration

Question 132: John, a 65-year-old male with a history of Type 2 diabetes mellitus, hypertension, and chronic kidney disease (CKD), presents with worsening shortness of breath and edema. Which of the following is the most significant risk factor contributing to his high mortality and morbidity?
A) Poor glycemic control
B) Uncontrolled hypertension
C) Chronic kidney disease
D) Congestive heart failure

Question 133: Emily, a 35-year-old patient, presents with symptoms of a urinary tract infection (UTI). As a Certified Clinical Medical Assistant (CCMA), you need to collect a clean-catch midstream urine specimen for analysis. Which step is crucial to ensure the accuracy of the specimen?
A) Instruct Emily to collect the first few drops of urine in the container.
B) Ensure Emily cleanses the genital area with antiseptic wipes before collecting the specimen.
C) Have Emily collect the entire stream of urine in the container.
D) Advise Emily to fast for 8 hours before collecting the urine sample.

Question 134: Which of the following is the most accurate method for determining a patient's forced vital capacity (FVC) during a spirometry test?
A) Instructing the patient to take a deep breath in and then exhale forcefully until no more air can be expelled
B) Asking the patient to exhale slowly and steadily after taking a deep breath
C) Having the patient perform multiple rapid inhalations and exhalations
D) Directly measuring lung volumes using body plethysmography

Question 135: Which of the following tasks is within the scope of practice for a Certified Clinical Medical Assistant (CCMA) to perform independently without direct supervision?
A) Administering intramuscular injections
B) Interpreting lab results
C) Prescribing medications
D) Diagnosing medical conditions

Question 136: When providing first aid for a deep

laceration with significant bleeding, what is the most appropriate initial step?
A) Apply a tourniquet above the wound.
B) Clean the wound with antiseptic solution.
C) Apply direct pressure to the wound with a clean cloth.
D) Elevate the injured limb above heart level.

Question 137: During an EKG recording, patient Mr. Smith's tracing shows a wandering baseline. Which of the following is the most likely cause of this artifact?
A) Patient movement
B) Electrical interference from nearby equipment
C) Loose electrodes
D) Respiratory activity

Question 138: Maria, a patient with chronic kidney disease, requires a referral to a nephrologist. As a Certified Clinical Medical Assistant (CCMA), what is your primary responsibility in ensuring that Maria's referral form is processed correctly?
A) Ensuring that all relevant patient information is accurately documented on the referral form.
B) Scheduling an appointment with the nephrologist before completing the referral form.
C) Sending the referral form directly to Maria's insurance company for approval.
D) Providing Maria with multiple options for nephrologists before completing the referral form.

Question 139: During a patient consultation, Maria, a Certified Clinical Medical Assistant (CCMA), needs to explain the importance of adhering to a new medication regimen to Mr. Johnson, who has recently been diagnosed with hypertension. Which of the following approaches best demonstrates clear and concise message relay?
A) "Mr. Johnson, it is crucial that you take your medication daily as prescribed by your doctor."
B) "Mr. Johnson, taking your medication regularly is important for managing your condition."
C) "Mr. Johnson, you must remember to take your pills every day without fail."
D) "Mr. Johnson, consistent medication intake is essential for controlling your blood pressure."

Question 140: Dr. Smith is prescribing medication for a patient named John using electronic prescribing software. Which feature of the software is crucial for ensuring that John's prescription does not interact negatively with his existing medications?
A) Automatic refill reminders
B) Drug-drug interaction alerts
C) Patient education materials
D) Electronic submission to pharmacy

Question 141: Emily, a medical assistant, is preparing to draw blood from Mr. Johnson. After collecting the sample, she needs to label it correctly to ensure accurate identification. Which of the following actions is the most appropriate step for Emily to take immediately after drawing the blood?
A) Label the tube with Mr. Johnson's name and date of birth before leaving the patient's side.
B) Label the tube with Mr. Johnson's name and date of birth at the nurse's station after completing all blood draws.
C) Ask Mr. Johnson to verify his name and date of birth after labeling the tube at her desk.
D) Label the tube with only Mr. Johnson's room number immediately after drawing the blood.

Question 142: Which of the following best defines "medical necessity" according to contemporary guidelines?

A) Medical necessity is defined as services or supplies needed for the diagnosis or treatment of a medical condition and meet accepted standards of medical practice.
B) Medical necessity is defined as any service or supply that a patient requests based on their personal preference.
C) Medical necessity is defined as services or supplies that are cost-effective and convenient for healthcare providers.
D) Medical necessity is defined as services or supplies that are experimental but show potential benefits in initial studies.

Question 143: When a claim is denied due to a lack of medical necessity, which step should a medical assistant take first to resolve the issue?
A) Submit an appeal with additional documentation supporting medical necessity.
B) Resubmit the claim without any changes.
C) Contact the patient to inform them of the denial.
D) File a complaint with the state insurance commissioner.

Question 144: During a busy flu season, Patient John presents with symptoms of fever, cough, and body aches. As a Certified Clinical Medical Assistant (CCMA), you must adhere to infection control guidelines while managing his care. Which of the following actions is MOST appropriate to prevent the spread of infection in this scenario?
A) Place John in an airborne isolation room immediately.
B) Provide John with a surgical mask and place him in a private room.
C) Instruct John to use hand sanitizer frequently and sit in the general waiting area.
D) Administer antiviral medication before conducting any further assessments.

Question 145: Which of the following is the correct placement for the V4 lead in a standard 12-lead EKG?
A) Fifth intercostal space at the left midclavicular line
B) Fourth intercostal space at the left midclavicular line
C) Fifth intercostal space at the left anterior axillary line
D) Fourth intercostal space at the left anterior axillary line

Question 146: During a patient consultation, Dr. Smith notes that Mr. Johnson has an inflammation of the liver. Which of the following medical terms correctly describes Mr. Johnson's condition?
A) Hepatitis
B) Hepatomegaly
C) Nephritis
D) Gastritis

Question 147: Mr. Johnson is scheduled for a minor surgical procedure to remove a benign skin lesion. As the medical assistant, which of the following aseptic techniques is most appropriate to ensure the prevention of infection during this procedure?
A) Hand washing with soap and water before donning sterile gloves.
B) Using alcohol-based hand sanitizer before donning sterile gloves.
C) Wearing non-sterile gloves after washing hands with soap and water.
D) Donning sterile gloves without any prior hand hygiene.

Question 148: Mr. Smith is a 65-year-old patient with diabetes and hypertension who requires coordinated outpatient services. As his medical assistant, you need to ensure he receives comprehensive care. Which of the following is the most effective initial step in coordinating his care?
A) Schedule an appointment with a dietitian for nutritional counseling.
B) Refer him to a diabetes educator for self-management training.

C) Arrange for a home health nurse to monitor his blood pressure.
D) Create a detailed care plan and communicate it with all his healthcare providers.

Question 149: During a routine check-up, the medical assistant notices that patient John Doe's medication list has not been updated with his recent prescription for hypertension. **Which function within the EHR/EMR system should the medical assistant use to ensure this information is accurately recorded?**
A) Medication Reconciliation
B) Clinical Decision Support
C) Order Entry
D) Patient Summary Update

Question 150: During a routine blood draw, Maria, a certified clinical medical assistant, encounters a patient named John who has small and difficult-to-locate veins. After applying the tourniquet and palpating the arm, she identifies a vein that appears suitable for venipuncture. What should Maria do next to ensure proper insertion technique?

A) Clean the site with an alcohol swab in a circular motion from the inside out.
B) Insert the needle at a 45-degree angle to ensure penetration of the vein.
C) Release the tourniquet immediately after needle insertion.
D) Ask John to make a fist and hold it tightly throughout the procedure.

ANSWER WITH DETAILED EXPLANATION SET [5]

Question 1: Correct Answer: D) Coordinate with her home health aide to monitor her daily activities.
Rationale: Coordinating with Mrs. Thompson's home health aide ensures continuous monitoring and support tailored to her specific needs, considering her cognitive impairment and physical limitations. While encouraging independence (A) is important, it may not be safe given her dementia. Regular physical therapy (B) is beneficial but secondary to ensuring daily safety and adherence. A pill organizer (C) aids medication adherence but does not address comprehensive daily monitoring required for someone in Mrs. Thompson's condition.

Question 2: Correct Answer: B) Isolating infected individuals to prevent further spread
Rationale: Isolating infected individuals is crucial in controlling the spread of highly contagious diseases by breaking the chain of transmission. Administering antivirals (Option A) is important but secondary to isolation. Distributing PPE (Option C) protects healthcare workers but does not directly control community spread. Mass vaccination (Option D) is effective for prevention but not an immediate response during an ongoing outbreak. Therefore, isolation is prioritized initially.

Question 3: Correct Answer: B) Inverting the collection tube gently after drawing blood
Rationale: Gently inverting the collection tube ensures proper mixing of blood with anticoagulants, preventing clot formation and hemolysis. Using a larger gauge needle (Option A) reduces hemolysis risk but is less critical than proper mixing. Allowing clotting before centrifugation (Option C) is relevant for serum samples but not directly related to hemolysis prevention. Storing at room temperature (Option D) can be appropriate depending on test requirements but does not directly prevent hemolysis. Thus, Option B is the most critical step.

Question 4: Correct Answer: A) Using manufacturer-specified calibration standards
Rationale: Using manufacturer-specified calibration standards is crucial because these standards are designed specifically for the equipment to ensure accuracy and reliability. Performing calibration checks biannually (Option B) is important but not as critical as using the correct standards. Documenting results (Option C) is necessary for record-keeping but does not directly impact accuracy. Cleaning equipment (Option D) is essential for infection control but not directly related to calibration accuracy. Thus, Option A ensures adherence to precise specifications essential for reliable performance.

Question 5: Correct Answer: B) This value indicates mild anemia.
Rationale: The normal hemoglobin range for an adult female is typically 12.0-15.5 g/dL. A hemoglobin level of 11.0 g/dL falls below this range, indicating mild anemia. Option A is incorrect as it falsely states that the value is normal. Option C is incorrect because polycythemia involves elevated hemoglobin levels, not decreased ones. Option D is incorrect because while the patient has anemia, it does not necessarily require immediate medical intervention unless accompanied by severe symptoms or other abnormal findings.

Question 6: Correct Answer: C) CCMA (Certified Clinical Medical Assistant)
Rationale: The CCMA credential indicates that Maria is qualified to perform both clinical and administrative tasks. Unlike other credentials, such as CMA or RMA, which may focus more on either clinical or administrative roles, the CCMA covers a broader scope. CMRS is specifically related to medical reimbursement and billing, making it less relevant for direct patient care and documentation. - Option A (CMA): While similar, CMA primarily focuses on clinical tasks but may not cover all administrative duties comprehensively. - Option B (RMA): Like CMA, RMA emphasizes clinical skills but doesn't explicitly cover the dual role as effectively as CCMA. - Option D (CMRS): This credential is specific to medical billing and reimbursement, not patient care or documentation tasks. The correct answer C) CCMA encompasses both clinical and administrative responsibilities, aligning with Maria's required duties in the scenario.

Question 7: Correct Answer: C) Labeling each specimen with the exact time of collection
Rationale: Accurate timing is critical in glucose tolerance tests to correlate glucose levels with specific time intervals. Option A is incorrect because fasting is required before starting but not during sampling. Option B is incorrect as samples are typically drawn at multiple intervals (e.g., 0, 30, 60 minutes). Option D is incorrect as using a tourniquet consistently does not directly impact timing accuracy. Proper labeling ensures precise tracking and interpretation of results.

Question 8: Correct Answer: D) Implementing standard precautions with all patients
Rationale: Implementing standard precautions with all patients is the most effective method for preventing the transmission of blood-borne pathogens because it assumes that every patient may be infectious, ensuring comprehensive protection. While using PPE (Option A), practicing proper hand hygiene (Option B), and disposing of needles and sharps correctly (Option C) are critical components, they are part of standard precautions. Standard precautions encompass all these practices and more, providing a broader and more consistent approach to infection control.

Question 9: Correct Answer: C) Apply a thin line of ointment inside the lower eyelid from inner to outer corner.
Rationale: The correct technique for administering eye ointment involves applying a thin line inside the lower eyelid from inner to outer corner (Option C). This ensures even distribution and maximizes therapeutic effect. Option A is incorrect because it suggests applying only to the inner corner, which doesn't cover the entire affected area. Option B is misleading as it suggests application only to the outer edge, missing most of the conjunctival sac. Option D is incorrect as applying a thick layer can cause blurred vision and discomfort without improving efficacy.

Question 10: Correct Answer: B) Appendix

Rationale: The appendix is most likely affected given the location of pain at McBurney's point and associated symptoms such as nausea and fever, which are indicative of appendicitis. The gallbladder (A) is located in the upper right abdomen and would not cause pain at McBurney's point. The pancreas (C) is situated behind the stomach and typically causes upper abdominal pain radiating to the back. The kidney (D), while it can cause lower abdominal pain, typically also presents with flank pain and urinary symptoms rather than localized tenderness at McBurney's point.

Question 11: Correct Answer: A) Physicians' Desk Reference (PDR)

Rationale: The Physicians' Desk Reference (PDR) is renowned for its detailed drug information, including FDA-approved indications, dosages, and side effects. It was traditionally available as a physical book but has transitioned to an online format. UpToDate is a clinical decision support resource, MedlinePlus provides general health information, and PubMed is a database of biomedical literature. These distinctions make PDR the correct answer.

Question 12: Correct Answer: A) Do not eat or drink anything except water for at least 8 hours before the test.

Rationale: Fasting blood glucose tests require patients to avoid all food and beverages except water for at least 8 hours to ensure accurate results. Option B is incorrect because avoiding only sugary foods and drinks does not suffice. Option C is incorrect because tea or coffee can affect glucose levels even without sugar. Option D is incorrect as fasting for 12 hours is unnecessary and may cause undue discomfort. The key difference lies in understanding the specific requirements of fasting protocols for accurate blood glucose measurement.

Question 13: Correct Answer: A) Projection

Rationale: Maria is exhibiting projection, where she attributes her own unacceptable feelings (inadequacy) onto others (colleagues). Displacement involves redirecting emotions to a safer outlet, which is not the case here. Rationalization refers to justifying behaviors with logical reasons, while reaction formation involves converting unwanted thoughts into their opposites. Thus, projection is the most accurate defense mechanism in this scenario.

Question 14: Correct Answer: A) Administer the IM injection as instructed by Dr. Smith.

Rationale: Medical Assistants are trained and permitted to administer intramuscular injections under the supervision of a licensed physician, which aligns with their scope of practice. Option B is incorrect because while preparation is within their scope, administering under supervision is also allowed. Option C is incorrect as documentation alone does not fulfill the task requirement. Option D is incorrect because it incorrectly suggests that MAs cannot administer injections at all, which misrepresents their scope of practice.

Question 15: Correct Answer: A) Supine with arms at sides

Rationale: The supine position with arms at the sides is ideal for an EKG as it minimizes muscle interference and allows for accurate electrode placement. Option B is incorrect because raising the arms can cause muscle tension and movement artifacts. Option C, while somewhat similar, is not optimal as the semi-Fowler's position can alter heart orientation and affect readings. Option D is incorrect because the prone position does not allow proper access to chest leads and can distort results.

Question 16: Correct Answer: B) Sphygmomanometer

Rationale: The sphygmomanometer is essential for accurately measuring blood pressure, which is crucial for assessing hypertension. While a stethoscope (Option A) is used in conjunction with the sphygmomanometer to listen to Korotkoff sounds, it cannot measure blood pressure alone. An otoscope (Option C) is used to examine the ears and does not relate to blood pressure measurement. A thermometer (Option D) measures body temperature and is not used for assessing blood pressure. Therefore, the sphygmomanometer (Option B) is the correct answer due to

its specific function in measuring blood pressure directly.

Question 17: Correct Answer: C) 35-37°C

Rationale: E. coli is a mesophilic bacterium that thrives best at body temperature, around 35-37°C. This temperature range supports its enzymatic activities and cellular processes efficiently. Option A (15-20°C) represents psychrophilic conditions, which are too cold for E. coli's optimal growth. Option B (20-25°C) is also below the optimal range and would slow down metabolic activities. Option D (45-50°C) is within the thermophilic range, which is too hot and would likely denature proteins and enzymes in E. coli, hindering its growth.

Question 18: Correct Answer: A) Ensuring the patient stands with feet flat and heels together.

Rationale: Ensuring the patient stands with feet flat and heels together is crucial for an accurate height measurement using a stadiometer. This position ensures proper alignment of the body. Option B is incorrect because looking down can alter spinal alignment. Option C is incorrect as shoes add extra height. Option D is partially correct but not as critical as proper stance for accuracy.

Question 19: Correct Answer: B) Document the missed inspections in the equipment log and inform the clinic manager.

Rationale: The correct answer is B. Documenting missed inspections ensures there is a record of non-compliance, which is critical for transparency and corrective actions. Informing the clinic manager allows for immediate administrative oversight and planning for necessary inspections. Option A focuses solely on scheduling without addressing documentation or managerial oversight. Option C involves performing checks without proper documentation or higher-level notification. Option D suggests updating logs without addressing past non-compliance or immediate managerial involvement.

Question 20: Correct Answer: B) Ensure she has non-slip socks and keep her call light within reach.

Rationale: While all options contribute to patient safety, ensuring Mrs. Johnson has non-slip socks and keeping her call light within reach (Option B) directly addresses immediate fall risks by providing traction and enabling easy access to assistance. Option A is important for awareness but doesn't provide immediate physical safety measures. Option C is proactive but may not prevent an immediate fall if she's unattended between rounds. Option D could be restrictive and potentially increase the risk of injury from climbing over side rails.

Question 21: Correct Answer: A) Reviewing the patient's current medication list for potential interactions.

Rationale: Reviewing the patient's current medication list for potential interactions is crucial because it directly impacts patient safety and treatment efficacy. While checking insurance information (B), ensuring accurate documentation of previous visits (C), and verifying contact information (D) are important administrative tasks, they do not have as immediate a clinical impact on patient care as identifying potential medication interactions. Medication review helps prevent adverse drug reactions and ensures that prescribed treatments are safe and effective.

Question 22: Correct Answer: D) Select the median cubital vein using a straight needle.

Rationale: The median cubital vein is typically larger and more stable, making it easier for venipuncture in patients with difficult access. A butterfly needle is less ideal for larger veins like the median cubital. Prolonged tourniquet application can cause hemoconcentration and discomfort. Repeated fist pumping can lead to inaccurate lab results due to hemolysis or increased potassium levels. Therefore, selecting the median cubital vein with a straight needle is optimal for minimizing discomfort and ensuring successful blood draw.

Question 23: Correct Answer: C) Claim Form (CMS-1500)

Rationale: The CMS-1500 form is essential for submitting claims to insurers and third-party payers to receive reimbursement. It includes all necessary information about the patient's diagnosis and the services provided. While the Explanation of Benefits (EOB) details what was paid by the insurer, it is not used for billing. A Superbill is an itemized form used by healthcare providers to reflect rendered services but does not directly facilitate reimbursement. The Patient Ledger keeps track of patient charges and payments but isn't submitted for insurance claims.

Question 24: Correct Answer: B) Intradermal Testing
Rationale: Intradermal testing involves injecting small amounts of allergens just under the skin and observing for an allergic reaction, typically a raised bump or redness. This method is more sensitive than scratch testing but carries a higher risk of systemic reactions. Patch testing (A) is used for diagnosing contact dermatitis by applying allergens on patches to the skin. Scratch testing (C), also known as prick testing, involves pricking the skin with allergens but is less sensitive than intradermal testing. RAST (D) is a blood test that measures specific IgE antibodies to identify allergies and does not involve direct skin exposure.

Question 25: Correct Answer: B) Real-Time Availability Updates
Rationale: Real-time availability updates are crucial for reducing patient wait times as they ensure that appointments are scheduled efficiently, and any changes or cancellations are immediately reflected. While automated appointment reminders (A) reduce no-shows, they don't directly impact wait times. Multiple provider scheduling (C) improves resource allocation but isn't directly linked to wait times. An integrated billing system (D) enhances financial operations but doesn't affect scheduling efficiency. Thus, real-time updates are the most critical feature for minimizing patient wait times in a busy practice.

Question 26: Correct Answer: A) To ensure consistency and accuracy across patient records
Rationale: Standardizing data fields in EHR is primarily aimed at ensuring consistency and accuracy across patient records. This standardization helps in maintaining uniformity, which is crucial for accurate diagnosis, treatment, and research. Option B is incorrect because while standardization may indirectly facilitate faster data entry, it is not the primary purpose. Option C is incorrect as standardization does not eliminate the need for patient consent. Option D is also incorrect because increasing storage capacity is unrelated to the standardization of data fields.

Question 27: Correct Answer: B) Office Manager
Rationale: The office manager usually has the authority to approve payment processing due to their oversight role in administrative and financial operations. While medical assistants (A) and registered nurses (C) play crucial roles in patient care and clinical tasks, they do not typically handle financial authorizations. A billing specialist (D) is involved in processing claims and payments but does not usually have the final approval authority. Therefore, option B is correct as it aligns with standard administrative practices.

Question 28: Correct Answer: C) Reviewing current medications and dosages
Rationale: Reviewing current medications and dosages is critical in ensuring accurate medication administration because it directly impacts patient safety. Verifying patient demographics (Option A) is essential but not specific to medication administration. Checking for allergies and adverse reactions (Option B) is important but secondary to knowing the exact medications being administered. Confirming upcoming appointments (Option D) is relevant for continuity of care but does not directly affect immediate medication accuracy.

Question 29: Correct Answer: C) Billing information
Rationale: Billing information, while essential for administrative purposes, is not considered a required component of medical records from a clinical perspective.

Patient demographics (A), progress notes (B), and consent forms (D) are crucial for providing comprehensive patient care and ensuring legal and ethical standards are met. Patient demographics include basic information like name, age, and contact details; progress notes document ongoing care and treatment; consent forms ensure that patients have agreed to procedures or treatments. Billing information pertains more to financial transactions rather than clinical documentation.

Question 30: Correct Answer: A) Scheduling patient appointments with specialists as needed.
Rationale: The correct answer is A because coordinating patient care often involves scheduling appointments with specialists to ensure continuity and comprehensive care. Option B, while important, focuses more on patient education than coordination. Option C is critical but pertains more to communication rather than coordination. Option D is essential for record-keeping but does not directly relate to coordinating care among departments. Thus, A best exemplifies Sarah's role in coordinating patient care in a multi-specialty clinic setting.

Question 31: Correct Answer: B) Adult day care
Rationale: Adult day care centers offer structured programs that provide social interaction, meals, and assistance with daily activities for seniors during the day. This option is ideal for Mrs. Johnson as it provides comprehensive support while her caregiver is unavailable. Home health aide services (Option A) focus more on in-home medical care rather than social engagement. Senior transportation services (Option C) only address mobility needs without offering daily activity support. Meals on Wheels (Option D) delivers food but does not provide the broader range of services needed for Mrs. Johnson's daily activities.

Question 32: Correct Answer: C) Integrated Care Team
Rationale: An Integrated Care Team is the most appropriate resource as it provides comprehensive support addressing both medical and mental health needs through a multidisciplinary approach. A Social Worker (A) focuses more on social services and less on direct medical care. A Psychiatrist (B) specializes in mental health but does not cover broader medical needs. A Case Manager (D) coordinates care but may not provide the integrated, multidisciplinary approach necessary for comprehensive support. Thus, an Integrated Care Team offers a holistic solution by combining expertise from various healthcare professionals.

Question 33: Correct Answer: C) Cleanse the site with alcohol, allow it to air dry, apply a tourniquet, perform venipuncture, and then use a light blue-top micro-tube first.
Rationale: The correct procedure involves cleansing the site with alcohol and allowing it to air dry completely before applying a tourniquet. The light blue-top micro-tube (containing sodium citrate) should be used first in the order of draw for coagulation studies. Options A) and D) suggest incorrect cleansing agents (iodine and chlorhexidine are not standard for routine phlebotomy). Option B) incorrectly places an EDTA tube first in the order of draw. Proper sequence prevents cross-contamination of additives between tubes.

Question 34: Correct Answer: B) Regularly auditing both electronic and paper records for accuracy
Rationale: Regularly auditing both electronic and paper records for accuracy ensures compliance with HIPAA regulations by maintaining the integrity and confidentiality of patient information. Encrypting only electronic records (A) or storing paper records securely without encrypting digital ones (C) fails to address all forms of data protection comprehensively. Shredding outdated paper records while keeping outdated electronic ones (D) does not align with best practices for data retention and disposal.

Question 35: Correct Answer: A) Reapply the electrodes and ensure they are securely attached.
Rationale: Wandering baseline often results from poor

electrode contact with the skin. Reapplying and securing the electrodes ensures proper contact, reducing artifacts. Increasing paper speed (B) might affect reading clarity but does not address electrode contact. Asking the patient to hold their breath (C) can reduce motion artifacts but is not a standard troubleshooting step for wandering baseline. Replacing the battery (D) is unnecessary unless there is a power issue, which would manifest differently than a wandering baseline.

Question 36: Correct Answer: B) Use a new batch of test strips and document the incident.

Rationale: According to CLIA-waived testing regulations, expired materials should never be used as they can compromise test accuracy. Sarah should use a new batch of test strips and document the incident for quality assurance purposes. Option A is incorrect because using expired materials violates regulatory standards. Option C is incorrect as reporting results from expired materials is not acceptable even with disclaimers. Option D suggests rescheduling, which is unnecessary if new strips are available immediately.

Question 37: Correct Answer: B) Patient Health Questionnaire-9 (PHQ-9)

Rationale: The PHQ-9 is the most commonly used tool for initial assessment of depression in primary care due to its brevity, ease of use, and strong validation in various populations. While the GAD-7 is a valid tool, it specifically screens for anxiety rather than depression. The Beck Depression Inventory is a longer, more detailed tool often used in clinical settings rather than primary care. The Hamilton Depression Rating Scale is typically used by clinicians for more detailed assessments rather than initial screenings. The PHQ-9's widespread use and validation make it the preferred choice for primary care depression screening.

Question 38: Correct Answer: B) Ask Mr. Smith to return after fasting for at least 12 hours.

Rationale: Fasting blood glucose tests typically require a minimum of 8-12 hours of fasting to ensure accuracy. Since Mr. Smith last ate at 10 PM, he has only fasted for 10 hours by 8 AM. The medical assistant should ask him to return after completing at least a full 12-hour fast to ensure reliable results. - Option A is incorrect because proceeding with the blood draw without completing the required fasting period could yield inaccurate results. - Option C is incorrect because rescheduling might be unnecessary if Mr. Smith can complete the required fasting soon. - Option D is irrelevant as water consumption does not affect fasting glucose levels significantly.

Question 39: Correct Answer: B) Intravenous

Rationale: The intravenous (IV) route is most appropriate for Mrs. Johnson as it provides rapid pain relief by delivering medication directly into the bloodstream. Oral administration is unsuitable due to her difficulty swallowing pills. Transdermal patches offer sustained release but are slower in onset compared to IV. Sublingual administration provides relatively quick absorption but may not be as effective for severe pain relief as IV.

Question 40: Correct Answer: A) Encouraging open communication through regular team meetings.

Rationale: Encouraging open communication through regular team meetings is essential for promoting teamwork and engagement as it allows for the exchange of ideas, problem-solving, and building trust. Option B focuses on individual performance rather than team cohesion, which can undermine teamwork. Option C emphasizes clear roles but neglects the importance of collaboration. Option D's competitive environment can create divisions rather than unity. Therefore, option A is the most comprehensive strategy for fostering teamwork and engagement.

Question 41: Correct Answer: B) Hypertension

Rationale: "HTN" is the standard abbreviation for hypertension, a condition characterized by high blood pressure. Hyperthyroidism (A) refers to an overactive thyroid gland, while hypotension (C) indicates low blood pressure. Hyperthermia (D) denotes an elevated body temperature. Each incorrect option involves terms that could easily be confused with "HTN" due to similar prefixes or contexts, but they refer to distinctly different medical conditions. Understanding these nuances is crucial for accurate medical documentation and patient care.

Question 42: Correct Answer: B) Elevate the ankle above heart level.

Rationale: Elevating the ankle above heart level helps reduce swelling and pain by decreasing blood flow to the injured area. Option A is incorrect because applying heat can increase swelling in the acute phase. Option C is incorrect as massaging can exacerbate inflammation initially. Option D is incorrect because while compression is useful, overly tight bandaging can impede circulation and worsen the injury. The correct answer aligns with contemporary research on effective initial treatment for sprains, emphasizing elevation as a key component of RICE protocol.

Question 43: Correct Answer: A) Review her medication list for any potential drug interactions.

Rationale: Reviewing Maria's medication list for potential drug interactions is crucial because it directly impacts her current treatment plan and safety. While checking lab results (B), verifying allergies (C), and assessing past medical history (D) are important, they do not immediately address potential adverse effects from current medications. Ensuring no harmful interactions can prevent complications, particularly given Maria's chronic conditions.

Question 44: Correct Answer: B) Ensuring logs are updated immediately after each temperature check

Rationale: Immediate updating ensures that any deviations are promptly addressed, maintaining medication efficacy and patient safety. Recording at the end of each day (A) may miss critical fluctuations. Weekly reviews (C) are insufficient for timely interventions. Automated systems (D), while useful, still require regular oversight and verification.

Question 45: Correct Answer: A) Oxygen availability

Rationale: Aerobic bacteria require oxygen for their metabolic processes, making oxygen availability the most critical factor for their optimal growth. While carbon dioxide concentration (Option B) can influence some bacteria, it is not as crucial as oxygen for aerobes. Light exposure (Option C) affects photosynthetic organisms more than aerobic bacteria. High salt concentration (Option D) is essential for halophiles but can inhibit many other bacteria, including aerobes. Thus, oxygen availability is the key factor distinguishing aerobic bacterial growth from other conditions.

Question 46: Correct Answer: C) Metabolism

Rationale: In patients with chronic liver disease, the liver's ability to metabolize drugs is often compromised. This can lead to increased drug levels and prolonged effects. While absorption, distribution, and excretion are also important pharmacokinetic processes, metabolism is most directly affected by liver function. Absorption occurs primarily in the gastrointestinal tract and is less influenced by liver disease. Distribution can be affected by changes in plasma proteins but not as significantly as metabolism. Excretion primarily involves renal function, which may be secondarily affected but not as directly as metabolism in liver disease patients.

Question 47: Correct Answer: A) Administering Metoprolol to Maria after confirming her identity using her medical record number.

Rationale: Option A ensures the "right patient" by confirming Maria's identity using her medical record number. This aligns with contemporary practices emphasizing patient safety through accurate identification. Option B is incorrect because administering medication based on a verbal order without written confirmation can lead to errors. Option C focuses on monitoring vital signs but does not address patient identification directly. Option D neglects the "right time," which is crucial for maintaining therapeutic drug levels and effectiveness. Thus, option A best exemplifies adherence to all key principles of medication administration rights.

Question 48: Correct Answer: C) Position Maria in the lithotomy position with her feet in stirrups and drape from her waist down, including over her legs.

Rationale: The lithotomy position is specifically used for pelvic examinations as it provides optimal access for the clinician while maintaining patient comfort. Draping from the waist down ensures privacy and modesty. The other options are incorrect due to improper positioning (A, B, D) or inadequate draping techniques (A, B). Option A does not provide necessary access; Option B does not fully cover or provide appropriate access; Option D is used for different procedures like shock management, not pelvic exams.

Question 49: Correct Answer: B) Pili

Rationale: Pili are hair-like structures on the surface of many bacteria that facilitate adherence to host tissues, which is crucial for establishing infections. Flagella are involved in motility, not adherence. Capsules can help in evading immune responses but are not primarily for adherence. Endospores are survival structures that protect the bacterium in harsh conditions but do not play a role in adherence. Understanding these distinctions is essential for recognizing how bacteria establish infections and evade host defenses.

Question 50: Correct Answer: B) A fee structure where patients are charged based on their ability to pay.

Rationale: A sliding scale fee structure adjusts charges based on a patient's income and financial situation, making healthcare more accessible to those with limited means. Option A is incorrect because it describes a fixed fee system. Option C is incorrect as it refers to government-funded programs rather than sliding scales. Option D is misleading because sliding scales apply regardless of insurance status. Thus, Option B correctly encapsulates the principle of adjusting fees based on financial capability, aligning with contemporary practices in healthcare affordability programs.

Question 51: Correct Answer: A) Cross-referencing the electronic schedule with the paper-based log at the end of each day.

Rationale: Cross-referencing ensures consistency between both systems, minimizing errors like missed or double-booked appointments. Option B is incorrect because relying solely on automated reminders doesn't address potential discrepancies between systems. Option C is close but doesn't account for verifying entries made throughout the day. Option D fails to proactively prevent conflicts, addressing them only reactively.

Question 52: Correct Answer: B) Providing comprehensive primary care

Rationale: A Patient-Centered Medical Home (PCMH) is designed to provide comprehensive primary care by focusing on the patient's overall health needs, including preventive services, chronic disease management, and coordination of specialty care. Option A is incorrect because while PCMHs do coordinate specialty care, their primary function is broader. Option C is incorrect as managing hospital admissions and discharges is typically a role of case management teams in hospitals. Option D is incorrect because emergency medical services are outside the scope of PCMHs, which focus on ongoing patient care rather than acute emergencies.

Question 53: Correct Answer: C) Use a gray-top tube containing sodium fluoride.

Rationale: Using a gray-top tube containing sodium fluoride is crucial as it inhibits glycolysis, ensuring accurate glucose levels. Storing at room temperature (A) can lead to glycolysis. Immediate centrifugation (B) is not specific for preventing glycolysis. A red-top tube (D) lacks necessary additives to inhibit glycolysis.

Question 54: Correct Answer: C) Recording weight in kilograms and height in centimeters for accurate BMI calculation

Rationale: The correct answer is C. Accurate BMI calculation depends on recording weight in kilograms and height in centimeters to apply the formula (weight in kg / height in meters squared). Option A is important but not critical for calculation accuracy. Option B is about proper technique but not directly related to BMI formula accuracy. Option D ensures accurate weight but doesn't address height measurement or unit conversion essential for BMI calculation. Thus, while all options are relevant, only C directly impacts the precision of BMI computation.

Question 55: Correct Answer: B) Keep digital medical records on a password-protected computer system with regular backups.

Rationale: Option B is correct because it ensures compliance with federal regulations by protecting patient information through password protection and regular backups. Option A, while partially correct, does not address digital records. Option C is incorrect as indefinite storage is not required and can lead to unnecessary data retention issues. Option D, although secure, does not specify the necessity of regular backups which are crucial for data integrity and compliance.

Question 56: Correct Answer: A) Greet the patient with a warm smile and maintain eye contact.

Rationale: Greeting the patient with a warm smile and maintaining eye contact is crucial for establishing trust and showing empathy, which are key components of professional presence. While using a calm tone (B) is important, it doesn't fully encompass the initial impact of appearance and demeanor. Clean scrubs (C) are necessary but don't address demeanor or tone. A neutral expression (D) may come off as indifferent rather than reassuring.

Question 57: Correct Answer: B) Blood Culture

Rationale: A blood culture is specifically designed to detect bacterial infections in the bloodstream by allowing bacteria present in the sample to grow and be identified. While a CBC can indicate an infection through elevated white blood cells, it does not identify the specific bacteria. A BMP assesses metabolic functions and electrolytes, which are not directly related to identifying infections. Urinalysis can detect infections in the urinary tract but not systemic bacterial infections. Thus, blood culture is the most appropriate test for diagnosing a bacterial infection.

Question 58: Correct Answer: B) Noise pollution

Rationale: Noise pollution is most strongly associated with increased rates of anxiety disorders in urban populations due to constant exposure to high noise levels, which can lead to chronic stress and sleep disturbances. While air pollution (Option A) can affect physical health and contribute indirectly to mental stress, it is less directly linked to anxiety disorders. Lack of green spaces (Option C) can contribute to poor mental health but is more associated with general well-being rather than specific anxiety disorders. High housing costs (Option D) are a significant socio-economic stressor but primarily impact financial stress rather than directly causing anxiety disorders.

Question 59: Correct Answer: A) Reposition the needle slightly by withdrawing it partially and then advancing it.

Rationale: Slightly repositioning the needle can help if it's against a vein wall or not fully within the vein lumen, improving blood flow. Applying more pressure with the tourniquet (Option B) may cause hemolysis or discomfort. Using a smaller gauge needle (Option C) is not typically effective once access is achieved. Releasing the tourniquet (Option D) might be necessary if repositioning fails, but it's not the first step. Understanding these nuances ensures optimal patient care and successful phlebotomy procedures.

Question 60: Correct Answer: C) Respectfully discuss alternative preventive measures with Mr. Ahmed and document his decision.

Rationale: Option C is correct because it respects Mr. Ahmed's religious beliefs while still addressing his health concerns by discussing alternative measures. This approach ensures unbiased care by valuing the patient's autonomy and providing informed choices. Option A is incorrect as insisting on administering the vaccine disregards the patient's beliefs and can be seen as coercive. Option B is partially correct but lacks engagement with the patient regarding alternatives, thus not fully addressing his concerns. Option D is incorrect because it delays care without addressing the immediate issue or providing alternative solutions, which may not respect the urgency of preventive measures.

Question 61: Correct Answer: D) Conducting annual staff training on HIPAA regulations.

Rationale: While ensuring EHRs are password-protected, updating consent forms, and implementing encryption are crucial, conducting annual staff training on HIPAA regulations is paramount. This ensures all staff are aware of current compliance requirements and can effectively protect patient information. Regular training addresses evolving threats and updates in regulations, making it the most comprehensive approach to maintaining HIPAA compliance. - Option A is important but only addresses one aspect of security. - Option B is essential but does not encompass overall compliance. - Option C is critical for data transmission but not sufficient alone. Conducting regular training ensures a holistic understanding and adherence to HIPAA standards across all areas.

Question 62: Correct Answer: B) Left ventricle

Rationale: The left ventricle is responsible for pumping oxygenated blood into systemic circulation via the aorta. If it is compromised, there would be a significant reduction in oxygenated blood reaching the body. The right atrium receives deoxygenated blood from the body, while the right ventricle pumps it to the lungs for oxygenation. The left atrium receives oxygenated blood from the lungs but does not pump it into systemic circulation. Thus, only compromise of the left ventricle directly affects systemic oxygenation levels.

Question 63: Correct Answer: C) Butterfly Method

Rationale: The Butterfly Method is ideal for patients with fragile veins because it allows for better control and reduced pressure during blood draw, minimizing the risk of vein collapse. The Evacuated Tube Method (A) can cause too much pressure, leading to vein collapse. The Syringe Method (B), while offering more control than the Evacuated Tube, still poses a higher risk compared to the Butterfly Method. Capillary Puncture (D) is not suitable for venipuncture as it is used for collecting smaller blood samples from capillaries rather than veins.

Question 64: Correct Answer: B) Use a gentle stream of warm water directed towards the upper wall of the ear canal.

Rationale: The correct technique for ear irrigation involves using a gentle stream of warm water directed towards the upper wall of the ear canal to avoid damaging the eardrum. Option A is incorrect because cold water can cause dizziness and aiming directly at the eardrum can cause injury. Option C is incorrect due to potential harm from direct pressure on the eardrum. Option D is incorrect because cold water can lead to discomfort and dizziness. Warm water helps soften cerumen without causing adverse reactions, and directing it towards the upper wall minimizes risks.

Question 65: Correct Answer: A) Patient's full name

Rationale: The patient's full name is essential for accurate patient identification on a provider request or requisition form. While other details like insurance number, address, and phone number are important, they do not provide the primary means of identifying the patient. Full names are used in conjunction with other identifiers to ensure that the correct patient receives the appropriate care and testing. Incorrect options are relevant but secondary identifiers compared to the full name, which is universally prioritized for initial identification purposes.

Question 66: Correct Answer: B) Supine

Rationale: The supine position refers to lying flat on the back with arms at the sides, which is what Dr. Smith requested. The prone position (Option A) involves lying face down, which is incorrect here. The lateral position (Option C) refers to lying on one side, not on the back. Fowler's position (Option D) involves sitting up at an angle, which does not match the description given in the scenario. Understanding these distinctions is critical for accurate patient positioning and care.

Question 67: Correct Answer: B) Check for a pulse and breathing.

Rationale: The first step in assessing an unresponsive patient is to check for a pulse and breathing to determine if CPR or other interventions are needed. This aligns with contemporary guidelines from organizations like the American Heart Association (AHA). Option A, beginning chest compressions immediately, is incorrect because it should only be done after confirming the absence of pulse/breathing. Option C, calling for help and retrieving an AED, is crucial but secondary to initial assessment. Option D, administering rescue breaths, is part of CPR but follows the assessment phase.

Question 68: Correct Answer: A) Activation of the sympathetic nervous system

Rationale: Anxiety primarily increases blood pressure through the activation of the sympathetic nervous system, which releases catecholamines like adrenaline and noradrenaline. These hormones increase heart rate and constrict blood vessels, raising blood pressure. Option B is incorrect because acetylcholine is associated with parasympathetic activity, which generally lowers heart rate. Option C is incorrect as parasympathetic stimulation typically reduces blood pressure. Option D is also incorrect because cortisol production usually increases under stress, not decreases. The correct answer reflects contemporary understanding of stress physiology and its effects on cardiovascular function.

Question 69: Correct Answer: C) Chemotherapy administration

Rationale: Chemotherapy administration is typically associated with oncology specialty clinics due to the specialized knowledge and equipment required. In contrast, immunizations (A) and routine physical exams (B) are standard services provided by general practices. Blood pressure monitoring (D) is also a common service in general practices and can be part of routine check-ups. Therefore, chemotherapy administration stands out as a service primarily found in specialty clinics, making it the correct answer.

Question 70: Correct Answer: B) Conducting a thorough review of current QC procedures and updating them as needed.

Rationale: According to COLA Accreditation Standards, addressing inconsistencies in quality control documentation requires a comprehensive review and update of existing procedures. This ensures that all aspects of QC are up-to-date and compliant with accreditation requirements. Option A focuses on implementing new protocols without reviewing existing ones, which may overlook underlying issues. Option C suggests retroactive documentation, which does not address future compliance. Option D assigns responsibility but does not ensure procedural adequacy or compliance. Therefore, Option B is the most aligned with ensuring continuous improvement and adherence to standards.

Question 71: Correct Answer: C) Blood culture bottles

Rationale: Blood culture tests specifically require blood culture bottles to detect bacterial or fungal infections in the bloodstream. Lavender-top tubes contain EDTA and are used for complete blood counts (CBCs). Light blue-top tubes contain sodium citrate and are used for coagulation studies. Red-top tubes are typically used for serum chemistry tests. Therefore, while all options involve phlebotomy supplies, only blood culture bottles are suitable for blood culture tests.

Question 72: Correct Answer: A) Compare the monitor's readings with a known standard pressure.

Rationale: Comparing the monitor's readings with a known standard pressure ensures accuracy by validating it against a reliable benchmark. Option B is incorrect because using an arbitrary value does not guarantee accuracy. Option C, while important for equipment maintenance, does not directly relate to calibration accuracy. Option D ensures operational readiness but not calibration precision. Therefore, A is correct as it directly addresses proper calibration methodology by using a known standard for comparison.

Question 73: Correct Answer: D) Information on alternative treatments

Rationale: Informed consent requires patients to be fully aware of their treatment options, including alternatives, to make an educated decision. Option A (the patient's full medical history) is important but not required in the consent form itself. Option B (a detailed description of the procedure) is necessary but not sufficient alone. Option C (the names of all healthcare providers involved) is relevant but not a critical element. Option D is correct because it ensures patients understand their choices.

Question 74: Correct Answer: D) Remain calm, listen actively, and validate his feelings before providing any information.

Rationale: Option D is correct because it prioritizes de-escalation by addressing the patient's emotional state first, which is crucial in defusing tension. Active listening and validation help build rapport and demonstrate empathy. Option A may seem considerate but doesn't address Mr. Johnson's emotions directly. Option B provides information but lacks emotional engagement. Option C offers a solution without first calming the patient, which could exacerbate his agitation. Therefore, option D is the most comprehensive approach based on contemporary communication theories emphasizing empathy and active listening in customer service settings.

Question 75: Correct Answer: A) Using a tourniquet for less than one minute before drawing blood

Rationale: The correct method to ensure accurate potassium levels is using a tourniquet for less than one minute before drawing blood (Option A). Prolonged use of a tourniquet can cause hemolysis, leading to falsely elevated potassium levels. Drawing blood from an intravenous line (Option B) can result in contamination with intravenous fluids. Collecting in a lavender-top tube (Option C) is incorrect because it contains EDTA, which binds calcium and could affect potassium levels. Allowing the patient to make a fist tightly (Option D) can also cause hemolysis and falsely elevated potassium levels.

Question 76: Correct Answer: B) Durable Power of Attorney

Rationale: A Durable Power of Attorney (DPOA) remains in effect even if the principal becomes incapacitated, allowing the designated agent to make medical decisions. A General POA (Option A) ceases to be effective upon incapacitation. A Limited POA (Option C) grants authority for specific tasks and may not cover medical decisions. A Springing POA (Option D) only comes into effect under specified conditions, usually requiring proof of incapacity, which might delay decision-making in urgent situations. - Option A (General Power of Attorney): Incorrect because it does not remain in effect if the principal becomes incapacitated. - Option C (Limited Power of Attorney): Incorrect because it typically covers specific tasks and may not include medical decision-making. - Option D (Springing Power of Attorney): Incorrect because it requires proof of incapacity before taking effect, which can delay urgent medical decisions. The correct option B is justified as it ensures continuous authority for medical decisions without interruption due to incapacitation.

Question 77: Correct Answer: C) Elevated blood pressure and rapid breathing

Rationale: Elevated blood pressure and rapid breathing are strong indicators of an adverse reaction that requires immediate attention. These signs suggest a significant physiological response that could lead to more severe complications if not promptly addressed. While mild pallor (A), a slight increase in respiration rate (B), and sweating (D) can also be symptoms of distress, they are less immediately critical compared to the combination of elevated BP and rapid breathing. - A) Mild pallor: This can indicate distress but is less critical than elevated BP and rapid breathing. - B) Slight increase in respiration rate: While important, it alone does not signify as severe a reaction as when combined with elevated BP. - D) Sweating: This is a common stress response but not as immediately alarming as elevated BP and rapid breathing. This question tests the candidate's ability to prioritize clinical signs based on their severity and urgency for intervention.

Question 78: Correct Answer: B) Listen actively to Mr. Johnson's concerns and acknowledge his frustration before explaining the scheduling policy.

Rationale: Listening actively and acknowledging Mr. Johnson's frustration shows empathy and helps de-escalate the situation by making him feel heard. It also allows for a calm explanation of clinic policies, which can reduce tension. Option A could escalate his anger by seeming dismissive. Option C is premature unless there's a threat of violence. Option D undermines clinic procedures and could set a problematic precedent.

Question 79: Correct Answer: C) Interpreting lab results for patients

Rationale: While MAs can administer injections, document patient information in the EHR, and conduct patient intake, interpreting lab results is outside their scope of practice. This responsibility typically falls to licensed healthcare providers such as physicians or nurse practitioners who have the necessary training and authority to interpret diagnostic data and provide clinical advice based on those interpretations.

Question 80: Correct Answer: C) Have the patient lie on their side with the affected ear facing up.

Rationale: Having the patient lie on their side with the affected ear facing up ensures that the medication stays in the ear canal and is properly absorbed. Option A is incorrect as pulling the earlobe down and back is appropriate for children, not adults. Option B is incorrect because ear drops should be at room temperature to avoid dizziness. Option D is partially correct but not as critical as ensuring proper positioning for absorption.

Question 81: Correct Answer: C) Using a cuff that is appropriately sized for the patient's arm.

Rationale: Using an appropriately sized cuff is crucial for accurate blood pressure measurement. An incorrect cuff size can lead to significant errors in readings. While other factors like caffeine intake, arm positioning, and resting time are important, they do not impact accuracy as directly as cuff size. Ensuring proper cuff size prevents overestimation or underestimation of blood pressure, which is vital for correct diagnosis and treatment. - Option A (Ensuring no caffeine intake): Important but less critical than cuff size. - Option B (Positioning arm at heart level): Necessary but secondary to correct cuff size. - Option D (Resting before measurement): Essential but does not directly affect accuracy as much as cuff size.

Question 82: Correct Answer: D) Self-adherent cohesive wrap

Rationale: The self-adherent cohesive wrap is ideal as it does not contain latex, reducing the risk of an allergic reaction, and it minimizes skin irritation due to its gentle adherence properties. Option A is incorrect because although latex-free, adhesive bandages can still irritate sensitive skin. Option B is incorrect as standard elastic bandages often contain latex. Option C is partially correct but hypoallergenic tape can still cause irritation in highly sensitive individuals. Thus, option D is the best choice for Emily's condition.

Question 83: Correct Answer: C) Call for help and retrieve the AED (Automated External Defibrillator).

Rationale: The first step in an emergency action plan when a patient collapses with no pulse or breathing is to call for help and retrieve the AED. This ensures that advanced life support can be initiated promptly. Starting chest compressions immediately (Option B) is critical but should follow calling for help and retrieving the AED. Administering epinephrine (Option A) is essential during anaphylaxis but not as an initial response in cardiac arrest without defibrillation readiness. Checking for airway obstruction (Option D) is important but secondary to initiating CPR and defibrillation procedures.

Question 84: Correct Answer: C) Opt for a butterfly needle and use a smaller gauge.

Rationale: Using a butterfly needle with a smaller gauge is recommended for patients with difficult veins as it provides better control and reduces the risk of vein collapse. Option A is incorrect because larger gauge needles can cause more trauma. Option B is incorrect as prolonged tourniquet application can lead to hemoconcentration. Option D is incorrect because inserting at a 45-degree angle increases the risk of going through the vein; an angle of 15-30 degrees is typically recommended.

Question 85: Correct Answer: B) Date and time of collection

Rationale: The date and time of collection are crucial for accurate laboratory analysis as they can impact test results significantly. While the patient's full name (A), type of specimen (C), and medical record number (D) are also important, they do not provide critical temporal information necessary for interpreting results accurately. Ensuring precise timing helps in tracking sample viability and correlating results with clinical events, making it indispensable in patient care.

Question 86: Correct Answer: A) Ensuring the patient has fasted for at least 8 hours before the test

Rationale: Ensuring that the patient has fasted for at least 8 hours is crucial for an accurate fasting glucose test result because food intake can significantly alter blood glucose levels. Option B is incorrect because EDTA tubes are used for hematology tests, not glucose tests. Option C is incorrect because transporting on ice is necessary for certain tests like lactic acid but not for glucose. Option D, while important, is less critical than fasting in this context.

Question 87: Correct Answer: B) 12 months

Rationale: The CDC recommends that the first dose of the MMR vaccine be administered at 12 months of age. This timing ensures optimal immunity development. Option A (6 months) is incorrect as it is generally too early for effective immunization unless in outbreak situations where an early dose might be given but not counted as part of the routine series. Option C (15 months) and D (18 months) are also incorrect as they delay protection against these diseases beyond the recommended timeframe, potentially leaving children vulnerable during a critical period.

Question 88: Correct Answer: A) High LDL cholesterol levels

Rationale: High LDL cholesterol levels are strongly associated with an increased incidence and prevalence of coronary artery disease (CAD). Elevated LDL cholesterol contributes to plaque buildup in arteries, leading to atherosclerosis. Regular physical activity (B) is protective against CAD, while low HDL cholesterol (C) is also a risk factor but not as strongly associated as high LDL. Moderate alcohol consumption (D) has been shown to have mixed effects on CAD risk and is less directly linked compared to high LDL levels.

Question 89: Correct Answer: B) Educate Mr. Johnson on recognizing early signs of heart failure.

Rationale: Educating Mr. Johnson on recognizing early signs of heart failure is crucial as it empowers him to take timely action and seek medical help, potentially preventing readmission. While scheduling follow-ups (A), coordinating with a dietitian (C), and arranging home health visits (D) are important aspects of care coordination, they do not directly address immediate self-management skills critical for preventing acute episodes. Recognizing symptoms early can

lead to prompt intervention, thus reducing complications and enhancing patient outcomes.

Question 90: Correct Answer: A) Review the appointment schedule to verify all patients seen have corresponding charges.

Rationale: The first step in ensuring accurate charge reconciliation is reviewing the appointment schedule to verify that all patients seen have corresponding charges entered in the EHR. This ensures no charges are missed. Entering charges based on memory (Option B) risks inaccuracies. Contacting each patient (Option C) is impractical and time-consuming. Adjusting accounts receivable balances based on estimated charges (Option D) can lead to financial discrepancies. Reviewing the appointment schedule is a systematic approach ensuring completeness and accuracy in charge entry.

Question 91: Correct Answer: C) Informed Consent

Rationale: The principle of informed consent ensures that a patient is fully informed about the potential risks, benefits, and alternatives before undergoing any medical procedure. This differs from autonomy (A), which refers to the patient's right to make their own decisions. Beneficence (B) involves acting in the patient's best interest, while confidentiality (D) pertains to keeping patient information private. Understanding these distinctions is crucial for ensuring ethical medical practice.

Question 92: Correct Answer: B) Asking John Doe to describe his current symptoms and concerns.

Rationale: While reviewing past medical history (A), conducting medication reconciliation (C), and measuring vital signs (D) are important components of the intake process, asking the patient to describe their current symptoms and concerns (B) is crucial for understanding the primary purpose of the visit. This step directly addresses why the patient is seeking care at this particular time and guides further assessment and treatment. The other options provide essential background information but do not directly elicit the patient's immediate health concerns.

Question 93: Correct Answer: B) Intravenous (IV)

Rationale: Intravenous (IV) administration is the most appropriate route for medications that need to bypass the gastrointestinal tract and provide a rapid onset of action. This method delivers the drug directly into the bloodstream, ensuring immediate effect. Oral administration (A) involves absorption through the digestive system, which delays onset. Subcutaneous (SC) (C) and Intramuscular (IM) (D) injections also bypass the GI tract but do not provide as rapid an onset as IV administration due to slower absorption rates into the bloodstream.

Question 94: Correct Answer: C) Ensure that the directive is documented in the patient's medical record.

Rationale: Ensuring that the advanced directive is documented in the patient's medical record is crucial for compliance. This ensures all healthcare providers are aware of and can follow the patient's wishes. Verifying with family members (A) can lead to conflicts if their understanding differs from what is documented. Consulting with a physician (B) is important but secondary to proper documentation. Following standard hospital protocol (D) may not respect individual patient wishes as outlined in their advanced directive. Proper documentation ensures legal and ethical adherence to patient autonomy.

Question 95: Correct Answer: B) Intravenous

Rationale: The intravenous (IV) route is the most appropriate for Mr. Johnson as it provides immediate pain relief and bypasses the gastrointestinal tract, which is compromised due to recent surgery. Oral administration is unsuitable due to his difficulty swallowing. Subcutaneous administration may not provide rapid relief required in this scenario. Rectal administration might be considered but is less efficient in delivering immediate relief compared to IV.

Question 96: Correct Answer: A) Open-ended question

Rationale: Open-ended questions are most effective for

gathering detailed information as they encourage patients to elaborate on their symptoms. In contrast, closed-ended questions elicit short responses and may miss important details. Screening questions are used to identify potential issues but do not provide in-depth information. Leading questions can bias the patient's responses. Thus, open-ended questions are essential for comprehensive patient interviews.

Question 97: Correct Answer: A) Labeling the specimen immediately after collection, before leaving the patient's side.
Rationale: Labeling the specimen immediately after collection, before leaving the patient's side, ensures that there is no mix-up or misidentification of samples. This practice minimizes errors and maintains patient safety. Option B is incorrect because verifying patient information should be done before labeling. Option C is misleading as pre-printed labels can be used but must still be verified against patient information at bedside. Option D is incorrect as it increases the risk of mixing up samples from different patients.

Question 98: Correct Answer: B) Cardiology
Rationale: Cardiology is the correct answer because Sarah's symptoms suggest a potential cardiac event, such as a myocardial infarction, which requires immediate evaluation by cardiology services. Radiology (A) could be useful for imaging but is not the priority in this acute scenario. Laboratory Services (C) are essential for blood tests but secondary to cardiology consultation. Physical Therapy (D) is irrelevant in this acute setting. Thus, cardiology provides the most direct and immediate assessment for her symptoms.

Question 99: Correct Answer: A) Respiratory system
Rationale: The respiratory system primarily regulates acid-base balance by controlling the levels of carbon dioxide (CO_2) in the blood. CO_2 combines with water to form carbonic acid, which dissociates into hydrogen ions and bicarbonate, thus influencing blood pH. The digestive system aids in nutrient absorption and waste elimination but is not directly involved in acid-base regulation. The integumentary system protects against environmental hazards and regulates temperature, while the nervous system coordinates body activities but does not directly regulate acid-base balance.

Question 100: Correct Answer: B) Document all patient interactions, including subjective complaints and objective findings.
Rationale: Comprehensive documentation involves recording all patient interactions, which includes both subjective complaints (what the patient says) and objective findings (what is observed/measured). This ensures a complete and accurate medical record. Option A is incorrect because it limits documentation to medications and dosages. Option C is incorrect as it suggests noting only significant changes, missing routine observations. Option D is incorrect as it focuses solely on physician's orders and treatment plans, omitting other crucial aspects of care.

Question 101: Correct Answer: A) Clean high-touch surfaces first using a disinfectant, then clean floors with a detergent solution.
Rationale: High-touch surfaces harbor more pathogens and should be cleaned first with a disinfectant to reduce infection risk. Floors are cleaned afterward with a detergent solution as they are less likely to contribute to direct transmission of pathogens. Option B incorrectly prioritizes floor cleaning, Option C uses an inappropriate product for high-touch surfaces initially, and Option D incorrectly uses disinfectants for floor cleaning first. Proper sequencing ensures effective infection control by targeting areas most likely to transmit infections initially.

Question 102: Correct Answer: A) Presence of a hemodialysis fistula
Rationale: A hemodialysis fistula is a critical vascular access point for dialysis patients, and performing

venipuncture on an arm with a fistula can damage it, leading to serious complications. Recent surgical incisions (Option B) and mild edema (Option C) are relative contraindications but not absolute. Previous history of phlebitis (Option D) may warrant caution but does not necessarily preclude venipuncture. Thus, the presence of a hemodialysis fistula is the definitive contraindication due to its vital role in patient care.

Question 103: Correct Answer: B) Providing additional training for staff on active listening techniques.
Rationale: Active listening is crucial for addressing patient concerns effectively, as it ensures patients feel heard and understood. Option A (standardized script) may lead to robotic interactions, Option C (follow-up calls) addresses post-consultation but not in-session issues, and Option D (reducing consultation duration) may exacerbate feelings of being unheard. Thus, enhancing active listening skills directly targets the core issue of patient concerns not being adequately addressed during consultations.

Question 104: Correct Answer: C) To verify that the procedure is medically necessary
Rationale: The primary purpose of obtaining pre-authorization is to verify that a procedure is medically necessary, ensuring it meets the insurer's criteria for coverage. Option A (ensuring patient eligibility) pertains to general insurance verification, not specific procedures. Option B (determining exact cost) involves billing, not authorization. Option D (confirming co-payment amount) relates to patient financial responsibility but not authorization criteria. Pre-authorization primarily focuses on medical necessity to control costs and avoid unnecessary procedures.

Question 105: Correct Answer: A) Documenting all observed hazards in a detailed report.
Rationale: Documenting all observed hazards in a detailed report is crucial as it ensures that all safety concerns are accurately recorded and can be addressed promptly. Discussing with colleagues (Option B) may delay action, while reporting directly to the patient (Option C) is inappropriate and unprofessional. Waiting until the end of the shift (Option D) could lead to further risks if immediate action is required. Proper documentation allows for systematic follow-up and resolution, aligning with best practices in clinical safety management.

Question 106: Correct Answer: C) Notify the healthcare provider about the potential interaction between warfarin and ciprofloxacin.
Rationale: Ciprofloxacin can enhance the effects of warfarin, increasing the risk of bleeding. The medical assistant should notify the healthcare provider to possibly adjust the warfarin dose or monitor John's INR more closely. Option A is incorrect because it ignores potential drug interactions. Option B is incorrect because increasing intake of green leafy vegetables, which are high in vitamin K, could counteract warfarin's effect. Option D is incorrect because antacids can interfere with ciprofloxacin absorption, reducing its efficacy.

Question 107: Correct Answer: A) Assisting a patient with suspected tuberculosis during an aerosol-generating procedure.
Rationale: An N95 respirator is required for protection against airborne pathogens like tuberculosis during aerosol-generating procedures. Option B (routine vaccinations) and D (routine physical exams) involve low-risk activities where standard surgical masks suffice. Option C (care for influenza patients in non-isolation rooms) typically requires surgical masks unless aerosol-generating procedures are involved. The key difference is that N95 respirators are specifically mandated for high-risk airborne pathogen exposure, especially during procedures that increase the risk of aerosolization.

Question 108: Correct Answer: C) Positioning the patient's arm at heart level while seated

Rationale: The most accurate blood pressure reading is obtained when the patient's arm is positioned at heart level while seated. This position ensures that hydrostatic pressure does not affect the measurement. Option A is incorrect because using a cuff covering 40% of arm circumference may not be appropriate for all patients; it should cover 80% of the arm's length. Option B is incorrect as physical activity can temporarily elevate blood pressure. Option D is less ideal than option C because readings can vary based on body position, and sitting provides a more standardized approach.

Question 109: Correct Answer: A) Hepatitis
Rationale: "Hepatitis" is derived from "hepat-" (liver) and "-itis" (inflammation), correctly describing liver inflammation. "Hepatomegaly" means liver enlargement, "Hepatosis" refers to any non-inflammatory liver disease, and "Hepatopathy" indicates a general liver disease. The key difference lies in the suffixes: "-itis" specifically denotes inflammation, making it the accurate choice for chronic liver inflammation.

Question 110: Correct Answer: A) Verifying the policy number with the insurance card
Rationale: Verifying the policy number with the insurance card is crucial because any error in this primary identifier can lead to significant issues in billing and claims processing. While entering provider names correctly (Option B), double-checking coverage details verbally (Option C), and cross-referencing data (Option D) are also important steps, they do not hold as much weight as ensuring that the policy number is accurate. The policy number serves as a unique identifier, making its verification paramount.

Question 111: Correct Answer: D) Care Coordinator
Rationale: The Care Coordinator is primarily responsible for coordinating patient care in a PCMH. They ensure comprehensive management of all aspects of the patient's health, facilitating communication among various healthcare providers. While physicians and nurse practitioners are involved in direct patient care and decision-making, they do not typically handle the overall coordination. Clinical Medical Assistants support clinical tasks but do not oversee comprehensive care coordination. Thus, understanding the distinct role of each team member is crucial for effective patient-centered care.

Question 112: Correct Answer: A) Using a fully integrated Electronic Health Record (EHR) system
Rationale: A fully integrated Electronic Health Record (EHR) system ensures the highest level of efficiency and accuracy by centralizing patient data, reducing errors, and facilitating real-time updates. Option B, maintaining a detailed paper-based ledger, is less efficient due to manual entry errors and difficulty in accessing historical data. Option C, combining electronic scheduling with manual backup, adds redundancy but can lead to inconsistencies. Option D, utilizing standalone software without integration, lacks the comprehensive data management provided by an integrated EHR system.

Question 113: Correct Answer: B) Label the sample with the patient's name, date of birth, and collection date.
Rationale: Proper labeling of the sample with the patient's name, date of birth, and collection date is crucial for maintaining sample integrity and ensuring accurate results. Incorrect labeling can lead to misidentification and erroneous test results. While placing samples in biohazard bags (Option A), using appropriate transport containers (Option C), and documenting collection details (Option D) are important steps, they do not directly prevent misidentification like proper labeling does. Accurate labeling ensures traceability and proper processing at the reference laboratory.

Question 114: Correct Answer: C) Avoid touching the dropper tip to any part of the eye or face.
Rationale: The correct step to prevent contamination is avoiding contact between the dropper tip and any part of the eye or face. This prevents transferring bacteria from these surfaces into the medication bottle. Option A (blinking rapidly) can cause loss of medication, Option B (placing dropper on sclera) increases contamination risk, and Option D (administering while lying flat) does not specifically address contamination prevention.

Question 115: Correct Answer: D) Using a butterfly needle with a syringe
Rationale: The butterfly needle (winged infusion set) is ideal for patients with fragile veins because it allows for more precise control and less pressure, reducing the risk of vein collapse. Combining it with a syringe further minimizes pressure compared to an evacuated tube system. Options A and C involve higher pressure from the vacuum in the tubes, increasing the risk of vein collapse. Option B lacks the precision control provided by the butterfly needle, making it less suitable for fragile veins.

Question 116: Correct Answer: A) Atrial Fibrillation
Rationale: Atrial fibrillation is characterized by an irregularly irregular rhythm without distinct P waves and a variable ventricular rate. Ventricular tachycardia typically presents with wide QRS complexes and a regular rhythm. Supraventricular tachycardia shows a rapid but regular rhythm with narrow QRS complexes. Sinus bradycardia is identified by a slow but regular heart rate with normal P waves preceding each QRS complex. Hence, the description provided in the question aligns best with atrial fibrillation.

Question 117: Correct Answer: C) Instruct the patient to call 911 immediately.
Rationale: The patient's symptoms indicate a potential myocardial infarction (heart attack), which requires immediate emergency medical intervention. While options A, B, and D involve some form of delayed response or less urgent action, option C is correct because it prioritizes immediate emergency care. Scheduling an appointment (A) or suggesting they come to the clinic (D) could delay critical treatment. Advising aspirin (B) is part of emergency care but does not address immediate transport to an emergency facility. Thus, instructing the patient to call 911 is essential for timely intervention.

Question 118: Correct Answer: A) Administrative
Rationale: The administrative category of the medical record includes non-clinical information such as patient demographics, insurance details, and consent forms. While billing (Option C) also deals with financial aspects, it focuses on charges and payments rather than the initial collection of insurance information. Clinical (Option B) pertains to medical history and treatment notes, whereas procedural (Option D) involves documentation of specific medical procedures. Thus, administrative is the correct category for updating insurance information.

Question 119: Correct Answer: A) Storing records in a locked cabinet accessible only to authorized personnel.
Rationale: Storing medical records in a locked cabinet accessible only to authorized personnel ensures both physical security and controlled access, complying with HIPAA regulations. Option B is incorrect because open shelves do not provide adequate security. Option C is incorrect as unrestricted access violates confidentiality principles. Option D is incorrect because while paper records are secure, digital records must also be protected with restricted access. Therefore, option A ensures comprehensive compliance with legal and ethical standards for medical record storage.

Question 120: Correct Answer: A) Empathizing with the patient's frustration and apologizing for the delay.
Rationale: Empathizing with the patient's frustration and apologizing for the delay (Option A) is considered best practice because it addresses emotional needs, demonstrating understanding and concern. Option B, while informative, may come off as defensive rather than empathetic. Option C fails to acknowledge the patient's feelings, which can exacerbate frustration. Option D might be practical but does not directly address immediate emotional

distress. Thus, empathy combined with an apology is most effective in de-escalating tension and maintaining a positive patient relationship.

Question 121: Correct Answer: D) Reposition Mrs. Johnson to a semi-Fowler's position.
Rationale: Repositioning Mrs. Johnson to a semi-Fowler's position can help improve her lung expansion and increase oxygenation. This is an immediate non-invasive intervention that can quickly enhance breathing without requiring additional equipment or orders. Increasing the oxygen flow rate (Option A) should be done cautiously and typically requires a physician's order. Notifying the attending physician (Option B) is important but not the immediate first step. Encouraging deep breathing exercises (Option C) can be beneficial but may not provide as immediate relief as repositioning in this acute situation.

Question 122: Correct Answer: B) Calories
Rationale: The "Calories" section on a food label indicates the total amount of energy provided by one serving of the product. While carbohydrates, fats, and proteins contribute to the total calorie count, they do not individually represent the total energy content. Carbohydrates (A), fats (C), and proteins (D) are macronutrients that each provide calories, but only the "Calories" section sums these contributions accurately. This makes option B correct as it directly provides the measure of energy per serving. Option A (Total Carbohydrates): This option is misleading because while carbohydrates do contribute to caloric intake, they are not the sole source of calories in food. Option C (Total Fat): Similar to carbohydrates, fats are another source of calories but do not represent total caloric content. Option D (Protein): Proteins also contribute to calories but again do not account for all sources of energy in food. By focusing on "Calories," candidates must recognize that this value encapsulates all sources of energy in a serving, making it distinct from individual macronutrient contributions.

Question 123: Correct Answer: C) Massage Therapy
Rationale: Massage therapy is the correct answer as it specifically involves the manipulation of the body's soft tissues to improve physical health and well-being. Acupuncture (A) involves inserting needles into specific points to balance energy flow. Chiropractic care (B) focuses on diagnosing and treating mechanical disorders of the musculoskeletal system, particularly the spine. Aromatherapy (D) uses essential oils for therapeutic benefits but does not involve physical manipulation. Therefore, while all options are forms of alternative therapies, only massage therapy directly involves soft tissue manipulation.

Question 124: Correct Answer: C) Medical Power of Attorney
Rationale: A Medical Power of Attorney specifically grants authority to an agent to make healthcare decisions for the principal if they become incapacitated. Unlike a General POA, which covers a broad range of financial and legal matters, or a Durable POA that remains in effect even after incapacitation but may not be limited to healthcare decisions, the Medical POA is exclusively focused on medical decisions. A Springing POA only takes effect upon a specific event (e.g., incapacitation), but it can cover various areas, not just healthcare. Thus, the correct answer is C) Medical Power of Attorney.

Question 125: Correct Answer: B) CPT
Rationale: The Current Procedural Terminology (CPT) code set is primarily used for reporting outpatient procedures. While ICD-10-CM codes are used for diagnoses (A), and HCPCS Level II codes (C) are used for services not covered by CPT, such as durable medical equipment, ICD-10-PCS (D) is used for inpatient hospital procedures. Understanding these distinctions ensures accurate documentation and billing in compliance with current guidelines.

Question 126: Correct Answer: C) Sudden onset of chest pain
Rationale: Sudden onset of chest pain during an EKG test is a critical sign of a potential myocardial infarction or other severe cardiac events, necessitating immediate intervention. Elevated blood pressure (A) and increased respiratory rate (B) can be signs of distress but are less specific. Mild dizziness (D) might indicate a less severe issue, such as orthostatic hypotension. Chest pain directly correlates with acute coronary syndromes, making it the most urgent symptom.

Question 127: Correct Answer: B) Using a sterile technique and disinfecting with chlorhexidine
Rationale: The correct procedure involves using a sterile technique and disinfecting the puncture site with chlorhexidine to reduce contamination risk. Option A is incorrect because alcohol alone is not sufficient. Option C is incorrect because, in most protocols, the aerobic bottle is filled first. Option D is incorrect as drawing directly into culture bottles without a syringe can increase contamination risk. Proper disinfection and sterile techniques are critical in obtaining accurate blood culture results.

Question 128: Correct Answer: B) Place it in a sharps container.
Rationale: Used needles must be disposed of in designated sharps containers to prevent needle-stick injuries and contamination. Biohazard bags (Option A) are for soft biohazardous waste like gauze and gloves. Discarding needles in regular trash (Option C), even if capped, poses significant health risks. Pharmaceutical waste containers (Option D) are for expired or unused medications, not sharp objects. This ensures compliance with OSHA and CDC guidelines, emphasizing safety and proper infection control practices.

Question 129: Correct Answer: C) Tachycardia
Rationale: Tachycardia refers to an abnormally rapid heart rate, which aligns with Sarah's symptoms. Bradycardia (Option A) is the opposite, indicating a slow heart rate. Tachypnea (Option B) involves rapid breathing but does not describe heart rate. Dyspnea (Option D) means difficulty breathing and is a symptom rather than a diagnosis of heart rate issues. The correct term, tachycardia (Option C), specifically addresses the condition of an elevated heart rate in this scenario.

Question 130: Correct Answer: A) Iron deficiency anemia
Rationale: John's lab results indicate microcytic anemia (low MCV). Iron deficiency anemia is characterized by low hemoglobin, hematocrit, and MCV, which aligns with John's values. Vitamin B12 deficiency typically causes macrocytic anemia with high MCV. Thalassemia minor can present similarly but often has a higher RBC count despite low MCV. Anemia of chronic disease usually shows normocytic or mildly microcytic anemia but not as pronounced as in iron deficiency. Thus, iron deficiency anemia is the most likely diagnosis given John's CBC results.

Question 131: Correct Answer: B) Asthma exacerbation
Rationale: Asthma exacerbation is most likely to cause a significant decrease in peak flow rate due to airway constriction and inflammation. Age can influence peak flow rates but does not typically cause sudden significant decreases. Recent physical exercise may temporarily affect readings but generally improves lung function. Adequate hydration does not directly impact peak flow rates significantly. This question tests the understanding of factors affecting peak flow rates and emphasizes the importance of recognizing acute clinical conditions like asthma exacerbation that directly impair respiratory function.

Question 132: Correct Answer: C) Chronic kidney disease
Rationale: Chronic kidney disease (CKD) is a major risk factor leading to high mortality and morbidity due to its association with cardiovascular diseases, electrolyte imbalances, and progression to end-stage renal disease. While poor glycemic control (A), uncontrolled hypertension (B), and congestive heart failure (D) are significant, CKD exacerbates these conditions by impairing renal function, making it the most critical factor in this scenario. Poor

glycemic control increases complications but is managed more effectively than CKD. Uncontrolled hypertension can lead to CKD but is not as immediately life-threatening. Congestive heart failure is severe but often secondary to CKD in this context.

Question 133: Correct Answer: B) Ensure Emily cleanses the genital area with antiseptic wipes before collecting the specimen.

Rationale: Proper cleansing of the genital area with antiseptic wipes is crucial to avoid contamination and ensure an accurate urine specimen. Option A is incorrect because collecting the first few drops may contain contaminants. Option C is incorrect as only a midstream sample is needed to avoid initial contaminants. Option D is irrelevant as fasting does not impact urine collection for UTI diagnosis. This highlights proper technique and rationale for clean-catch midstream collection.

Question 134: Correct Answer: A) Instructing the patient to take a deep breath in and then exhale forcefully until no more air can be expelled

Rationale: Option A is correct because it describes the standard procedure for measuring FVC during spirometry, which involves a maximal inhalation followed by a forceful, complete exhalation. Option B is incorrect because it describes slow vital capacity (SVC), not FVC. Option C is incorrect as multiple rapid breaths do not accurately measure FVC. Option D, while used for lung volume measurements, does not specifically measure FVC but rather total lung capacity (TLC) and residual volume (RV).

Question 135: Correct Answer: A) Administering intramuscular injections

Rationale: Administering intramuscular injections is within the CCMA's scope of practice and can be performed independently after proper training. Interpreting lab results, prescribing medications, and diagnosing medical conditions require advanced medical knowledge and licensure beyond the CCMA's training. Option B is incorrect as interpreting lab results should be done by a licensed healthcare provider. Option C is incorrect because prescribing medications is outside the CCMA's legal authority. Option D is incorrect since diagnosing medical conditions requires a licensed physician or advanced practice provider's expertise.

Question 136: Correct Answer: C) Apply direct pressure to the wound with a clean cloth.

Rationale: Applying direct pressure with a clean cloth is crucial in controlling bleeding for a deep laceration. This method effectively reduces blood flow from the wound site. Option A (applying a tourniquet) is typically reserved for severe arterial bleeding when direct pressure fails. Option B (cleaning the wound with antiseptic solution) should be done after controlling bleeding to prevent infection. Option D (elevating the injured limb) can assist in reducing blood flow but is secondary to applying direct pressure. Thus, option C is the most appropriate initial step in this scenario.

Question 137: Correct Answer: D) Respiratory activity

Rationale: Respiratory activity is a common cause of a wandering baseline in EKG recordings due to changes in thoracic impedance as the patient breathes. While patient movement (A), electrical interference (B), and loose electrodes (C) can also cause artifacts, they typically present differently (e.g., muscle tremors, 60-cycle interference, or abrupt signal loss). Recognizing respiratory patterns allows for accurate identification and correction of this specific artifact.

Question 138: Correct Answer: A) Ensuring that all relevant patient information is accurately documented on the referral form.

Rationale: The primary responsibility of a CCMA in processing a referral form is to ensure that all relevant patient information is accurately documented. This includes patient demographics, medical history, reason for referral, and any pertinent clinical findings. Option B is incorrect because scheduling an appointment should occur after ensuring proper documentation. Option C is incorrect as referrals are typically sent to specialists first, not directly to insurance companies. Option D is incorrect because providing options can be part of patient education but does not precede accurate documentation.

Question 139: Correct Answer: A) "Mr. Johnson, it is crucial that you take your medication daily as prescribed by your doctor."

Rationale: Option A is the most effective because it provides specific instructions ("take your medication daily") and emphasizes the importance of following the doctor's prescription. Option B is less specific about the frequency and lacks emphasis on adherence to the doctor's orders. Option C uses a commanding tone ("you must remember"), which may not be well-received by patients. Option D is informative but less direct about the necessity of daily intake and adherence to medical advice.

Question 140: Correct Answer: B) Drug-drug interaction alerts

Rationale: Drug-drug interaction alerts are critical as they help prevent adverse interactions between new prescriptions and existing medications, ensuring patient safety. Automatic refill reminders (Option A) help with adherence but do not address interactions. Patient education materials (Option C) provide valuable information but do not offer real-time safety checks. Electronic submission to pharmacy (Option D) ensures efficient delivery but does not check for interactions. Therefore, Option B is the most relevant feature for preventing negative drug interactions.

Question 141: Correct Answer: A) Label the tube with Mr. Johnson's name and date of birth before leaving the patient's side.

Rationale: The correct practice is to label the tube with Mr. Johnson's name and date of birth before leaving his side (Option A). This ensures immediate verification and reduces errors. Option B is incorrect because delaying labeling increases error risk. Option C is incorrect as verification should occur before labeling, not after. Option D is incorrect because using only a room number lacks sufficient patient identification details and can lead to misidentification.

Question 142: Correct Answer: A) Medical necessity is defined as services or supplies needed for the diagnosis or treatment of a medical condition and meet accepted standards of medical practice.

Rationale: Option A is correct because it aligns with established guidelines, emphasizing services required for diagnosis/treatment and adherence to accepted standards. Option B is incorrect as it prioritizes patient preference over clinical need. Option C is misleading by focusing on cost-effectiveness and convenience rather than clinical appropriateness. Option D incorrectly suggests experimental treatments qualify without established efficacy. The correct definition requires alignment with both clinical need and accepted medical standards, distinguishing it from other options which lack these essential criteria.

Question 143: Correct Answer: A) Submit an appeal with additional documentation supporting medical necessity.

Rationale: The first step in resolving a denial due to lack of medical necessity is to submit an appeal with additional documentation supporting why the service was necessary. Resubmitting the claim without changes (Option B) will likely result in another denial. Contacting the patient (Option C) is important but not the immediate first step. Filing a complaint with the state insurance commissioner (Option D) is premature at this stage and should be considered only if appeals are exhausted.

Question 144: Correct Answer: B) Provide John with a surgical mask and place him in a private room.

Rationale: The correct action is to provide John with a surgical mask and place him in a private room. This adheres to infection control guidelines by minimizing the risk of droplet transmission. Option A is incorrect because airborne isolation is unnecessary for flu symptoms, which are typically droplet-spread. Option C fails to isolate the patient, increasing the risk of spreading the virus. Option D addresses treatment rather than immediate infection control measures. Thus, option B is most appropriate for preventing the spread of infection while managing John's care effectively.

Question 145: Correct Answer: A) Fifth intercostal space at the left midclavicular line

Rationale: The V4 lead is placed in the fifth intercostal space at the left midclavicular line. This position ensures accurate monitoring of electrical activity in this specific region of the heart. Option B is incorrect because it specifies the fourth intercostal space instead of the fifth. Option C is incorrect as it places V4 at the anterior axillary line rather than the midclavicular line. Option D combines both errors from B and C, placing it in both an incorrect intercostal space and an incorrect anatomical line.

Question 146: Correct Answer: A) Hepatitis

Rationale: The term "Hepatitis" is derived from "hepato-" meaning liver and "-itis" meaning inflammation, thus correctly describing an inflammation of the liver. "Hepatomegaly" (Option B) means enlargement of the liver, not inflammation. "Nephritis" (Option C) refers to inflammation of the kidney, not the liver. "Gastritis" (Option D) refers to inflammation of the stomach lining, not the liver. Understanding these distinctions is crucial for accurate medical documentation and diagnosis.

Question 147: Correct Answer: A) Hand washing with soap and water before donning sterile gloves.

Rationale: Hand washing with soap and water before donning sterile gloves (Option A) is the most appropriate technique to ensure asepsis during a minor surgical procedure. This method effectively removes transient microorganisms and reduces resident flora, providing a higher level of infection control. Option B, using alcohol-based hand sanitizer, is effective but not as thorough as soap and water in removing all types of contaminants. Option C, wearing non-sterile gloves, does not provide the necessary sterility required for surgical procedures. Option D, donning sterile gloves without hand hygiene, fails to remove potential contaminants from hands that could compromise sterility.

Question 148: Correct Answer: D) Create a detailed care plan and communicate it with all his healthcare providers.

Rationale: Creating a detailed care plan and communicating it with all healthcare providers ensures that everyone involved in Mr. Smith's care is on the same page, which is crucial for managing multiple chronic conditions effectively. While scheduling appointments with specialists (A), referring to educators (B), and arranging home health services (C) are important steps, they are components of the broader care plan that needs to be established first. A comprehensive care plan ensures coordinated efforts and avoids fragmented care.

Question 149: Correct Answer: A) Medication Reconciliation

Rationale: The correct answer is A) Medication Reconciliation. This function ensures that all medications a patient is taking are accurately documented and updated in their medical record. Clinical Decision Support (B) provides alerts and recommendations based on clinical data but does not update medication lists directly. Order Entry (C) is used for placing orders for tests or treatments but not for updating medication records. Patient Summary Update (D) involves general updates to the patient's summary but lacks the specific focus on medications required for accurate reconciliation.

Question 150: Correct Answer: A) Clean the site with an alcohol swab in a circular motion from the inside out.

Rationale: Cleaning the site with an alcohol swab in a circular motion from inside out is crucial for maintaining aseptic technique and preventing infection. Option B is incorrect because inserting at a 45-degree angle can cause unnecessary pain and damage; the correct angle is usually 15-30 degrees. Option C is incorrect because releasing the tourniquet immediately may cause difficulty in blood flow into the collection tube; it should be released once blood flow is established. Option D is incorrect because having John hold his fist tightly throughout can cause hemoconcentration and affect sample quality; he should relax his hand once blood flow starts.

Made in United States
Troutdale, OR
11/17/2024

24961114R00095